Maternal Care

A health professional's guide to pregnancy and childbirth

Developed by the Perinatal Education Programme

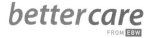

bettercare
FROM EBW

We have taken every care to ensure that drug dosages and related medical advice in this book are accurate. However, drug and disinfectant dosages can change and are updated often, so always double-check dosages and procedures against a reliable, up-to-date formulary and the given drug's documentation before administering it.

Maternal Care: A health professional's guide to pregnancy and childbirth

First published in 2010 by Bettercare, a division of Electric Book Works. Updated 25 Mar 2011, 1 Aug 2011 (layout), 15 Aug 2012, 31 Mar 2014, 11 Aug 2014, 23 Feb 2015 (layout). This version produced on 23 September 2015.

Text © Perinatal Education Programme

ISBN (paperback): 978-1-920218-27-0
ISBN (PDF ebook): 978-1-920218-45-4
ISBN (reflowable ebook): 978-1-920218-89-8

Contents

Tests

Acknowledgements

Maternal Care has been edited from the Maternal Care manual of the Perinatal Education Programme. This learning programme for professionals is developed by the Perinatal Education Trust and funded by Eduhealthcare.

We acknowledge all the participants of the Perinatal Education Programme who have made suggestions and offered constructive criticism over the years. It is only through constant feedback from colleagues and participants that the content of the Perinatal Education Programme courses can be improved.

Contributors to *Maternal Care*: Prof H van C de Groot, Dr D Greenfield, Ms H Louw, Ms M Petersen, Dr N Rhoda, Prof G Theron, Prof D Woods

Bettercare would like to acknowledge Dr Kenneth Beviss-Challinor for his contribution towards the proofreading of this book.

Editor-in-Chief of the Perinatal Education Programme: Prof D Woods

Editor of *Maternal Care*: Prof G Theron

Introduction

About the Bettercare series

Bettercare publishes an innovative series of distance-learning books for healthcare professionals, developed by the Perinatal Education Trust, Eduhealthcare, the Desmond Tutu HIV Foundation, the Desmond Tutu TB Centre, the Perinatal Mental Health Project, the Academic Unit for Infection Prevention and Control at Stellenbosch University, and the Infection Control Africa Network, with contributions from numerous experts.

Our aim is to provide appropriate, affordable and up-to-date learning material for healthcare workers in under-resourced areas, so that they can learn, practise and deliver excellent patient care.

The Bettercare series is built on the experience of the Perinatal Education Programme (PEP), which has provided learning opportunities to over 60 000 nurses and doctors in South Africa since 1992. Many of the educational methods developed by PEP are now being adopted by the World Health Organisation (WHO).

Why decentralised learning?

Continuing education for health workers traditionally consists of courses and workshops run by formal trainers at large central hospitals. These courses are expensive to attend, often far away from the health workers' families and places of work, and the content frequently fails to address the biggest healthcare challenges of poor, rural communities.

To help solve these many problems, a self-help decentralised learning method has been developed which addresses the needs of professional healthcare workers, especially those in under-resourced regions.

Books in the Bettercare series

Adult HIV

Adult HIV covers an introduction to HIV infection, management of HIV-infected adults at primary-care clinics, preparing patients for antiretroviral (ARV) treatment, ARV drugs, starting and maintaining patients on ARV treatment and an approach to opportunistic infections. *Adult HIV* was developed by doctors and nurses with wide experience in the care of adults with HIV, in collaboration with the Desmond Tutu HIV Foundation.

Birth Defects

Birth Defects was written for healthcare workers who look after individuals with birth defects, their families, and women who are at increased risk of giving birth to an infant with a birth defect. Special attention is given to modes of inheritance, medical genetic counselling, and birth defects due to chromosomal abnormalities, single gene defects, teratogens and multifactorial inheritance. This book is being used in the Genetics Education Programme, which trains healthcare workers in genetic counselling in South Africa.

Breast Care

Breast Care was written for nurses and doctors who manage the health needs of women from childhood to old age. It covers breast examination, the assessment and management of benign breast conditions, the diagnosis and management of breast cancer and palliative care.

Child Healthcare

Child Healthcare addresses all the common and important clinical problems in children, including immunisation, history and examination, growth and nutrition, acute and chronic infections, parasites, skin conditions, and difficulties in the home and society. *Child Healthcare* was developed for use in primary-care settings.

Childhood HIV

Childhood HIV enables nurses and doctors to care for children with HIV infection. It addresses an introduction to HIV in children, the clinical and immunological diagnosis of HIV infection, management of children with and without antiretroviral treatment, antiretroviral drugs, opportunistic infections and end-of-life care.

Childhood TB

Childhood TB was written to enable healthcare workers to learn about the primary care of children with tuberculosis. The book covers an introduction to TB infection, and the clinical presentation, diagnosis, management and prevention of tuberculosis in children and HIV/TB co-infection. *Childhood TB* was developed in collaboration with the Desmond Tutu TB Centre.

Ebola Prevention and Control

Ebola Prevention and Control was written for all healthcare workers and administrators managing, preventing and controlling viral haemorrhagic diseases. Chapters cover virology and epidemiology, patient management, protection of healthcare workers, support services and documentation, and communication and community engagement. There is a strong emphasis on the protection of healthcare workers in the field, particularly in resource-limited settings.

Infection Prevention and Control

Infection Prevention and Control was written for nurses, doctors and health administrators working in the field of infection prevention and control, particularly in resource-limited settings. It includes chapters on IPC programmes, risk management, health facility design, outbreak surveillance and antimicrobial stewardship.

Intrapartum Care

Intrapartum Care was developed for doctors and advanced midwives who care for women who deliver in level 2 hospitals. It contains theory and skills chapters adapted from the labour chapters of *Maternal Care*. Particular attention is given to the care of the mother, the management of labour and monitoring the wellbeing of the fetus. *Intrapartum Care* was written to support and complement the national protocol of intrapartum care and the essential steps to manage obstetric emergencies (ESMOE) in South Africa.

Maternal Care

Maternal Care addresses all the common and important problems that occur during pregnancy, labour, delivery and the puerperium. It covers the antenatal and postnatal care of healthy women with normal pregnancies, monitoring and managing the progress of labour, specific medical problems during pregnancy, labour and the puerperium, family planning, and regionalised perinatal care. Skills chapters teach clinical examination in pregnancy and labour, routine screening tests, the use of an antenatal card and partogram, measuring blood pressure, detecting proteinuria, and performing and repairing an episiotomy. *Maternal Care* is aimed at health workers in level 1 hospitals or clinics.

Maternal Mental Health

Maternal Mental Health was written for doctors, nurses and social workers caring for women before and after birth. It includes an introduction to maternal mental health and illness, making referrals for maternal mental illness, helping mothers with mental health problems and special issues in maternal mental health. It includes a resource section for assessing, referring and supporting mothers in the perinatal period.

Mother and Baby Friendly Care

Mother and Baby Friendly Care describes gentler, kinder, evidence-based ways of caring for women during pregnancy, labour and delivery. It also presents improved methods of providing infant care with an emphasis on kangaroo mother care and exclusive breastfeeding.

Newborn Care

Newborn Care was written for health workers providing special care for newborn infants in level 2 hospitals. It covers resuscitation at birth, assessing infant size and gestational age, routine care and feeding of both normal and high-risk infants, the prevention, diagnosis and management of hypothermia, hypoglycaemia, jaundice, respiratory distress, infection, trauma, bleeding and congenital abnormalities, as well as communication with parents. Skills chapters address resuscitation, size measurement, history, examination and clinical notes, nasogastric feeds, intravenous infusions, use of incubators, measuring blood glucose concentration, insertion of an umbilical vein catheter, phototherapy, apnoea monitors, and oxygen therapy.

Perinatal HIV

Perinatal HIV enables midwives, nurses and doctors to care for pregnant women and their infants in communities where HIV infection is common. Special emphasis has been placed on the prevention of mother-to-infant transmission of HIV. It covers the basics of HIV infection and screening, antenatal and intrapartum care of women with HIV infection, care of HIV-exposed newborn infants, and parent counselling.

Primary Maternal Care

Primary Maternal Care addresses the needs of health workers who provide antenatal and postnatal care, but do not conduct deliveries. It is adapted from theory and skills chapters from *Maternal Care*. This book is ideal for midwives and doctors providing primary maternal care in level 1 district hospitals and clinics, and complements the national protocol of antenatal care in South Africa.

Primary Newborn Care

Primary Newborn Care was written specifically for nurses and doctors who provide primary care for newborn infants in level 1 clinics and hospitals. *Primary Newborn Care* addresses the care of infants at birth, care of normal infants, care of low-birth-weight infants, neonatal emergencies, and common minor problems in newborn infants.

Saving Mothers and Babies

Saving Mothers and Babies was developed in response to the high maternal and perinatal mortality rates found in most developing countries. Learning material used in this book is based on the results of the annual confidential enquiries into maternal deaths and the Saving Mothers and Saving Babies reports published in South Africa. It addresses the basic principles of mortality audit, maternal mortality, perinatal mortality, managing mortality meetings, and ways of reducing maternal and perinatal mortality rates. This book should be used together with the Perinatal Problem Identification Programme (PPIP).

Well Women

Well Women was written for primary health workers who manage the everyday health needs of women. It covers reproductive health, family planning and infertility, common genital infections, vaginal bleeding, and the abuse of women.

Format of the courses

Objectives

The learning objectives are clearly stated at the start of each chapter. They help the participant to identify and understand the important lessons to be learned.

Pre- and post-tests

There is a multiple-choice test of 20 questions for each chapter at the end of the book. Participants are encouraged to take a pre-test before starting each chapter to benchmark their current knowledge, and a post-test after each chapter to assess what they have learned. Self-assessment allows participants to monitor their own progress through the course.

Question-and-answer format

Theoretical knowledge is presented in a question-and-answer format, which encourages the learner to actively participate in the learning process. In this way, the participant is led step by step through the definitions, causes, diagnosis, prevention, dangers and management of a particular problem.

Participants should cover the answer for a few minutes with a piece of paper while thinking about the correct reply to each question. This method helps learning.

Simplified flow diagrams are also used, where necessary, to indicate the correct approach to diagnosing or managing a particular problem.

Each question is identified with the number of the chapter, followed by the number of the question, for example 5-23.

Important practical lessons are emphasised like this.

NOTE
Additional, non-essential information is provided for interest and given in notes like this. These facts are not used in the case studies or included in the multiple-choice questions.

Case studies

Each chapter closes with a few case studies which encourage the participant to consolidate and apply what was learned earlier in the chapter. These studies give the participant an opportunity to see the problem as it usually presents itself in the clinic or hospital. The participant should attempt to answer each question in the case study before reading the correct answer. Case studies without the correct answers are also used at the start of some chapters to identify common clinical problems that need to be addressed.

Practical skills

Some Bettercare books include chapters on practical skills that need to be practised, preferably in groups. These skills chapters list essential equipment and present step-by-step instructions on how to perform each task, often with pictures. If participants are not familiar with a practical skill, they should ask an appropriate medical or nursing colleague to demonstrate the clinical skill to them. In this way, senior personnel are encouraged to share their skills with their colleagues.

Final examination

On completion of each course, participants can take a 75-question, self-managed multiple-choice examination.

All the exam questions will be taken from the multiple-choice tests from the book. The content of the skills chapters will not be included in the examination.

Participants need to achieve at least 80% in the examination in order to successfully complete the course. Successful candidates will be sent a certificate which states that they have successfully completed that course. South African doctors can earn CPD points on the successful completion of the CPD test at the end of each chapter.

Contributors

The developers of our learning materials are a multi-disciplinary team of nurses, midwives, obstetricians, neonatologists, general paediatricians and other medical specialists. The development and review of all course material is overseen by the Editor-in-Chief, emeritus Professor Dave Woods, a previous head of neonatal medicine at the University of Cape Town who now consults to UNICEF and the WHO.

Perinatal Education Trust

Books developed for the Perinatal Education Programme are provided as cheaply as possible. Writing and updating the programme is both funded and managed on a non-profit basis by the Perinatal Education Trust.

Eduhealthcare

Eduhealthcare is a non-profit organisation based in South Africa. It aims to improve health and wellbeing, especially in poor communities, through affordable education for healthcare workers. To this end it provides financial support for the development and publishing of the Bettercare series.

The Desmond Tutu HIV Foundation

The Desmond Tutu HIV Foundation at the University of Cape Town, South Africa, is a centre of excellence in HIV medicine, building capacity through training and enhancing knowledge through research.

The Desmond Tutu TB Centre

The Desmond Tutu TB Centre at Stellenbosch University, South Africa, strives to improve the health of vulnerable groups through the education of healthcare workers and community members, and by influencing policy based on research into the epidemiology of childhood tuberculosis, multi-drug-resistant tuberculosis, HIV/TB co-infection and preventing the spread of TB and HIV in southern Africa.

Perinatal Mental Health Project

The Perinatal Mental Health Project of the Centre for Public Mental Health in the Department of Psychiatry and Mental Health at the University of Cape Town, South Africa, aims to improve the mental health of women during pregnancy and in the months afterwards. The project targets women in low-resource settings who are at risk of depression and anxiety.

The Infection Control Africa Network

The Infection Control Africa Network (ICAN) promotes and facilitates the establishment of infection control programmes. This includes promotion of surveillance for and reduction of healthcare-associated infections, and antimicrobial stewardship activities through education. ICAN works with infection prevention structures in Africa and other international health-related associations.

Updating the course material

Bettercare learning materials are regularly updated to keep up with developments and changes in healthcare protocols. Course participants can make important contributions to the continual improvement of Bettercare books by reporting factual or language errors, by identifying sections that are difficult to understand, and by suggesting additions or improvements to the contents. Details of alternative or better forms of management would be particularly appreciated. Please send any comments or suggestions to the Editor-in-Chief, Professor Dave Woods.

Contact information

Bettercare

- Website: www.bettercare.co.za
- Email: info@bettercare.co.za
- Phone: +27 (0)21 671 1278
- Fax: +27 (0)86 219 8093

Perinatal Education Programme

- Editor-in-Chief: Professor Dave Woods
- Website: www.pepcourse.co.za
- Email: pepcourse@mweb.co.za
- Phone/fax: +27 (0)21 786 5369
- Post: Perinatal Education Programme, 70 Dorries Drive, Simon's Town, 7975

Exams

- exams@bettercare.co.za

1

Antenatal care

Take the chapter test before and after you read this chapter.

Objectives

When you have completed this unit you should be able to:

- List the goals of good antenatal care.
- Diagnose pregnancy.
- Know what history should be taken and examination done at the first visit.
- Determine the duration of pregnancy.
- List and assess the results of the side-room and screening tests needed at the first visit.
- Identify low-, intermediate- and high-risk pregnancies.
- Plan and provide antenatal care that is problem orientated.
- List what specific complications to look for at 28, 34 and 41 weeks.
- Provide health information during antenatal visits.
- Manage pregnant women with HIV infection.

Goals of good antenatal care

1-1 What are the aims and principles of good antenatal care?

The aims of good antenatal care are to ensure that pregnancy causes no harm to the mother and to keep the fetus healthy during the antenatal period. In addition, the opportunity must be taken to provide health education. These aims can usually be achieved by the following:

1. Antenatal care must follow a definite plan.
2. Antenatal care must be problem oriented.

3. Possible complications and risk factors that may occur at a particular gestational age must be looked for at these visits.
4. The fetal condition must be repeatedly assessed.
5. Healthcare education must be provided.

All information relating to the pregnancy must be entered on a patient-held antenatal card. The antenatal card can also serve as a referral letter if a patient is referred to the next level of care and therefore serves as a link between the different levels of care as well as the antenatal clinic and labour ward.

The antenatal card is an important source of information during the antenatal period and labour.

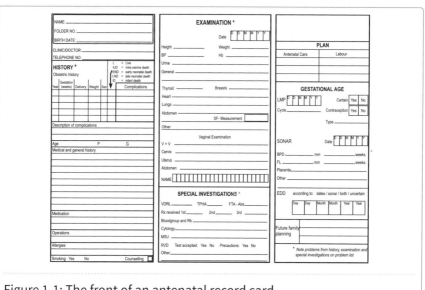

Figure 1-1: The front of an antenatal record card

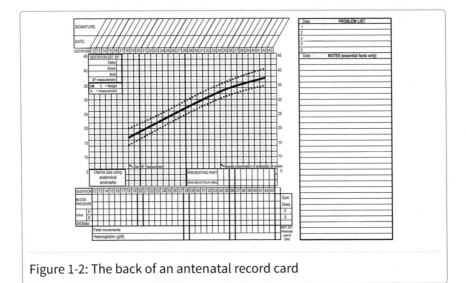

Figure 1-2: The back of an antenatal record card

Diagnosing pregnancy

1-2 How can you confirm that a patient is pregnant?

The common symptoms of pregnancy are amenorrhoea (no menstruation), nausea, breast tenderness and urinary frequency. If the history suggests that a patient is pregnant, the diagnosis is easily confirmed by testing the urine with a standard pregnancy test. The test becomes positive by the time the first menstrual period is missed.

A positive pregnancy test is produced by both an intra-uterine and an extra-uterine pregnancy. Therefore, it is important to establish whether the pregnancy is intra-uterine or not.

> Confirm that the patient is pregnant before beginning antenatal care.

1-3 How do you diagnose an intra-uterine pregnancy?

The characteristics of an intra-uterine pregnancy are:

1. The size of the uterus is appropriate for the duration of pregnancy.
2. There is no lower abdominal pain or vaginal bleeding.
3. There is no tenderness of the lower abdomen.

1-4 How do you diagnose an extra-uterine pregnancy?

The characteristics of an extra-uterine (ectopic) pregnancy are:

1. The uterus is smaller than expected for the duration of pregnancy.
2. Lower abdominal pain and vaginal bleeding are usually present.
3. Tenderness over the lower abdomen is usually present.

The first antenatal visit

This visit is usually the patient's first contact with medical services during her pregnancy. She must be treated with kindness and understanding in order to gain her confidence and to ensure her future co-operation and regular attendance. This opportunity must be taken to book the patient for antenatal care and thereby ensure the early detection and management of treatable complications.

1-5 At what gestational age (duration of pregnancy) should a patient first attend an antenatal clinic?

As early as possible, preferably when the second menstrual period has been missed, i.e. at a gestational age of 8 weeks. Note that for practical reasons the gestational age is measured from the first day of the last normal menstrual period. Antenatal care should start at the time that the pregnancy is confirmed.

It is important that all pregnant women book for antenatal care as early as possible.

1-6 What are the aims of the first antenatal visit?

1. A full history must be taken.
2. A full physical examination must be done.
3. The duration of pregnancy must be established.
4. Important screening tests must be done.
5. Some high-risk patients can be identified.

1-7 What history should be taken?

A full history, containing the following:

1. The previous obstetric history.
2. The present obstetric history.
3. A medical history.
4. HIV status.
5. History of medication and allergies.
6. A surgical history.
7. A family history.
8. The social circumstances of the patient.

1-8 What is important in the previous obstetric history?

1. Establish the number of pregnancies (gravidity), the number of previous pregnancies reaching viability (parity) and the number of miscarriages and ectopic pregnancies that the patient may have had. This information may reveal the following important factors:
   - Grande multiparity (i.e. five or more pregnancies which have reached viability).
   - Miscarriages: 3 or more successive first-trimester miscarriages suggest a possible genetic abnormality in the father or mother. A previous midtrimester miscarriage suggests a possible incompetent internal cervical os.
   - Ectopic pregnancy: ensure that the present pregnancy is intra-uterine.
   - Multiple pregnancy: non-identical twins tend to recur.

2. The birth weight, gestational age, and method of delivery of each previous infant as well as of previous perinatal deaths are important.
   ○ Previous low-birth-weight infants or spontaneous preterm labours tend to recur.
   ○ Previous large infants (4 kg or more) suggest maternal diabetes.
   ○ The type of previous delivery is also important: a forceps delivery or vacuum extraction may suggest that a degree of cephalopelvic disproportion had been present. If the patient had a previous Caesarean section, the indication for the Caesarean section must be determined.
   ○ The type of incision in the uterus is also important (this information must be obtained from the patient's folder) as only patients with a transverse lower segment incision should be considered for a possible vaginal delivery.
   ○ Having had one or more perinatal deaths places the patient at high risk of further perinatal deaths. Therefore, every effort must be made to find out the cause of any previous deaths. If no cause can be found, then the risk of a recurrence of perinatal death is even higher.

3. Previous complications of pregnancy or labour.
   ○ In the antenatal period, e.g. pre-eclampsia, preterm labour, diabetes, and antepartum haemorrhage. Patients who develop pre-eclampsia before 34 weeks gestation have a greater risk of pre-eclampsia in further pregnancies.
   ○ First stage of labour, e.g. a long labour.
   ○ Second stage of labour, e.g. impacted shoulders.
   ○ Third stage of labour, e.g. a retained placenta or a postpartum haemorrhage.

Complications in previous pregnancies tend to recur in subsequent pregnancies. Therefore, patients with a previous perinatal death are at high risk of another perinatal death, while patients with a previous spontaneous preterm labour are at high risk of preterm labour in their next pregnancy.

1-9 What information should be asked for when taking the present obstetric history?

1. The first day of the last normal menstrual period must be determined as accurately as possible.
2. Any medical or obstetric problems which the patient has had since the start of this pregnancy, for example:
   - Pyrexial illnesses (such as influenza) with or without skin rashes.
   - Symptoms of a urinary tract infection.
   - Any vaginal bleeding.

3. Attention must be given to minor symptoms which the patient may experience during her present pregnancy, for example:
   - Nausea and vomiting.
   - Heartburn.
   - Constipation.
   - Oedema of the ankles and hands.

4. Is the pregnancy planned and wanted, and was there a period of infertility before she became pregnant?
5. If the patient is already in the third trimester of her pregnancy, attention must be given to the condition of the fetus.

1-10 What important facts must be considered when determining the date of the last menstrual period?

1. The date should be used to measure the duration of the pregnancy only if the patient had a regular menstrual cycle.
2. Were the date of onset and the duration of the last period normal? If the last period was shorter in duration and earlier in onset than usual, it may have been an implantation bleed. Then the previous period must be used to determine the duration of pregnancy.
3. Patients on oral or injectable contraception must have menstruated spontaneously after stopping contraception, otherwise the date of the last period should not be used to measure the duration of pregnancy.

1-11 Why is the medical history important?

Some medical conditions may become worse during pregnancy, e.g. a patient with heart valve disease may go into cardiac failure while a hypertensive patient is at high risk of developing pre-eclampsia.

Ask the patient if she has had any of the following:

1. Hypertension.
2. Diabetes mellitus.
3. Rheumatic or other heart disease.
4. Epilepsy.
5. Asthma.
6. Tuberculosis.
7. Psychiatric illness.
8. Any other major illness.

It is important to ask whether the patient knows her HIV status. If she had an HIV test, both the date and result need to be noted. If she is HIV positive, record whether she is on ARV treatment and which drugs she is taking. If she is not on ARV treatment, note whether she knows her CD4 count and when it was done.

1-12 Why is it important to ask about any medication taken and a history of allergy?

1. Ask about the regular use of any medication. This is often a pointer to an illness not mentioned in the medical history.
2. Certain drugs, such as retinoids which are used for acne, and efavirenz (Stocrin) which is used in ARV treatment, can be teratogenic (damaging to the fetus) during the first trimester of pregnancy.
3. Some drugs, such as Warfarin, can be dangerous to the fetus if they are taken close to term.
4. Allergies are also important and the patient must be specifically asked if she is allergic to penicillin.

1-13 What previous operations may be important?

1. Operations on the urogenital tract, e.g. Caesarean section, myomectomy, a cone biopsy of the cervix, operations for stress incontinence, and vesicovaginal fistula repair.
2. Cardiac surgery, e.g. heart valve replacement.

1-14 Why is the family history important?

Close family members with a condition such as diabetes, multiple pregnancy, bleeding tendencies or mental retardation increases the risk of these conditions in the patient and her unborn infant. Some birth defects are inherited.

1-15 Why is information about the patient's social circumstances very important?

1. Ask if the woman smokes cigarettes or drinks alcohol. Smoking may cause intra-uterine growth restriction (fetal growth restriction) while alcohol may cause both intra-uterine growth restriction and congenital malformations.
2. An unmarried mother may need help to plan for the care of her infant.
3. Unemployment, poor housing, and overcrowding increase the risk of tuberculosis, malnutrition, and intra-uterine growth restriction. Patients living in poor social conditions need special support and help.

1-16 To which systems must you pay particular attention when doing a physical examination?

1. The general appearance of the patient is of great importance as it can indicate whether or not she is in good health.
2. A woman's height and weight may reflect her past and present nutritional status.
3. In addition, the following systems or organs must be carefully examined:
   - The thyroid gland.
   - The breasts.
   - Lymph nodes in the neck, axillae (armpits) and inguinal areas.
   - The respiratory system.
   - The cardiovascular system.

- The abdomen.
- Both external and internal genitalia.

1-17 What is important in the examination of the thyroid gland?

1. A thyroid gland which is visibly enlarged is possibly abnormal and must be examined by a doctor.
2. A thyroid gland which on palpation is only slightly diffusely enlarged is normal in pregnancy.
3. An obviously enlarged gland, a single palpable nodule, or a nodular goitre is abnormal and needs further investigation.

1-18 What is important in the examination of the breasts?

1. Inverted or flat nipples must be diagnosed and treated so that the patient will be more likely to breastfeed successfully.
2. A breast lump or a blood-stained discharge from the nipple must be investigated further as it may indicate the presence of a tumour.
3. Whenever possible, patients should be advised and encouraged to breastfeed. Teaching the advantages of breastfeeding is an essential part of antenatal care and must be emphasised in the following groups of women:
   - HIV-negative women.
   - Women with unknown HIV status.
   - HIV-positive women who have elected to exclusively breastfeed.

1-19 What is important in the examination of the respiratory and cardiovascular systems?

1. Look for any signs which suggest that the patient has difficulty breathing (dyspnoea).
2. The blood pressure must be measured and the pulse rate counted.

1-20 How do you examine the abdomen at the booking visit?

1. The abdomen is palpated (felt) for enlarged organs or masses.
2. The height of the fundus above the symphysis pubis is measured.

1-21 What must be looked for when the external and internal genitalia are examined?

1. Signs of sexually transmitted diseases which may present as single or multiple ulcers, a purulent discharge or enlarged inguinal lymph nodes.
2. Carcinoma of the cervix is the commonest form of cancer in most communities. Advanced stages of this disease present as a wart-like growth or an ulcer on the cervix. A cervix which looks normal does not exclude the possibility of an early cervical carcinoma.

1-22 When must a cervical smear be taken when examining the internal genitalia (gynaecological examination)?

1. All patients aged 30 years or more who have not previously had a cervical smear that was reported as normal.
2. All patients who have previously had a cervical smear that was reported as abnormal.
3. All patients who have a cervix that looks abnormal.
4. All HIV-positive patients who did not have a cervical smear reported as normal within the last year.

A cervix that looks normal may have an early carcinoma.

Determining the duration of pregnancy

All available information is now used to assess the duration of pregnancy as accurately as possible:

1. Last normal menstrual period.
2. Size of the uterus on bimanual or abdominal examination up to 18 weeks.
3. Height of the fundus at or after 18 weeks.
4. The result of an ultrasound examination (ultrasonology).

> An accurate assessment of the duration of pregnancy is of great importance, especially if the woman develops complications later in her pregnancy.

1-23 When is the duration of pregnancy calculated from the last normal menstrual period?

When there is certainty about the accuracy of the dates of the last normal menstrual period. The duration of pregnancy is then calculated from the first day of that period.

1-24 How does the size of the uterus indicate the duration of pregnancy?

1. Up to 12 weeks the size of the uterus, assessed by bimanual examination, is a reasonably accurate method of determining the duration of pregnancy. Therefore, if there is uncertainty about the duration of pregnancy before 12 weeks the patient should be referred for a bimanual examination.
2. From 13 to 17 weeks, when the fundus of the uterus is still below the umbilicus, the abdominal examination is the most accurate method of determining the duration of pregnancy.
3. From 18 weeks, the symphysis-fundus (SF) height measurement is the more accurate method.

1-25 How should you determine the duration of pregnancy if the uterine size and the menstrual dates do not indicate the same gestational age?

1. If the fundus is below the umbilicus (in other words, the patient is less than 22 weeks pregnant).
   - If the dates and the uterine size differ by 3 weeks or more, the uterine size should be considered as the more accurate indicator of the duration of pregnancy.
   - If the dates and the uterine size differ by less than 3 weeks, the dates are more likely to be correct.
2. If the fundus is at or above the umbilicus (in other words, the patient is 22 weeks or more pregnant).
   - If the dates and the uterine size differ by 4 weeks or more, the uterine size should be considered as the more accurate indicator of the duration of pregnancy.
   - If the dates and the uterine size differ by less than 4 wccks, the dates are more likely to be correct.

1-26 How should you use the symphysis-fundus height measurement to determine the duration of pregnancy?

From 18 weeks gestation, the symphysis-fundus (SF) height measurement in cm is plotted on the 50th centile of the SF growth curve to determine the duration of pregnancy. For example, a SF measurement of 26 cm corresponds to a gestation of 27 weeks.

> A difference between the gestational age according to the menstrual dates and the size of the uterus is usually the result of incorrect dates.

1-27 What conditions other than incorrect menstrual dates cause a difference between the duration of pregnancy calculated from menstrual dates and the size of the uterus?

1. A uterus bigger than dates suggests:
   - Multiple pregnancy.

- Polyhydramnios.
- A fetus which is large for the gestational age.
- Diabetes mellitus.

2. A uterus smaller than dates suggests:
   - Intra-uterine growth restriction.
   - Oligohydramnios.
   - Intra-uterine death.
   - Rupture of the membranes.

Side-room and special screening investigations

1-28 Which side-room examinations must be done routinely?

1. A haemoglobin estimation at the first antenatal visit and again at 28 and 36 weeks.
2. A urine test for protein and glucose is done at every visit.

1-29 What special screening investigations should be done routinely?

1. A laboratory serological screening test for syphilis such as a VDRL, RPR or TPHA test. An on-site RPR card test or syphilis rapid test can be performed in the clinic, if a laboratory is not within easy reach of the hospital or clinic.
2. Determining whether the patient's blood group is Rh positive or negative. A Rh card test can be done in the clinic.
3. A rapid HIV screening test after health worker initiated counselling and preferably after written consent.
4. A smear of the cervix for cytology if it is indicated.
5. If possible, all patients should have a midstream urine specimen examined for asymptomatic bacteriuria. The best test is bacterial culture of the urine.
6. Where possible, an ultrasound examination when the patient is 18–22 weeks pregnant can be arranged

1-30 Is it necessary to do an ultrasound examination on all patients who book early enough for antenatal care?

With well-trained ultrasonographers and adequate ultrasound equipment, it is of great value to:

1. Accurately determine the gestational age if the first ultrasound examination is done at 24 weeks or less. With uncertain gestational age the fundal height will measure less than 24 cm.
2. Diagnose multiple pregnancies early.
3. Identify the site of the placenta.
4. Diagnose severe congenital abnormalities.

If it is not possible to provide ultrasound examinations to all antenatal patients before 24 weeks gestation, the following groups of patients may benefit greatly from the additional information which may be obtained:

1. Patients with a gestational age of 14 to 16 weeks:
   - Patients aged 37 years or more because of their increased risk of having a fetus with a chromosomal abnormality (especially Down syndrome). A patient who would agree to termination of pregnancy if the fetus was abnormal, should be referred for amniocentesis.
   - Patients with a previous history or family history of congenital abnormalities. The nearest hospital with a genetic service should be contacted to determine the need for amniocentesis.

2. Patients with a gestational age of 18 to 22 weeks:
   - Patients needing elective delivery (e.g. those with two previous Caesarean sections, a previous perinatal death, a previous vertical uterine incision or hysterotomy, and diabetes).
   - Gross obesity when it is often difficult to determine the duration of pregnancy.
   - Previous severe pre-eclampsia or preterm labour before 34 weeks. As there is a high risk of recurrence of either complication, accurate

determination of the duration of pregnancy greatly helps in the management of these patients.

- ○ Rhesus sensitisation where accurate determination of the duration of pregnancy helps in the management of the patient.

> **An ultrasound examination done after 24 weeks is too unreliable to be used to estimate the duration of pregnancy.**

1-31 What is the assessment of risk after booking the patient?

Once the patient has been booked for antenatal care, it must be assessed whether she or her fetus have complications or risk factors present, as this will decide when she should be seen again. At the first visit some patients should already be placed in a high-risk category.

1-32 If no risk factors are found at the booking visit, when should the patient be seen again?

She should be seen again when the results of the screening tests are available, preferably 2 weeks after the booking visit. However, if no risk factors were noted and the screening tests were normal the second visit is omitted.

1-33 If there are risk factors noted at the booking visit, when should the patient be seen again?

1. A patient with an underlying illness must be admitted for further investigation and treatment.
2. A patient with a risk factor is followed up sooner if necessary:
   - ○ The management of a patient with chronic hypertension would be planned and the patient would be seen a week later.
   - ○ An HIV-positive patient with an unknown CD4 count must be seen a week later to assess the state of her immune system.

1-34 How should you list risk factors?

All risk factors must be entered on the problem list on the back of the antenatal card. The gestational age when management is needed should be entered opposite the gestational age at the top of the card, e.g. vaginal examination must be done at each visit from 26 to 32 weeks if there is a risk of preterm labour.

The clinic checklist (Figure 1-3) for the first visit could now be completed. If all the open blocks for the first visit can be ticked off, the visit is completed and all important points have been addressed. The checklist should again be used during further visits to make sure that all problems have been considered (i.e. it should be used as a quality control tool).

Clinic Checklist – Classifying (first) visit

Name of patient _____

Clinic record number | | | | | | |

Address _____

Telephone _____

_____

Cell _____

INSTRUCTIONS: Answer all the following questions by placing a cross mark in the corresponding box

Obstetric History

		No	Yes
1.	Previous stillbirth or neonatal loss?		▨
2.	History of three or more consecutive spontaneous abortions		
3.	Birth weight of last baby < 2500g?		▨
4.	Birth weight of last baby > 4500g?		▨
5.	Last pregnancy: hospital admission for hypertension or pre-eclampsia/eclampsia?		▨
6.	Previous surgery on reproductive tract (Caesarean section, myomectomy, cone biopsy, cervical cerclage,)		▨

Current pregnancy

		No	Yes
7.	Diagnosed or suspected multiple pregnancy		▨
8.	Age < 16 years		▨
9.	Age > 40 years		▨
10.	Isoimmunisation Rh (-) in current or previous pregnancy		▨
11.	Vaginal bleeding		▨
12.	Pelvic mass		▨
13.	Diastolic blood pressure 90 mmHg or more at booking		▨
14.	AIDS		▨

General medical

		No	Yes
15.	Diabetes mellitus on insulin or oral hypoglycaemic treatment		▨
16.	Cardiac disease		▨
17.	Renal disease		▨
18.	Epilepsy		▨
19.	Asthmatic on medication		▨
20.	Tuberculosis		▨
21.	Known substance abuse (including heavy alcohol drinking)		▨
22.	Any other severe medical disease or condition		▨

Please specify _____

A yes to any ONE of the above questions (i.e. ONE shaded box marked with a cross) means that the woman is not eligible for the basic component of antenatal care.

Is the woman eligible (circle)   Yes   No

If NO, she is referred to _____

Date_____   Name _____   Signature _____
                      (Staff responsible for antenatal care)

Figure 1-3: The front of a clinic checklist

Clinic Checklist: Follow-up visits
(Back page of first visit checklist)

	VISITS				
First visit for all women at first contact with clinics, regardless of gestational age. If first visit later than recommended, carry out activities up to that time	1	2	3	4	5
DATE :					
Approximate Gest. Age.	___	(20) ___	(26-28) ___	(32) ___	(38) ___
Classifying form which indicates eligibility for BANC					
History taken					
Clinical examination					
Estimated date of delivery calculated					
Blood pressure taken					
Maternal height/weight					
Haemoglobin test					
RPR performed					
Urine tested					
Rapid Rh performed					
Counselled and voluntary testing for HIV					
Tetanus toxoid given					
Iron and folate supplementation provided					
Calcium supplementation provided					
Information for emergencies given					
Antenatal card completed and given to woman					
AZT and NVP given (if required) – Check each visit if AZT sufficient					
Clinical examination for anaemia					
Urine test for protein					
Uterus measured for excessive growth (twins), poor growth (IUGR)					
Instructions for delivery /transport to institution					
Recommendations for lactation and contraception					
Detection of breech presentation and referral					
Complete antenatal card and remind woman to bring it when in labour					
Give follow-up visit date for 41 weeks at referring institution					
Initials of staff member responsible					

Additional Visits		
Date	Reason	Action/Treatment

Figure 1-4: The back of a clinic checklist

The second antenatal visit

1-35 What are the aims of the second antenatal visit?

If the results of the screening tests were not available by the end of the first antenatal visit, a second visit should be arranged 2 weeks later. The aims of this second visit are:

1. To review and act on the results of the special screening investigations done at the booking visit.
2. To perform the second assessment for risk factors.

If possible, all the results of the screening tests should be obtained at the first visit.

Assessing the results of the special screening investigations

1-36 How should you interpret the results of the VDRL or RPR screening tests for syphilis?

The correct interpretation of the results is of the greatest importance:

1. If either the VDRL (Venereal Disease Research Laboratory),or RPR (Rapid Plasmin Reagin)testis negative, then the patient does not have syphilis and no further tests for syphilis are needed.
2. If the VDRL or RPR titre is 1:16 or higher, the patient has syphilis and must be treated.
3. If theVDRL or RPR titre is 1:8 or lower (or the titre is not known), the laboratory should test the same blood sample by means of the TPHA (Treponema pallidum hemagglutination assay) or FTA (Fluorescent Treponemal Antibody) test:
   ○ If the TPHA or FTA is also positive, the patient has syphilis and must be fully treated.

- If the TPHA or FTA is negative, then the patient does not have syphilis and, therefore, need not be treated.
- If a TPHA or FTA test cannot be done, and the patient has not been fully treated for syphilis in the past 3 months, she must be given a full course of treatment.

A syphilis rapid test can be done instead of a TPHA or FTA test.

> **A VDRL or RPR titre of less than 1 in 16 may be caused by syphilis.**

NOTE

The VDRL, RPR or rapid syphilis test may still be negative during the first few weeks after infection with syphilis as the patient has not yet had enough time to form antibodies. The VDRL and RPR tests detect regain antibodies which indicate present syphilis infection while the TPHA, FTA and syphilis rapid tests detect spirochaetal antibodies which indicate syphilis at any time in that person's life.

1-37 How should the results of the on-site RPR card test and syphilis rapid test be interpreted?

If either test is negative the patient does not have syphilis.

1. If the PRP card test is strongly positive the patient most likely has syphilis and treatment should be started. However, a blood specimen must be sent to the laboratory to confirm the diagnosis, and the patient must be seen again 1 week later. Further treatment will depend on the result of the laboratory test. It is important to explain to the patient that the result of the card test needs to be checked with a laboratory test. If the test is weakly positive a blood specimen must still be sent to the laboratory and the patient seen 1 week later. Any treatment will depend on the result of the laboratory test.

2. If the syphilis rapid test is positive the person either has active (untreated) syphilis or was infected in the past and no longer has active disease. The diagnosis of active syphilis must be confirmed or rejected by a VDRL or RPR test. It is advisable that treatment for syphilis be started immediately while waiting for the result of the RPR or VDRL

test. A TPHA can be used as a screening test in the same way as the syphilis rapid test.

1-38 What is the treatment of syphilis in pregnancy?

The treatment of choice is penicillin. If the patient is not allergic to penicillin, she is given benzathine penicillin (Bicillin LA or Penilente LA) 2.4 million units intramuscularly weekly for 3 weeks. At each visit 1.2 million units is given into each buttock. This is a painful injection so the importance of completing the full course must be impressed on the patient.

Benzathine penicillin crosses the placenta and also treats the fetus.

If the patient is allergic to penicillin, she is given erythromycin 500 mg 6-hourly orally for 14 days. This may not treat the fetus adequately, however. Tetracycline is contraindicated in pregnancy as it may damage the fetus.

1-39 How should the results of the rapid HIV test be interpreted?

1. If the rapid HIV test is *negative*, there is a very small chance that the patient is HIV positive. The patient should be informed about the result and given counselling to help her to maintain her negative status.
2. If the rapid HIV test is *positive*, a second rapid test should be done with a kit from another manufacturer. If the second test is also positive, then the patient is HIV positive. The patient should be given the result, and post-test counselling for an HIV-positive patient should be provided.
3. If the first rapid test is positive and the second negative, the patient's HIV status is uncertain. This information should be given to the patient and blood should be taken and sent to the nearest laboratory for an ELISA test for HIV.
    ○ If the ELISA test is negative, there is only a very small chance that the patient is HIV positive.
    ○ If the ELISA test is positive, the patient is HIV positive.

1-40 What should you do if the cervical cytology result is abnormal?

1. A patient whose smear shows an infiltrating cervical carcinoma must immediately be referred to the nearest gynaecological oncology clinic

(level 3 hospital). The duration of pregnancy is very important, and this information (determined as accurately as possible) must be available when the unit is phoned.

2. A patient with a smear showing a low grade CIL (cervical intra-epithelial lesion) such as CIN I (cervical intra-epithelial neoplasia), atypia or only condylomatous changes is checked after 9 months, or as recommended on the cytology report.

3. A patient with a smear showing a high grade CIL, such as CIN II or III or atypical condylomatous changes, must get an appointment at the nearest gynaecology or cytology clinic.

4. Abnormal vaginal flora is only treated if the patient is symptomatic.

NOTE

A colposcopy will be done at the referral clinic. If there are no signs of infiltrating cervical carcinoma, the patient can deliver normally and receive further treatment six weeks after birth. A patient with a macroscopically normal cervix, who comes from an area which does not have access to a gynaecological or cytology clinic, must have her smear repeated at 32 weeks gestation. If the result is unchanged, the patient may deliver normally and receive further treatment six weeks after delivery. Biopsies must be taken from areas which are macroscopically suspicious of cervical carcinoma to exclude infiltrating carcinoma.

NOTE

The latest information from the Cochrane Library indicates that treating bacterial vaginosis does not reduce the risk of preterm labour.

It is essential to record on the antenatal card the plan that has been decided upon, and to ensure that the patient is fully treated after delivery.

1-41 What should you do if the patient's blood group is Rh negative?

Between 5 and 15% of patients are Rhesus negative (i.e. they do not have the Rhesus D antigen on their red cells). The blood grouping laboratory will look for Rhesus anti-D antibodies in these patients. If the Rh card test was used, blood must be sent to the blood grouping laboratory to confirm the result and look for Rhesus anti-D antibodies.

1. If there are no anti-D antibodies present, the patient is not sensitised. Blood must be taken at 26, 32 and 38 weeks of pregnancy to determine if the patient has developed anti-D antibodies since the first test was done.
2. If anti-D antibodies are present, the patient has been sensitised to the Rhesus D antigen. With an anti-D antibody titre of 1:16 or higher, she must be referred to a centre which specialises in the management of this problem. If the titre is less than 1:16, the titre should be repeated within 2 weeks or as directed by the laboratory.

1-42 What is the importance of atypical antibodies?

The presence of these antibodies indicates that the patient has been sensitised to a red-cell antigen other than the Rhesus D antigen. The husband's blood must be examined to determine if he has the antigen which gave rise to the development of these maternal antibodies.

1. If this is the case, then these atypical antibodies may endanger the fetus, and the laboratory or referral hospital must be consulted as to the further management of the patient.
2. If not, then the atypical antibodies are usually the result of an incompatible blood transfusion which the patient has had, and they will not endanger the fetus.

1-43 What should you do if the ultrasound findings do not agree with the patient's dates?

Between 18 and 22 weeks:

1. If the duration of pregnancy, as suggested by the patient's menstrual dates, falls within the range of the duration of pregnancy as given by the

ultrasonographer (usually 3 to 4 weeks), the dates should be accepted as correct.

2. However, if the dates fall outside the range of the ultrasound assessment, then the dates must be regarded as incorrect.

If the ultrasound examination is done in the first trimester (14 weeks or less), the error in determining the gestational age is only 1 week (range 2 weeks).

Remember, if the patient is more than 24 weeks pregnant, ultrasonology cannot be used to determine the gestational age.

1-44 What action should you take if an ultrasound examination at 18 to 22 weeks shows a placenta praevia?

In most cases the placenta will move out of the lower segment as pregnancy progresses, as the size of the uterus increases more than the size of the placenta. Therefore, a follow-up ultrasound examination must be arranged at 32 weeks, where a placenta praevia type II or higher has been diagnosed, to assess whether the placenta is still praevia.

1-45 What should you do if the ultrasound examination shows a possible fetal abnormality?

The patient must be referred to a level 3 hospital for detailed ultrasound evaluation and a decision about further management.

Grading the risk

Once the results of the special investigations have been obtained, all patients must be graded into a risk category. (A list of risk factors and the level of care needed is given in appendix 1). A few high-risk patients would have already been identified at the first antenatal visit while others will be identified at the second visit.

1-46 What are the risk categories?

There are three risk categories:

1. Low (average) risk
2. Intermediate risk
3. High risk

A low-risk patient has no maternal or fetal risk factors present. These patients can receive primary care from a midwife.

An intermediate-risk patient has a problem which requires some, but not continuous, additional care. For example, a grande multipara should be assessed at her first or second visit for medical disorders, and at 34 weeks for an abnormal lie. She also requires additional care during labour and postpartum. She, therefore, is at an increased risk of problems only during part of her pregnancy, labour and puerperium. Most of the antenatal care in these patients can be given by a midwife.

A high-risk patient has a problem which requires continuous additional care. For example, a patient with heart valve disease or a patient with a multiple pregnancy. These patients usually require care by a doctor.

Subsequent visits

General principles:

1. The subsequent visits must be problem oriented.
2. The visits at 28, 34 and 41 weeks are more important visits. At these visits, complications specifically associated with the duration of pregnancy are looked for.
3. From 28 weeks onwards the fetus is viable and the fetal condition must, therefore, be regularly assessed.

1-47 When should a patient return for further antenatal visits?

If a patient books in the first trimester, and is found to be at low risk, her subsequent visits can be arranged as follows:

1. Every 8 weeks until 28 weeks.

2. The next visit is six weeks later at 34 weeks.
3. Primigravidas are then seen every 2 weeks from 36 weeks and multigravidas from 38 weeks. However, multigravidas are also seen again at 36 weeks if a breech presentation was found at their 34 week visit.
4. Thereafter primigravidas are seen at 40 weeks while multigravidas are seen at 41 weeks, if they have not yet delivered.

In some rural areas it may be necessary to see low-risk patients less often because of the large distances involved. The risk of complications with less frequent visits in these patients is minimal. Visits may be scheduled as follows: after the first visit (combining the booking and second visit), the follow-up visits at 28, 34 and 41 weeks.

1-48 Which patients should have more frequent antenatal visits?

If a complication develops, the risk grading will change. This change must be clearly recorded on the patient's antenatal card. Subsequent visits will now be more frequent, depending on the nature of the risk factor.

Primigravidas, whenever possible, must be seen every 2 weeks from 36 weeks, even if it is only to check the blood pressure and test the urine for protein, because they are a high-risk group for developing pre-eclampsia.

A waiting area (obstetric village), where cheap accommodation is available for patients, provides an ideal solution for some intermediate-risk patients, high-risk patients and the above-mentioned primigravidas, so that they can be seen more regularly.

The visit at 28 weeks

1-49 What important complications of pregnancy should be looked for?

1. Antepartum haemorrhage becomes a very important high-risk factor from 28 weeks.
2. Early signs of pre-eclampsia may now be present for the first time, as it is a problem which develops in the second half of pregnancy. Therefore,

the patient must be assessed for proteinuria and a rise in the blood pressure.
3. Cervical changes in a patient who is at high risk for preterm labour, e.g. a patient with multiple pregnancy, a history of previous preterm labour, or polyhydramnios.
4. If the symphysis-fundus height measurement is below the 10th centile, assess the patient for causes of poor fundal growth.
5. If the symphysis-fundus height measurement is above the 90th centile, assess the patient for the causes of a uterus larger than dates.
6. Anaemia may be detected for the first time during pregnancy.
7. Diabetes in pregnancy may present now with glycosuria. If so, a random blood glucose concentration must be measured.

1-50 Why is an antepartum haemorrhage a serious sign?

1. Abruptio placentae causes many perinatal deaths.
2. It may also be a warning sign of placenta praevia.

1-51 How should you monitor the fetal condition?

1. All women should be asked about the frequency of fetal movements and warned that they must report immediately if the movements suddenly decrease or stop.
2. If a patient has possible intra-uterine growth restriction or a history of a previous fetal death, then she should count fetal movements once a day from 28 weeks and record them on a fetal-movement chart.

The visit at 34 weeks

1-52 Why is the 34 weeks visit important?

1. All the risk factors of importance at 28 weeks (except for preterm labour) are still important and must be excluded.
2. The lie of the fetus is now very important and must be determined. If the presenting part is not cephalic, then an external cephalic version must be attempted at 36 weeks if there are no contraindications. A grande

multipara who goes into labour with an abnormal lie is at high risk of rupturing her uterus.

3. Patients who have had a previous Caesarean section must be assessed with a view to the safest method of delivery. A patient with a small pelvis, a previous classical Caesarean section, as well as other recurrent causes for a Caesarean section must be booked for an elective Caesarean section at 39 weeks.

4. The patient's breasts must be examined again for flat or inverted nipples, or eczema of the areolae which may impair breastfeeding. Eczema should be treated.

5. If the first HIV screen was negative, it should be repeated around 32 weeks gestation to detect any late infections.

The visit at 41 weeks

1-53 Why is the visit at 41 weeks important?

A patient whose pregnancy extends beyond 42 weeks has an increased risk of developing the following complications:

1. Intrapartum fetal distress.
2. Meconium aspiration.
3. Intra-uterine death.

1-54 How should you manage a patient who is 41 weeks pregnant?

1. A patient with a complication such as intra-uterine growth restriction (retardation) or pre-eclampsia must have labour induced.

2. A patient who booked early and was sure of her last menstrual period and where, at the booking visit, the size of the uterus corresponded to the duration of pregnancy by dates must have the labour induced on the day she reaches 42 weeks. The same applies to a patient whose duration of pregnancy was confirmed by ultrasound examination before 24 weeks.

3. A patient who is unsure of her dates, or who booked late, must have an ultrasound examination on the day she reaches 42 weeks to determine the amount of amniotic fluid present.
   - If the amniotic fluid index (AFI) is more than 5 (or if the largest pool of liquor measures 3 cm or more) and the patient reports good fetal movement, she should be reassessed in 1 week's time.
   - If the AFI is less than 5 (or if the largest pool of liquor measures less than 3 cm), the pregnancy must be induced.

NOTE

The amniotic fluid index measures the largest vertical pool of liquor in the each of the 4 quadrants of the uterus and adds them together.

Remember that the commonest cause of being post-term is wrong dates.

NOTE

If the patient is to be induced, a surgical induction of labour may be performed if the cervix is favourable and the patient is HIV negative. With an unfavourable cervix or HIV-positive patient, provide a medical induction of labour with misoprostol (Cytotec) 50 μg (a quarter of a tablet) every 4 hours orally until a total of 4 doses (total = 200 μg). Prostaglandin E2 (Prepidil gel 0.5 mg or Prandin 1 mg) can also be used. Induction of labour should take place in a hospital with facilities for Caesarean section.

It is very important that the above problems are actively looked for at 28, 34 and 41 weeks. It is best to memorise these problems and check then one by one at each visit.

1-55 How should the history, clinical findings and results of the special investigations be recorded in low-risk patients?

There are many advantages to a hand-held antenatal card which records all the patient's antenatal information. It is simple, cheap, and effective. It is uncommon for patients to lose their records. The clinical record is then always available wherever the patient presents for care. The clinic need only record the patient's personal details such as name, address and age together with the dates of her clinic visits and the result of any special investigations.

On the one side of the card are recorded the patient's personal details, history, estimated gestational age, examination findings, results of the special investigations, plan of management, and proposed future family planning. On the other side are recorded all the maternal and fetal observations made during pregnancy.

It is important that all antenatal women have a hand-held antenatal card.

1-56 What topics should you discuss with patients during the health education sessions?

The following topics must be discussed:

1. Danger symptoms and signs.
2. Dangerous habits, e.g. smoking or drinking alcohol.
3. Healthy eating.
4. Family planning.
5. Breastfeeding.
6. Care of the newborn infant.
7. The onset of labour and labour itself must also be included when the patient is a primigravida.
8. Avoiding HIV infection or getting counselling if HIV positive.

1-57 What symptoms or signs, which may indicate the presence of serious complications, must be discussed with patients?

1. Symptoms and signs that suggest abruptio placentae:
   ◦ Vaginal bleeding.

- Persistent, severe abdominal pain.
- Decreased fetal movements.

2. Symptoms and signs that suggest pre-eclampsia:
   - Persistent headache.
   - Flashes before the eyes.
   - Sudden swelling of the hands, feet or face.

3. Symptoms and signs that suggest preterm labour:
   - Rupture of the membranes.
   - Regular uterine contractions before the expected date of delivery.

Managing pregnant women with HIV infection

1-58 What is HIV infection and AIDS?

AIDS (Acquired Immune Deficiency Syndrome) is a severe chronic illness caused by the human immunodeficiency virus (HIV). Women with HIV infection can remain clinically well for many years before developing signs of the disease. Severe HIV disease is called AIDS. These patients have a damaged immune system and often die of other opportunistic infections such as tuberculosis.

1-59 Is AIDS an important cause of maternal death?

As the HIV epidemic spreads, the number of pregnant women dying of AIDS has increased dramatically. In some countries, such as South Africa, AIDS is now the commonest cause of maternal death. Therefore all pregnant women must be screened for HIV infection.

NOTE
The Second, Third and Forth Interim Report on Confidential Enquiries into Maternal Deaths in South Africa showed that AIDS was the commonest cause of maternal death. Many additional AIDS deaths may have been missed, as HIV testing is often not done.

> All pregnant women must be screened for HIV infection as AIDS is the commonest cause of maternal death in South Africa.

1-60 Does pregnancy increase the risk of progression from asymptomatic HIV infection to AIDS?

Pregnancy appears to have little or no effect on the progression from asymptomatic to symptomatic HIV infection. However, in women who already have symptomatic HIV infection, pregnancy may lead to a more rapid progression to AIDS.

1-61 How is the severity of HIV infection classified?

The severity and progression of HIV infection during pregnancy can be monitored by:

1. Assessing the clinical stage of the disease
   - Stage 1: Clinically well.
   - Stage 2: Mild clinical problems.
   - Stage 3: Moderate clinical problems.
   - Stage 4: Severe clinical problems (i.e. AIDS).

2. Measuring the CD4 count in the blood. A falling CD4 count is an important marker of progression in HIV infection. It is an indicator of the degree of damage to the immune system. The normal adult CD4 count is 700 to 1100 cells/mm^3. A CD4 count equal or below 350 cells/mm^3 indicates severe damage to the immune system.

> The CD4 count is an important marker of the severity and progression of HIV infection during pregnancy.

1-62 What clinical signs suggest stage 1 and 2 HIV infection?

1. Persistent generalised lymphadenopathy is the only clinical sign of stage 1 HIV infection.
2. Signs of stage 2 HIV infection include:
   - Repeated or chronic mouth or genital ulcers.

- Extensive skin rashes.
- Repeated upper respiratory tract infections such as otitis media or sinusitis.
- Herpes zoster (shingles).

1-63 What are important features suggesting stage 3 or 4 HIV infection?

1. Features of stage 3 HIV infection include:
   - Unexplained weight loss.
   - Oral candidiasis (thrush).
   - Cough, fever and night sweats suggesting pulmonary tuberculosis.
   - Cough, fever and shortness of breath suggesting bacterial pneumonia.
   - Chronic diarrhoea or unexplained fever for more than 1 month.
   - Pulmonary tuberculosis

2. Features of stage 4 HIV infection include:
   - Severe weight loss.
   - Severe or repeated bacterial infections, especially pneumonia.
   - Severe HIV-associated infections such as oesophageal candidiasis (which presents with difficulty swallowing) and Pneumocystis pneumonia (which presents with cough, fever and shortness of breath).
   - Malignancies such as Kaposi's sarcoma.
   - Extrapulmonary tuberculosis (TB).

1-64 How should pregnant women with a positive HIV screening test be managed?

It is very important to identify women with HIV infection as soon as possible in pregnancy so that they can be carefully assessed and their management can be planned. The HIV management should be integrated into the rest of the antenatal care. All women with a positive HIV screening test must have their CD4 count determined as soon as the HIV screening result is obtained.

Determine and note the clinical stage of the disease on the antenatal record.

1-65 What are the indications for antiretroviral prophylaxis in pregnancy?

All pregnant women who are HIV positive should have either ARV prophylaxis or treatment.

All pregnant women who are HIV positive should receive either antiretroviral prophylaxis or treatment.

1-66 What is antiretroviral prophylaxis?

ARV prophylaxis aims at reducing the risk of the mother infecting her fetus and newborn infant with HIV (prevention of mother-to-child transmission or PMTCT). It is not aimed at treating the mother's HIV infection and therefore is given to HIV positive women who are clinically well with a CD4 count above 350 cells/mm3. With prophylaxis the women stop their ARVs once they have stopped breastfeeding and there is no further risk of mother-to-child transmission (WHO option B). ARV prophylaxis should be started at 14 weeks or as soon as possible thereafter. It will reduce the risk of HIV transmission from mother to infant to 2%, compared to 30% without prophylaxis.

For prophylaxis a fixed dose combination (FDC) pill is taken daily, usually at bedtime.

NOTE
WHO option A , which is no longer used in South Africa, consists of zidovudine (AZT) 300 mg orally twice daily from 14 weeks gestation. In addition a single dose of nevirapine 200mg is given to the mother at the onset of labour and AZT 300mg 3 hourly is given during labour. In addition a single dose of Truvada, a combination of tenofovir (TNF) and emtricitabine (FTC), must be given to the mother during or immediately after labour to prevent nevirapine resistance in the mother.

1-67 What are the indications for antiretroviral treatment in pregnancy?

The indications for ARV treatment instead of ARV prophylaxis are any of the following:

1. Clinical signs of stage 3 or 4 HIV infection.
2. A CD4 count equal or below 350 cells/mm^3.
3. Tuberculosis.

The difference between ARV prophylaxis and treatment is that women on treatment continue their ARVs for life and do not stop once breast feeding is completed. In future all pregnant women who are HIV positive will probably be given treatment with ARVs for life (WHO option B+).

1-68 What is antiretroviral treatment?

The aim of ARV treatment is to lower the viral load and allow the immune system to recover. This will both reduce the risk of HIV transmission to the infant and to treat the mother's HIV infection. ARV treatment consists of taking TDF, FTC and EFV as a FDC tablet daily. The use of FDC during pregnancy is the same for both prophylaxis and treatment.

Women who are already on ARV treatment when they book for antenatal care should continue on their ARV treatment during the pregnancy. If not already on FDC, their ARV's may be changed to FDC by a special HIV clinic.

> A fixed dose combination of antiretroviral drugs is used for HIV prophylaxis and treatment during pregnancy.

1-69 Can an HIV-positive woman be cared for in a primary-care clinic?

Most women who are HIV positive are clinically well with a normal pregnancy. Others may only have minor problems (stage 1 or 2). These women can usually be cared for in a primary-care clinic throughout their pregnancy, labour, and puerperium provided they remain well and their pregnancy is normal. Women with a pregnancy complication should be referred to hospital as would be done with HIV-negative patients. Women with severe (stage 3 or 4) HIV-related problems or severe treatment side effects will need to be referred to a special HIV clinic or hospital.

> **Most HIV-positive women can be managed at a primary-care clinic during pregnancy.**

1-70 How are pregnant women with HIV infection managed at a primary-care clinic?

The management of pregnant women with HIV infection is very similar to that of non-pregnant adults with HIV infection. The most important step is to identify those pregnant women who are HIV positive.

The principles of management of pregnant women with HIV infection at a primary-care clinic are:

1. Make the diagnosis of HIV infection by offering HIV screening to all pregnant women at the start of their antenatal care.
2. Assess the CD4 count in all HIV-positive women as soon as their positive HIV status is known.
3. Screen for clinical signs of HIV infection and clinical staging at each antenatal visit.
4. Screen for symptoms of TB.
5. Good diet. Nutritional support may be needed.
6. Emotional support and counselling.
7. Start ARV prophylaxis or treatment when indicated.
8. Early referral if there are pregnancy or HIV complications.

1-71 What preparation is needed for antiretroviral treatment?

Preparing a patient to start ARV treatment is very important. This requires education, counselling and social assessment before ARV treatment can be started. These patients must have regular clinic attendance and must learn about their illness and the importance of excellent adherence (taking their ARV drugs at the correct time every day). They also need to know the side effects of ARV drugs and how to recognise them. Careful general examination and some blood tests are also needed before starting ARV treatment. ARV management should start as soon as possible, preferably within a few days.

1-72 How should pregnant women on antiretroviral treatment be managed?

The national drug protocol using a FDC should be followed. It is very important that staff at the antenatal clinic are trained to manage women with HIV infection. They should work together with the local ARV clinic or HIV service of the local hospital.

1-73 What drugs are used in the fixed dose combination pill?

A fixed dose combination regimen of three drugs is usually used as first line treatment in South Africa. The FDC consists of tenofovir (TDF) 300 mg, emtricitabine (FTC) 200 mg and efavirenz (EFV) 600 mg.

1-74 What are the side effects of antiretroviral drugs?

Pregnant women on ARV prophylaxis or treatment may experience side effects to the ARV drugs. These are usually mild and occur during the first six weeks of treatment. However, side effects may occur at any time that patients are taking ARV drugs. It is important that the staff at primary-care clinics are aware of these side effects and that they ask for symptoms and look for signs at each clinic visit.

Common early side effects during the first few weeks of starting ARV drugs include:

1. Lethargy, tiredness and headaches.
2. Nausea, vomiting and diarrhoea.
3. Muscle pains and weakness.

These mild side effects usually disappear on their own. They can be treated symptomatically. It is important that ARVs are continued even if there are mild side effects.

EFV may cause insomnia (cannot sleep), abnormal dreams and rarely psychiatric symptoms.

More severe side effects may be fatal.

TDF may cause decreased renal function. Less common dangerous side effects of ARV drugs include severe skin rashes, anaemia, hepatitis and lactic acidosis which presents with weight loss, tiredness, nausea, vomiting, abdominal pain and shortness of breath.

Staff at primary-care clinics must be aware and look out for these very important side effects.

1-75 Is HIV/TB co-infection common in pregnancy?

Tuberculosis (TB) is common in patients with HIV who have a weakened immune system. Therefore co-infection with both HIV and TB bacilli is common during pregnancy in communities with a high prevalence of HIV and TB.

Symptomatic screening for TB must be done at each visit by weighing the patient, to check for weight loss, and by asking her about a chronic cough, fever or profuse night sweats. If any one of these are present further investigations for TB are required.

TB is treated with four drugs (rifampicin, isoniazid, pyrazinamide and ethambutol) which may interact and increase the adverse effects of ARV drugs. Treatment of both HIV and tuberculosis should be integrated with routine antenatal care whenever possible.

NOTE
> The negative predictive value of symptomatic screening is 97%. Therefore a negative screen reliably excludes TB. Further investigations for TB include sputum for microscopy and culture as well as a single posterior-anterior chest X-ray with the fetus screened off with a lead apron.

Case study 1

A 36-year-old gravida 4 para 3 patient presents at her first antenatal clinic visit. She does not know the date of her last menstrual period. The patient says that she had hypertension in her last two pregnancies. The symphysis-fundus height measurement suggests a 32-week pregnancy. At her second visit, the report of the routine cervical smear states that she has a low-grade cervical intra-epithelial lesion.

1. Why is her past obstetric history important?

Because hypertension in a previous pregnancy places her at high risk of hypertension again in this pregnancy. She must be carefully examined for hypertension and proteinuria at this visit and at each subsequent visit. This case stresses the importance of a careful history at the booking visit.

2. How accurate is the symphysis-fundus height measurement in determining that the pregnancy is of 32 weeks duration?

This is the most accurate clinical method to determine the size of the uterus from 18 weeks gestation. If the uterine growth, as determined by symphysis-fundus measurement, follows the curve on the antenatal card, the gestational age as determined at the first visit is confirmed.

3. Why would an ultrasound examination not be helpful in determining the gestational age?

Ultrasonology is accurate in determining the gestational age only up to 24 weeks. Thereafter, the range of error is virtually the same as that of a clinical examination.

4. What should you do about the result of the cervical smear?

The cervical smear must be repeated after 9 months. It is important to write the result in the antenatal record and to indicate what plan of management has been decided upon.

Case study 2

At booking, a patient has a positive VDRL test with a titre of 1:4. She has had no illnesses or medical treatment during the past year. By dates and abdominal palpation she is 26 weeks pregnant.

1. What does the result of this patient's VDRL test indicate?

The positive VDRL test indicates that the patient may have syphilis. However, the titre is below 1:16 and, therefore, a definite diagnosis of syphilis cannot be made without a further blood test.

2. What further test is needed to confirm or exclude a diagnosis of syphilis?

If possible, the patient must have a TPHA or FTA or rapid syphilis test. A positive result of any of these tests will confirm the diagnosis of syphilis. If these tests are not available, the patient must be treated for syphilis.

3. Why is the fetus at risk of congenital syphilis?

Because the spirochaetes that cause syphilis may cross the placenta and infect the fetus.

4. What treatment is required if the patient has syphilis?

The patient should be given 2.4 million units of benzathine penicillin (Bicillin LA or Penilente LA) intramuscularly weekly for 3 weeks. Half of the dose is given into each buttock. Benzathine penicillin will cross the placenta and also treat the fetus.

5. What other medical conditions is this patient likely to suffer from?

She may have other sexually transmitted diseases such as HIV.

Case study 3

A healthy primigravida patient of 18 years booked for antenatal care at 22 weeks pregnant. Her rapid syphilis and HIV tests were negative. Her Rh blood group is positive according the Rh card test. She is classified as at low risk for problems during her pregnancy.

1. What is the best time for a pregnant woman to attend an antenatal-care clinic for the first time?

If possible, all pregnant women should book for antenatal care within the first 12 weeks. The duration of pregnancy can then be confirmed with reasonable accuracy on physical examination, medical problems can be diagnosed early, and screening tests can be done as soon as possible.

2. When should this patient return for her next antenatal visit?

She should attend at 28 weeks.

3. What important complications should be looked for in this patient at her 28 week visit?

Anaemia, early signs of pre-eclampsia, a uterus smaller than expected (suggesting intra-uterine growth restriction), or a uterus larger than expected (suggesting multiple pregnancy). A history of antepartum haemorrhage should also be asked for.

4. When should she attend antenatal clinic in the last trimester if she and her fetus remain normal?

The next visit should be at 34 weeks, and then every 2 weeks until 41 weeks.

Case study 4

A 24-year-old gravida 2 para 1 attends the booking antenatal clinic and is seen by a midwife. The previous obstetric history reveals that she had a Caesarean section at term because of poor progress in labour. She is sure of her last menstrual period and is 14 weeks pregnant by dates. On abdominal palpation the height of the uterine fundus is halfway between the symphysis pubis and the umbilicus.

1. What further important information must be obtained about the previous Caesarean section?

The exact indication for the Caesarean section must be found in the patient's hospital notes. In addition, the type of uterine incision made must be established, i.e. whether it was a transverse lower segment or a vertical incision.

2. Why is it important to obtain this additional information?

If the patient had a Caesarean section for a non-recurring cause and she had a transverse lower segment incision, she may be allowed a trial of labour.

3. In which risk category would you place this patient?

She should be placed in the intermediate category.

4. How must you plan this patient's antenatal care?

Her next visit must be arranged at a hospital. If possible, the hospital where she had the Caesarean section so that the required information may be obtained from her folder. Then she may continue to receive her antenatal care from the midwife at the clinic until 36 weeks gestation. From then on the patient must again attend the hospital antenatal clinic where the decision about the method of delivery will be made.

5. Which of the two estimations of the duration of pregnancy is the correct one?

A fundal height measurement midway between the symphysis pubis and the umbilicus suggests a gestational age of 16 weeks. According to her dates, the patient is 14 weeks pregnant. As the difference between these two estimations is less than 3 weeks, the duration of pregnancy as calculated from the patient's dates must be accepted as the correct one.

Skills: General examination at the first antenatal visit

Objectives

When you have completed this skills chapter you should be able to:

- Take an adequate history.
- Perform a good general examination.
- Test the patient's urine.
- Perform and interpret a pregnancy test.

History taking

The purpose of taking a history is to assess the past and present obstetrical, medical and surgical problems in order to detect risk factors for the patient and her fetus.

A. The last normal menstrual period (LMP)

Does the patient have a normal and regular menstrual cycle? When did she last have a *normal* menstrual period?

It may be difficult to establish the LMP when she has an irregular cycle.

If the patient is uncertain of her dates, it is often helpful to relate the onset of pregnancy to some special event, e.g. Christmas or school holidays. For example 'How many periods have you had since your birthday?' or 'How many periods had you missed before New Year?'.

The expected date of delivery (EDD) must now be estimated as accurately as possible. A quick estimate can be made by taking the date of the LMP and adding 9 months and 1 week. Therefore, if the LMP was on 2-2-2009, the EDD will be on 9-11-2009. If the LMP is 27-10-2009, the EDD will be 3-8-2010.

B. Past obstetric history

It is important to know how many pregnancies the patient has lost. Patients often forget about miscarriages and ectopic pregnancies, and may also not mention previous pregnancies from another husband or boyfriend. Questions which need to be asked are:

1. *How many times have you been pregnant?* Ask specifically about miscarriages and ectopic pregnancies.
2. *How many children do you have?* This can bring to light the fact that she has had twins.
3. *How many children do you have who are still alive?* If a child has died, one needs to know approximately at what age the child died, and the cause of death, e.g. 'died at 15 months from diarrhoea'. If the death occurred before delivery or during the neonatal period (first 28 days), information about the cause of death is of particular importance. Approximate birth weights of previous children, and the approximate period of gestation, if the infant was small or preterm, are useful. Low birth weight suggests either growth restriction or preterm delivery, and heavy infants should alert one to the possibility of maternal diabetes.
4. *Were you well during your previous pregnancies?* In addition, asking about any episodes of hospitalisation can be helpful.
5. *How long were you in labour?* It is important to know if she has had a long labour, as this may indicate cephalopelvic disproportion.

6. *The type of delivery* is important. Any form of assisted delivery, including a Caesarean section, suggests that there may have been cephalopelvic disproportion. The patient should always be asked if she knows the reason for having had a Caesarean section. Information about the type of incision made in the uterus must be obtained from the hospital where the patient had her Caesarean section. A history of impacted shoulders is important as it suggests that the infant was very large.
7. *A retained placenta or postpartum haemorrhage* in previous pregnancies should also specifically be asked about.

All these findings should be recorded briefly on the antenatal clinic record.

HISTORY *

Obstetric history

L = Live
IUD = intra-uterine death
END = early neonatal death
LND = late neonatal death
ID = infant death

Year	Gestation (weeks)	Delivery	Weight	Sex		Complications
92	40	N	3 200	F	L	Gastroenteritis
98	36	C/S	2 000	M	IUD	Cong. Abnor.
03	38	N	2 900	F	L	

Description of complications

Figure 1A-1: Recording past obstetric history

C. Medical history

Patients must be asked about diabetes, epilepsy, hypertension, renal disease, heart valve disease and tuberculosis. Also ask about any other illnesses which she may have had. Asking about allergies and medication often brings to light a problem which the patient may have forgotten, or thought not to be of significance. Always ask whether she has ever had an operation or has been admitted to hospital and, if so, where and why.

Any abnormal findings in the medical history should be recorded, with a brief comment, on the antenatal record.

D. Family planning

The patient's family planning needs and wishes should be discussed at the first antenatal visit. She (and her partner) should be encouraged to plan the number and spacing of their children. The contraceptive methods used should also be in keeping with these plans. The patient's wishes should be respected. The outcome of these discussions should be recorded on the antenatal record.

Examination of the patient

E. General examination

The following should be assessed:

1. *Height* – measured in cm. This does not require special equipment. A tape measure stuck to the wall, or a wall marked at 1 cm intervals is adequate. The patient should not wear shoes when her height is measured.
2. *Weight* – measured in kilograms. The patient should only wear light clothing while her weight is being measured. The scale should be periodically checked for accuracy, and, if necessary, re-calibrated. Latest research indicates that poor weight gain, no weight gain or excessive weight gain during pregnancy is not important. Worldwide there is a swing away from weighing patients except at the first antenatal visit.
3. *General appearance*:
   - Is the patient thin or overweight?
   - Is there evidence of recent weight loss?
   - The presence of pallor, oedema, jaundice and enlarged lymph nodes should be specifically looked for.

F. Examination of the thyroid gland

This can be difficult when the patient has a short, thick neck, or when she is obese. Look for an obviously enlarged thyroid gland (a goitre). The patient should be referred for further investigation when there is obvious enlargement of the thyroid, the thyroid feels nodular, or a single nodule can be felt. A normal thyroid gland is usually slightly enlarged during pregnancy.

G. Examination of the breasts

The patient must be undressed in order for the breasts to be examined properly. The breasts should be examined with the patient both sitting and lying on her back, with her hands above her head.

1. *Look*: There may be obvious gross abnormalities. Particularly look for any distortion of the breasts or nipples. The nipples should be specifically examined with regard to their position and deformity (if any), discharge, and whether or not they are inverted. Note any eczema of the areola.
2. *Feel*: Feel for lumps, using the flat hand rather than the fingers.

H. Examination of the lymph nodes

When the thyroid is examined, the neck should also be thoroughly examined for enlarged lymph nodes. The areas above the clavicles and behind the ears must be palpated. The axillae and inguinal areas should also be examined for enlarged lymph nodes.

Patients with AIDS usually have enlarged lymph nodes in all these areas.

I. Examination of the chest

The patient must be undressed. Look for any of the following signs:

1. Any deformities or scars.
2. Any abnormality of the spine.
3. Any difficulty breathing (dyspnoea).

J. Examination of the cardiovascular system

1. *Pulse.* The rate is important. A rapid heart rate is almost always an indication that the patient is anxious or ill.
2. *Blood pressure.* It is important that the blood pressure is recorded correctly.

Testing the patient's urine

Urine is most conveniently tested using reagent strips. Some strips, such as Lenstrip-5, will measure pH, glucose, ketones, protein and blood while others, such as Multistix and Combi-9, will also measure bilirubin, specific gravity, urobilinogen, nitrite and leucocytes. However, measuring glucose and protein are most important and, therefore, only glucose and protein need to be measured in routine antenatal screening. You can use Uristix for this. This is the cheapest method and the cost can be reduced even further by cutting the strips in two, longitudinally.

The strips should be kept in their containers, away from direct sunlight, and at a temperature of less than 30 °C. A cool dry cupboard is satisfactory. The strips should only be removed from their containers one at a time immediately before use, and the container should be closed immediately.

K. Procedure for testing urine

1. The patient should pass a fresh specimen of urine. If the specimen is more than 1 hour old the test results may be unreliable.
2. The specimen should be collected in a clean, dry container.
3. Dip the reagent strip in the urine so that all the reagent areas are covered, and then remove it immediately. If the strip is left in the urine, the reagents dissolve out of the strip, giving a false reading.
4. Draw the edge of the reagent strip across the edge of the urine container to remove excess urine, and hold the strip horizontally.
5. Hold the strip close to the colour chart on the container label (but not touching it). It is important to compare the colours of the test strip with those on the chart at the correct times. Most of the test results are read between 30 and 60 seconds after dipping the strip in urine:
   ○ Lenstrip-5: All the tests are read after 30–60 seconds.
   ○ Multistix: The times for reading the individual tests are on the chart.
   ○ Combi-9: All the tests are read after 60 seconds.
6. After 2 minutes the colours on the reagent strips no longer give a reliable result.

The patient's urine should be tested at every antenatal visit, and the results recorded on the antenatal chart. Proteinuria of 1+ or more is abnormal while glycosuria must be investigated further.

Doing a pregnancy test

L. Indications for a pregnancy test

This test is usually done when a patient has missed 1 or more menstrual periods and when, on clinical examination, one is uncertain whether or not she is pregnant.

The test is based on the detection of human chorionic gonadotrophin in the patient's urine.

The earliest that the test can be expected to be positive is 10 days after conception. The test will be positive by the time a pregnant woman first misses her period. If the test is negative and the woman has not missed her period yet, the test should be repeated after 48 hours.

NOTE
Modern pregnancy tests, which use reagent strips, are very accurate and become positive when the β-hCG concentration in the urine reaches 20 mIU/ml.

M. Storage of test kit

The test which is described in this unit is the U-test β-hCG strip foil. If another pregnancy test is used, the method of doing the test and reading the results must be carefully studied in the instruction booklet. All these kits can be stored at room temperature. However, do not expose to direct sunlight, moisture or heat.

N. Method of performing a pregnancy test

The patient should bring a fresh urine specimen.

1. Open the foil wrapper and remove the test strip.

2. Hold the blue end of the test strip so that the blue arrow points downwards. Dip the test strip into the urine, as far as the point of the arrow, for 5 seconds.
3. Place the test strip on a flat surface and read after 30 seconds. The result is not reliable if the test strip is read more than 10 minutes after it was dipped into the urine.

O. Reading the result of the pregnancy test

1. *Negative* if only the control band nearest the upper blue part of the test strip becomes pink.
2. *Positive* if 2 pink bands are visible. Between the control band and the blue part of the test strip another pink band is seen.
3. *Uncertain* if no pink bands are seen. Either the test was not performed correctly or the test strip is damaged. Repeat the test with another test strip.

Skills: Examination of the abdomen in pregnancy

Objectives

When you have completed this skills chapter you should be able to:

- Determine the gestational age from the size of the uterus.
- Measure the symphysis-fundus height.
- Assess the lie and the presentation of the fetus.
- Assess the amount of liquor present.
- Listen to the fetal heart.
- Assess fetal movements.
- Assess the state of fetal wellbeing.

General examination of the abdomen

There are two main parts to the examination of the abdomen:

1. General examination of the abdomen.
2. Examination of the uterus and the fetus.

A. Preparation of the patient for examination

1. The patient should have an empty bladder.
2. She should lie comfortably on her back with a pillow under her head. She should *not* lie slightly turned to the side, as is needed when the blood pressure is being taken.

B. General appearance of the abdomen

The following should be specifically looked for and noted:

1. The presence of obesity.
2. The presence or absence of scars. When a scar is seen, the reason for it should be specifically asked for (e.g. what operation did you have?), if this has not already become clear from the history.
3. The apparent size and shape of the uterus.
4. Any abnormalities.

C. Palpation of the abdomen

1. The liver, spleen, and kidneys must be specifically palpated.
2. Any other abdominal mass should be noted.
3. The presence of an enlarged organ, or a mass, should be reported to the responsible doctor, and the patient should then be assessed by the doctor.

Examination of the uterus and the fetus

D. Palpation of the uterus

1. Check whether the uterus is lying in the midline of the abdomen. Sometimes it is rotated either to the right or the left.
2. Feel the wall of the uterus for irregularities. An irregular uterine wall suggests either:
   - The presence of myomas (fibroids) which usually enlarge during pregnancy and may become painful.
   - A congenital abnormality such as a bicornuate uterus.

E. Determining the size of the uterus before 18 weeks gestation

1. Anatomical landmarks, i.e. the symphysis pubis and the umbilicus, are used.
2. Gently palpate the abdomen with the left hand to determine the height of the fundus of the uterus:
   - If the fundus is palpable just above the symphysis pubis, the gestational age is probably 12 weeks.
   - If the fundus reaches halfway between the symphysis and the umbilicus, the gestational age is probably 16 weeks.
   - If the fundus is at the same height as the umbilicus, the gestational age is probably 22 weeks (1 finger under the umbilicus = 20 weeks and 1 finger above the umbilicus = 24 weeks).

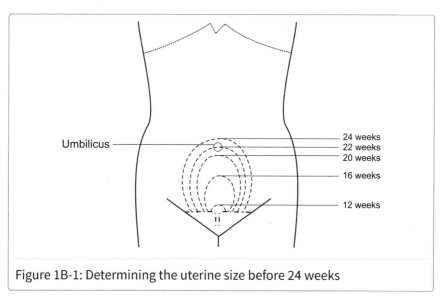

Figure 1B-1: Determining the uterine size before 24 weeks

F. Determining the height of the fundus from 18 weeks gestation

The symphysis-fundus height should be measured as follows:

1. *Feel for the fundus of the uterus.* This is done by starting to gently palpate from the lower end of the sternum. Continue to palpate down the abdomen until the fundus is reached. When the highest part of the fundus has been identified, mark the skin at this point with a pen. If the

uterus is rotated away from the midline, the highest point of the uterus will not be in the midline but will be to the left or right of the midline. Therefore, also palpate away from the midline to make sure that you mark the highest point at which the fundus can be palpated. Do not move the fundus into the midline before marking the highest point.

2. *Measure the symphysis-fundus (SF) height.* Having marked the fundal height, hold the end of the tape measure at the top of the symphysis pubis. Lay the tape measure over the curve of the uterus to the point marking the top of the uterus. The tape measure must not be stretched while doing the measurement. Measure this distance in centimetres from the symphysis pubis to the top of the fundus. This is the symphysis-fundus height.

3. If the uterus does not lie in the midline but, for example, lies to the right, then the distance to the highest point of the uterus must still be measured *without* moving the uterus into the midline.

Having determined the height of the fundus, you need to assess whether the height of the fundus corresponds to the patient's dates, and to the size of the fetus. From 18 weeks, the SF height must be plotted on the SF growth curve to determine the gestational age. This method is, therefore, only used once the fundal height has reached 18 weeks. In other words, when the SF height has reached 2 fingers width under the umbilicus.

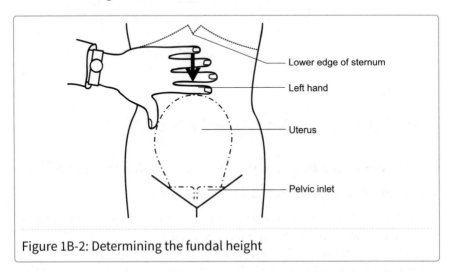

Figure 1B-2: Determining the fundal height

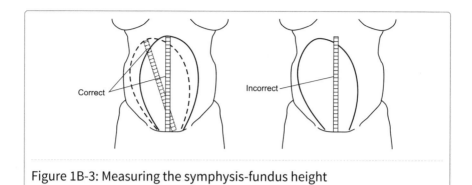

Figure 1B-3: Measuring the symphysis-fundus height

G. Palpation of the fetus

The lie and presenting part of the fetus only becomes important when the gestational age reaches 34 weeks.

The following must be determined:

1. *The lie of the fetus.* This is the relationship of the long axis of the fetus to that of the mother. The lie may be longitudinal, transverse, or oblique.
2. *The presentation of the fetus.* This is determined by the presenting part:
   - If there is a breech, it is a breech presentation.
   - If there is a head, it is a cephalic presentation.
   - If no presenting part can be felt, it is a transverse or oblique lie.
3. *The position of the back of the fetus.* This refers to whether the back of the fetus is on the left or right side of the uterus, and will assist in determining the position of the presenting part.

H. Methods of palpation

There are four specific steps for palpating the fetus. These are performed systematically. With the mother lying comfortably on her back, the examiner faces the patient for the first three steps, and faces towards her feet for the fourth.

1. *First step.* Having established the height of the fundus, the fundus itself is gently palpated with the fingers of both hands, in order to discover which pole of the fetus (breech or head) is present. The head feels hard

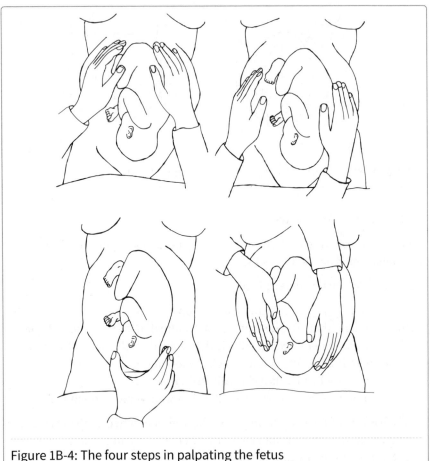

Figure 1B-4: The four steps in palpating the fetus

and round, and is easily movable and ballotable. The breech feels soft, triangular and continuous with the body.

2. *Second step.* The hands are now placed on the sides of the abdomen. On one side there is the smooth, firm curve of the back of the fetus, and on the other side, the rather knobbly feel of the fetal limbs. It is often difficult to feel the fetus well when the patient is obese, when there is a lot of liquor, or when the uterus is tight, as in some primigravidas.

3. *Third step.* The examiner grasps the lower portion of the abdomen, just above the symphysis pubis, between the thumb and fingers of one hand.

The objective is to feel for the presenting part of the fetus and to decide whether the presenting part is loose above the pelvis or fixed in the pelvis. If the head is loose above the pelvis, it can be easily moved and balloted. The head and breech are differentiated in the same way as in the first step.

4. *Fourth step.* The objective of this step is to determine the amount of head palpable above the pelvic brim, if there is a cephalic presentation. The examiner faces the patient's feet, and with the tips of the middle 3 fingers palpates deeply in the pelvic inlet. In this way the head can usually be readily palpated, unless it is already deeply in the pelvis. The amount of the head palpable above the pelvic brim can also be determined.

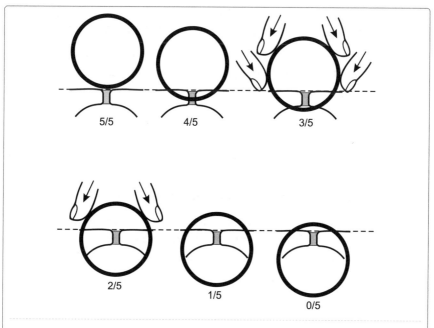

Figure 1B-5: An accurate method of determining the amount of head palpable above the brim of the pelvis

I. Special points about the palpation of the fetus

1. When you are palpating the fetus, always try to assess the size of the fetus itself. Does the fetus fill the whole uterus, or does it seem to be smaller than you would expect for the size of the uterus and the duration of pregnancy? A fetus which feels smaller than you would expect for the duration of pregnancy, suggests intra-uterine growth restriction, while a fetus which feels smaller than expected for the size of the uterus, suggests the presence of a multiple pregnancy.
2. If you find an abnormal lie when you palpate the fetus, you should always consider the possibility of a multiple pregnancy. When you suspect that a patient might have a multiple pregnancy, she should have an ultrasound examination.

J. Special points about the palpation of the fetal head

1. *Does the head feel too small for the size of the uterus?* You should always try to relate the size of the head to the size of the uterus and the duration of pregnancy. If it feels smaller than you would have expected, consider the possibility of a multiple pregnancy.
2. *Does the head feel too hard for the size of the fetus?* The fetal head feels harder as the pregnancy gets closer to term. A relatively small fetus with a hard head suggests the presence of intra-uterine growth restriction.

K. Assessment of the amount of liquor present

This is not always easy to feel. The amount of liquor decreases as the pregnancy nears term. The amount of liquor is assessed clinically by feeling the way that the fetus can be moved (balloted) while being palpated.

1. If the liquor volume is reduced (oligohydramnios), it suggests that:
   - There may be intra-uterine growth restriction.
   - There may be a urinary tract obstruction or some other urinary tract abnormality in the fetus. This is uncommon.

2. If the liquor volume is increased (polyhydramnios), it suggests that one of the following conditions may be present:
   - Multiple pregnancy.

- Maternal diabetes.
- A fetal abnormality such as spina bifida, anencephaly or oesophageal atresia.

In many cases, however, the cause of polyhydramnios is unknown. However, serious problems can be present and the patient should be referred to a hospital where the fetus can be carefully assessed. The patient needs an ultrasound examination by a trained person to exclude multiple pregnancy or a congenital abnormality in the fetus.

L. Assessment of uterine irritability

This means that the uterus feels tight, or has a contraction, while being palpated. Uterine irritability normally only occurs after 36 weeks of pregnancy, i.e. near term. If there is an irritable uterus before this time, it suggests either that there is intra-uterine growth restriction or that the patient may be in, or is likely to go into, preterm labour.

M. Listening to the fetal heart

1. *Where should you listen?* The fetal heart is most easily heard by listening over the back of the fetus. This means that the lie and position of the fetus must be established by palpation before listening for the fetal heart.
2. *When should you listen to the fetal heart?* You need only listen to the fetal heart if a patient has not felt any fetal movements during the day. Listening to the fetal heart is, therefore, done to rule out an intra-uterine death.
3. *How long should you listen for?* You should listen long enough to be sure that what you are hearing is the fetal heart and not the mother's heart. When you are listening to the fetal heart, you should, at the same time, also feel the mother's pulse.

N. Assessment of fetal movements

The fetus makes two types of movement:

1. *Kicking* movements, which are caused by movement of the limbs. These are usually quick movements.
2. *Rolling* movements, which are caused by the fetus changing position.

When you ask a patient to count her fetal movements, she must count both types of movement.

If there is a reason for the patient to count fetal movements and to record them on a fetal-movement chart, it should be done as follows:

1. *Time of day.* Most patients find that the late morning is a convenient time to record fetal movements. However, she should be encouraged to choose the time which suits her best. She will need to rest for an hour. It is best that she use the same time every day.
2. *Length of time.* This should be for 1 hour per day, and the patient should be able to rest and not be disturbed for this period of time. Sometimes the patient may be asked to rest and count fetal movements for 2 or more half-hour periods a day. The patient must have access to a watch or clock, and know how to measure half- and 1-hour periods.
3. *Position of the patient.* She may either sit or lie down. If she lies down, she should lie on her side. In either position she should be relaxed and comfortable.
4. *Recording of fetal movements.* The fetal movements should be recorded on a chart as shown in Table 1B-1.

Table 1B-1: Chart for recording fetal movements

Date	Time		Total
3 July	8–9	√√√√√√	6
4 July	11–12	√√√√√√√√√	9
5 July	8–9	√√√	3

The chart records that:

- *Between 08:00 and 09:00 on 3 July the fetus moved 6 times.*
- *Between 11:00 and 12:00 on 4 July the fetus moved 9 times.*
- *Between 08:00 and 09:00 on 5 July the fetus moved 3 times.*

Every time the fetus moves, the patient must make a tick on the chart so that all the movements are recorded. The time and day should be marked on the chart. If the patient is illiterate, the nurse giving her the chart can fill in the day (and times if the chart is to be used more than once a day). It is important to explain to the patient exactly how to use the chart. Remember that a patient who is resting can easily fall asleep and, therefore, miss fetal movements.

O. Assessment of the state of fetal wellbeing

It is very important to assess the state of fetal wellbeing at the end of *every* abdominal palpation. This is done by taking into account all the features mentioned in this skills chapter.

1C

Skills: Vaginal examination in pregnancy

Objectives

When you have completed this skills chapter you should be able to:

- List the indications for a vaginal examination.
- Insert a bivalve speculum.
- Perform a bimanual vaginal examination.
- Take a cervical smear.

Indications for a vaginal examination

A vaginal examination is the most intimate examination a woman is ever subjected to. It must never be performed without:

1. A careful explanation to the patient about the examination.
2. Asking permission from the patient to perform the examination.
3. A valid reason for performing the examination.

A. Indications for a vaginal examination in pregnancy

1. *At the first visit:*
   - The diagnosis of pregnancy during the first trimester.
   - Assessment of the gestational age.
   - Detection of abnormalities in the genital tract.
   - Investigation of a vaginal discharge.
   - Examination of the cervix.
   - Taking a cervical (Papanicolaou) smear.

2. *At subsequent antenatal visits:*
   ○ Investigation of a threatened abortion.
   ○ Confirmation of preterm rupture of the membranes with a sterile speculum.
   ○ To confirm the diagnosis of preterm labour.
   ○ Detection of cervical effacement and/or dilatation in a patient with a risk for preterm labour e.g. multiple pregnancy, a previous midtrimester abortion, preterm labour or polyhydramnios.
   ○ Assessment of the ripeness of the cervix prior to induction of labour.
   ○ Identification of the presenting part in the pelvis.
   ○ Performance of a pelvic assessment.
3. *Immediately before labour:*
   ○ Performance of artificial rupture of the membranes to induce labour.

B. Contraindications to a vaginal examination in pregnancy

1. *Antepartum haemorrhage.* However, there are two exceptions to this rule:
   ○ A cephalic presentation with the fetal head palpable 2/5 or less above the pelvic brim (i.e. engaged), thereby, excluding a placenta praevia.
   ○ Obvious signs and symptoms of abruptio placentae.
2. Preterm and prelabour rupture of the membranes without contractions (except with a sterile speculum to confirm or exclude rupture of the membranes).

Method of vaginal examination

C. Preparation for vaginal examination

1. The bladder must be empty.

2. The procedure must be carefully explained to the patient.
3. The patient is put in the dorsal or lithotomy position:
   - The *dorsal* position is more comfortable and less embarrassing than the lithotomy position and does not require any equipment. This is the position most often used.
   - The *lithotomy* position provides better access to the genital tract than the dorsal position. Lithotomy poles and stirrups are required.

> A vaginal examination must always be preceded by an abdominal examination.

D. Examination of the vulva

The vulva must be carefully inspected for any abnormalities, such as scars, warts, varicosities, congenital abnormalities, ulcers or discharge.

E. Speculum examination

1. A speculum examination is always performed at the first antenatal visit. At subsequent antenatal visits this examination is only done when indicated, e.g. to investigate a vaginal discharge or in the case of preterm or prelabour rupture of the membranes.
2. The Cusco or bivalve speculum is the one most commonly used.

F. Insertion of a bivalve speculum

1. The procedure must be explained to the patient.
2. The labia are parted with the fingers of the gloved left hand.
3. The patient is asked to bear down.
4. The closed speculum is gently inserted posteriorly into the vagina. Great care must be taken to avoid undue contact with the anterior vaginal wall at the introitus as this causes great discomfort, or even pain, from pressure on the urethra.
5. As soon as the speculum has passed through the vaginal opening, the blades must be slightly opened. The speculum is now inserted deeper into the vagina. When the cervix is reached, the speculum is fully opened. This method allows for inspection of the vaginal walls during insertion and ensures that the cervix is found.

6. Any vaginal discharge must be identified. Where needed, a sample is taken with a wooden spatula.
7. The vagina is inspected for congenital abnormalities such as a vaginal septum, a vaginal stenosis or a double vagina and cervix.
8. The cervix is inspected for any laceration or tumour. A smooth red area surrounding the external os that retains the normal smooth surface is normal during the reproductive years and is called ectopy.
9. If there is a history of rupture of the membranes, the presence of liquor is noted and tested for.
10. A cervical (Papanicolaou) smear must be taken if a smear has not been taken recently.
11. At the end of the examination the speculum is gently withdrawn, keeping it slightly open, so that the vaginal walls can again be inspected all the way out.

G. Taking a cervical smear

1. A cervical (Papanicolaou) smear is taken to detect abnormalities of the cervix, e.g. human papilloma virus infection, cervical intra-epithelial neoplasia or carcinoma of the cervix.
2. Ideally the first cervical smear should be taken when the patient becomes sexually active. In practice the first smear is usually taken when the patient first attends a family planning or antenatal clinic.
3. If the cervical smear is normal, it should be repeated at 30, 40 and 50 years of age.
4. The technique of taking a cervical smear is as follows:
   ○ The name, folder number and date must be written on the slide with a pencil beforehand. Also make sure that a spray can is close at hand to fix the slide.
   ○ A vaginal speculum is inserted.
   ○ The cervix must be clearly seen and is carefully inspected.
   ○ A suitable spatula is inserted into the cervix and rotated through 360 degrees, making sure that the whole circumference is gently scraped. It is important that the smear is taken from the inside of the cervical canal as well as from the surface of the cervix. An Ayres (Aylesbury) or tongue spatula must be used and not a brush with sharp or long points such as a Cervibrush or Cytobrush.

- The material obtained is smeared onto a glass slide and *immediately* sprayed with Papanicolaou's fixative.
- When the slide is dry, it is sent to the laboratory for examination.

H. Performing a bimanual examination

1. First 1 and then, where possible, 2 gloved and lubricated fingers are gently inserted into the vagina.
2. If a vaginal septum or stenosis is present, the patient should be referred to a doctor to decide whether delivery will be interfered with.
3. The cervix is palpated and the following are noted:
   - Any dilatation.
   - The length of the cervix in cm, i.e. whether the cervix is effaced or not.
   - The surface should be smooth and regular.
   - The consistency, which will become softer during pregnancy.

4. Special care must be taken, when performing a bimanual examination *late* in pregnancy and in the presence of a high presenting part, not to damage a low-lying placenta. If the latter is suspected, a finger must not be inserted into the cervical canal. Instead, the presenting part is gently palpated through all the fornices. If any bogginess is noted between the fingers of the examining hand and the presenting part, the examination must be immediately abandoned and the patient must be referred urgently for ultrasonography.
5. Where possible the presenting part is identified.
6. A most important part of the bimanual examination is the determination of the gestational age, by estimating the size of the uterus and comparing it with the period of amenorrhoea. This is only really accurate in the first trimester. Thereafter, the fundal height and the size of the fetus must be determined by abdominal examination.
7. The uterine wall is palpated for any irregularity, suggesting the presence of a congenital abnormality (e.g. bicornuate uterus) or myomata (fibroids).
8. Lastly, the fornices are palpated to exclude any masses, the commonest of which is an ovarian cyst or tumour.

I. Explanation to the patient

Do not forget to explain to the patient, after the examination is completed, what you have found. It is especially important to tell her how far pregnant she is, if that can be determined, and to reassure her, if everything appears to be normal.

1D

Skills: Screening tests for syphilis

Objectives

When you have completed this skills chapter you should be able to:

- Screen a patient for syphilis with the syphilis rapid test and the RPR card test.
- Interpret the results of the screening tests.

Syphilis screening

At the first antenatal visit each woman should be screened for syphilis. This could be done at the clinic with the syphilis rapid test (Determine Syphilis TP) or RPR card test. If syphilis is diagnosed, the patient must be informed and treatment must be started immediately at the antenatal clinic. Positive rapid screening tests must be confirmed with a laboratory RPR or VDRL test. The syphilis rapid test or RPR card test can be used in any antenatal clinic, as no sophisticated equipment is required.

Syphilis rapid test

The syphilis rapid test is a specific test for syphilis and will become positive when there are antibodies against Treponema pallidum (the organism that causes syphilis) in the blood. The test result corresponds to that of a TPHA or FTA test which are also specific tests for syphilis.

A. Equipment needed to perform a syphilis rapid test

1. The Abbott Determine TB Whole Blood Essay. Each kit contains 10 cards with 10 tests. The Chase Buffer (2.5 ml bottle) is supplied with the kit.
2. EDTA capillary tubes marked to indicate 50 μl, lancets, alcohol swabs and sterile gauze swabs. These are not supplied with the kit.

The kit needs to be stored at room temperature between 2 °C and 30 °C. Storage in a fridge is required during summer time. The kit must not be used after the expiry date.

B. Performing the syphilis rapid test

1. Clean the patient's fingertip with an alcohol swab and allow the finger to dry.
2. Remove a test strip from the foil cover.
3. Prick the skin of the fingertip with a lancet. Wipe the first drop of blood away with a sterile gauze swab.
4. Collect the next drop of blood into the EDTA tube. Either side of the tube can be used to collect blood. Fill the tube from the tip to the first black circle (i.e. 50 μl blood). Avoid the collection of air bubbles.
5. Apply the 50 μl of blood from the EDTA tube onto the sample pad marked with an arrow on the test strip.
6. Wait until all the blood has been absorbed into the sample pad and then apply 1 drop of Chase Buffer. The bottle must be held vertically (upside down) above the test strip when a drop of the buffer is dropped onto the sample pad.
7. Wait a minimum of 15 minutes and then read the result. The maximum waiting time for reading the test is 24 hours. After 24 hours the test becomes invalid.

C. Reading the results of the syphilis rapid test

1. *Positive*: A red bar will appear within both the Control window and the Patient window on the test strip. Any visible red bar in the Patient window must be regarded as positive.

2. *Negative*: A red bar will appear within the Control window but no red bar is seen in the Patient window.
3. *Invalid*: If no red bar appears in the Control window, even if a red bar is visible in the Patient window, the result is invalid and the test must be repeated.

D. The interpretation of the syphilis rapid test

1. A positive test indicates that a person has antibodies against syphilis. This means that the person either has active (untreated) syphilis or was infected in the past and no longer has the disease.
2. A negative test indicates that a person does not have antibodies and cannot have syphilis, either in the present or past, unless the person was infected very recently and has not yet formed antibodies.

E. Management if the syphilis rapid test is positive

1. Explain to the patient that the screening test for syphilis is positive but that this should be confirmed or rejected by a laboratory test (RPR or VDRL test).
2. It is advisable, however, that treatment with penicillin be started immediately so that the fetus can be treated while waiting for the result of the laboratory test.
3. Ask the patient to return in 1 week for the result of the laboratory test.

F. Interpretation of the RPR or VDRL test when the syphilis rapid test is positive

1. If the RPR or VDRL is negative the patient does not have syphilis. Treatment can be stopped.
2. If the RPR or VDRL titre is 1:16 or higher the patient has syphilis and must be treated with a full course of 3 doses of benzathine penicillin (Bicillin LA of Penilente LA).
3. If the RPR of VDRL titre is 1:8 or lower and the patient and her partner have been fully treated in the past 3 months, treatment can be stopped. Otherwise, a full course of 3 doses of benzathine penicillin must be given.

The RPR card test

The RPR card test is a non-specific test that will become positive if the patient has syphilis. The result corresponds to that of a laboratory RPR and VDRL test which are also non-specific tests for syphilis.

G. Collecting a blood sample

A 3 ml sample of venous blood is needed for the test. Place the blood in a test tube for clotted blood (red-topped tube).

H. Equipment needed to perform a RPR card test

1. The carbon antigen suspension.
2. The antigen dispenser attached to the special calibrated needle with a blunt tip.
3. The special stirrers (Dispenstirs).
4. The white RPR card.
5. The test tube holder.

Except for the test tube holder, all the necessary equipment comes with the RPR card kit.

If many tests are to be done each day and the container with the carbon antigen will be used up within 3 weeks, it is not necessary to keep the container in a fridge. However, the container should be kept in a fridge if it is to be used for more than 3 weeks.

NOTE
> A number of different commercial companies manufacture RPR card tests. (A RPR kit can be obtained from Davies Diagnostics at the toll-free number 0800 110 509 in South Africa).

I. The method of performing the RPR card test

1. Keep the test tube containing 3 ml of clotted blood in an upright position. It is important to remove the stopper when the blood is placed in the tube.
2. Place the test tube in the test tube stand for 30 minutes so that the serum can be expressed from the clotted blood.

3. Use the special stirrer to transfer *1* drop of serum from the test tube to the card. Squeeze the hollow stirrer between your thumb and forefinger while the tip of the stirrer is in the serum. Now relax your grip on the stirrer and a sample will be sucked up.
4. Place the tip of the stirrer above the test card and again squeeze the stirrer so that 1 drop falls onto the centre of the circle. If the serum of more than one patient is tested at the same time, the test tube of clotted blood must be numbered and the same number must be written on the card with a soft pen. Make sure that the number on the test tube always corresponds to the number on the card.
5. Using the flat end of the stirrer, spread the drop of serum over the whole area within the circle.
6. Shake the antigen dispenser containing the antigen suspension well. Use the dispenser with the attached calibrated needle to place *1* drop (50 μl) of antigen onto the serum in the circle.
7. The card must now be gently rocked by hand so that the serum and the antigen suspension are well mixed, while the fluid on the card remains within the circle. If available, an electrical rotator can be used to rock the card.
8. After 4 minutes of hand rocking or 8 minutes of electronic rocking the test can be read.

J. Reading the results of the RPR card test

1. *A positive test*: Obvious clumping takes place (flocculation). Definite black particles form which are clearly seen with the naked eye. While the particles cover the whole area of the spread-out droplet, they tend to gather around the edge of the droplet.
2. *A negative test*: *No* clumping takes place. The small black particles of the carbon antigen tend to collect at the centre of the spread-out droplet where they form a black dot. They do not collect around the rim of the droplet as is seen in a positive test.

K. Interpretation of the results of the RPR card test

1. *A positive test*: Explain to the patient that the screening test for syphilis is positive, but that this should be confirmed or rejected by a laboratory test. It is advisable, however, that treatment with penicillin be started

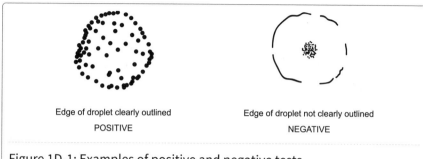

Edge of droplet clearly outlined

POSITIVE

Edge of droplet not clearly outlined

NEGATIVE

Figure 1D-1: Examples of positive and negative tests

immediately so that the fetus can be treated. If possible, send a sample of clotted blood to the laboratory for a RPR or VDRL test and ask the patient to return in 1 week for the result.

NOTE

When the RPR card test is clearly positive the laboratory RPR or VDRL is almost always positive with a titre of 1:8 or more. If the laboratory RPR or VDRL is negative, the patient does not have syphilis and the treatment can be stopped.

2. *A negative test*. The patient can be reassured that she does not have syphilis. No treatment is needed.

NOTE

It is advisable that 1 out of every 20 negative RPR tests be checked with a laboratory VDRL test in order that quality control can be observed.

If it cannot be decided whether clumping of particles is present or not, a sample of the patient's blood must be sent to the laboratory for a VDRL test. The patient must be seen again as soon as the results are available and treatment given according to the laboratory results. If the patient cannot come back for the result or if it is not possible to get a laboratory VDRL, start treatment immediately.

1E

Skills: Screening tests for HIV

Objectives

When you have completed this skills chapter you should be able to:

- Screen a patient for HIV.
- Interpret the results of the screening test.

HIV screening

At the first antenatal visit each woman should be offered screening for HIV. An HIV rapid test can be used in any antenatal clinic as no sophisticated equipment is required. Prior to testing, provider-initiated counselling must be given and consent must be obtained.

A. Equipment needed to perform an HIV rapid test

1. The Abbott Determine HIV-1/2 Whole Blood Essay. Each kit contains 10 cards with 10 tests. The Chase Buffer (2.5 ml bottle) is supplied with the kit.
2. EDTA capillary tubes marked to indicate 50 µl, lancets, alcohol swabs and sterile gauze swabs. These are not supplied with the kit.

The kit needs to be stored at room temperature between 2 ℃ and 30 ℃. Storage in a fridge is required during summer time. The kit cannot be used after the expiry date.

B. The method of performing the HIV rapid test

1. Clean the patient's fingertip with an alcohol swab and allow the finger to dry.
2. Remove a test strip from the foil cover.
3. Prick the skin of the fingertip with a lancet. Wipe the first drop of blood away with a sterile gauze swab.
4. Collect the next drop of blood with the EDTA tube. Either side of the tube can be used to collect blood. Fill the tube from the tip to the first black circle (i.e. 50 µl of blood). Avoid the collection of air bubbles.
5. Apply the 50 µl of blood from the EDTA tube onto the sample pad marked with an arrow on the test strip.
6. Wait 1 minute until all the blood has been absorbed into the sample pad and then apply 1 drop of Chase Buffer. The bottle must be held vertically (upside down) above the test strip when a drop of the buffer is dropped on the sample pad.
7. Wait a minimum of 15 minutes and then read the results. The maximum waiting time for reading the test is 24 hours. After 24 hours the test becomes invalid.

C. Reading the results of the HIV rapid test

1. *Positive*: A red bar will appear within both the Control window and the Patient window on the test strip. Any visible red bar in the Patient window must be regarded as positive. The result is positive even if the patient bar appears lighter or darker than the control bar.
2. *Negative*: A red bar will appear within the Control window and but no red bar is seen in the Patient window.
3. *Invalid*: If no red bar appears in the Control window, even if a red bar is visible in the Patient window, the result is invalid and the test must be repeated.

D. The interpretation of the HIV rapid test

The test is a specific test for HIV and will become positive when there are antibodies against HIV (the virus that causes AIDS) in the blood.

1. A positive test indicates that a person has antibodies against HIV. Therefore the person is infected with HIV (and is HIV positive).
2. A negative test indicates that a person does not have antibodies against HIV. Therefore the person is not infected with HIV, unless they were infected very recently and the HIV antibodies have not appeared yet.

E. Management if the HIV rapid test is positive

1. Explain to the patient that the first screening test for HIV is positive but that this should be confirmed with a second test.
2. Proceed with a second test using a different kit.
3. If the second test is also positive, the patient is HIV positive.
4. Proceed with post-test counselling for a patient with a positive test.

F. Management if the first HIV rapid test is positive but the second is negative

1. A blood sample for a confirming HIV test must be sent to the laboratory.
2. The patient must be informed that the results of the HIV rapid tests are inconclusive and that a laboratory test is required to determine her HIV status.
3. If the laboratory test is positive, the patient is HIV positive.
4. If the laboratory test is negative, the patient is HIV negative.
5. Proceed with appropriate counselling.

Skills: Examination of the breasts

Objectives

When you have completed this skills chapter you should be able to:

- Take an adequate history for breast conditions.
- Perform a good breast examination.
- Perform an examination of the supraclavicular and axillary lymph nodes.

History taking

The purpose of taking a family, past and present history is to assess whether there are any warning symptoms of serious breast conditions, especially cancer.

A. The importance of asking the woman's age

Breast cancer becomes more common as a woman gets older. While breast cancer is rare under 20 years of age it becomes more common over the age of 40 years.

B. The importance of a positive family history of breast cancer

Has any member of the mother or father's family or a sibling had breast or ovarian cancer? A positive family history, especially of her mother or sisters, increases the chance that the woman will develop breast cancer

C. The importance of a past history of breast or ovarian cancer

A woman who has had breast cancer before has a much higher chance of having breast cancer again.

D. Any present history of breast changes or complaints

Always ask about:

- One breast becoming larger than the other or changing shape
- Any new breast lumps or lumps that are getting bigger
- Any nipple changes, especially watery or bloody nipple discharge, a nipple which becomes inverted (pulled in) or a new rash on the nipple or areola
- Any rash or redness of a breast

Examination of the breasts

E. Preparation for a breast examination

The woman should undress down to her waist and put on a gown. The examination must be done somewhere private and well lit. Always explain what you are going to do. It is very important to be able to have a good look at both breasts.

F. Step-by-step examination of the breast

The examination consists of both looking (inspection) and feeling (palpating). Wherever possible, the examination should be done in a standardized step-by-step manner. Once you have done a few breast examinations, it will become quite quick and easy.

G. Inspection of the breasts is usually done in three positions with the woman sitting up

Ask the woman to sit down on the examining couch facing you with her arms relaxed at her sides. Look at her breasts asymmetry, nipple inversion, skin changes and redness. You may even be able to see a breast lump.

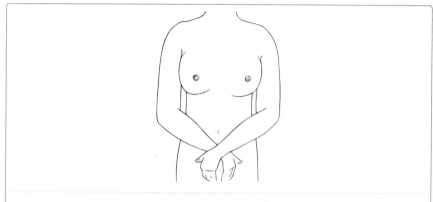

Figure 1F-1: Position during inspection of breasts.

Next ask her to raise both her arms above her head. Look for any skin puckering (skin pulled in). This will help identify a lump that is attached to the skin.

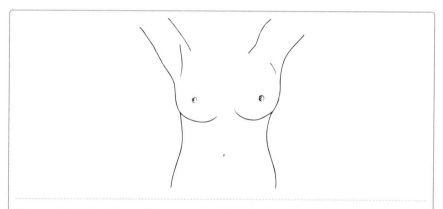

Figure 1F-2: Position with arms raised while looking for a lump or skin puckering.

Finally ask the woman to put her hands on her hips and squeeze (push her hands towards each other). This will tighten her chest muscles. Look and see if an area of skin is puckering due to being attached (tethered) to underlying muscle. This may indicate the site of a breast lump.

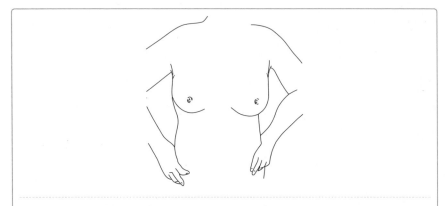

Figure 1F-3: Position with hands on hips while looking for tethering to underlying muscle

H. Palpation for enlarged supraclavicular lymph nodes

While the woman is still sitting it is a good opportunity to palpate for enlarged lymph nodes. Start by palpating above her clavicles (collar bones) for an enlarged supraclavicular lymph node. Breast cancers towards the centre of the chest may spread to this site.

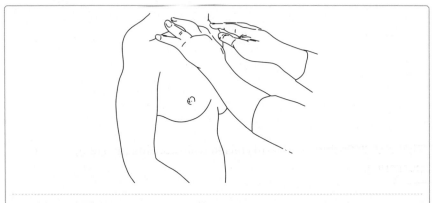

Figure 1F-4: Position for supraclavicular node examination.

I. Palpation for enlarged axillary lymph nodes

To examine the (axillae) armpits properly the woman must be relaxed. If she is very ticklish it helps to press more firmly. The best way to get a woman to relax her muscles is by asking her to extend her arms and rest them on your shoulders while you examine the armpits.

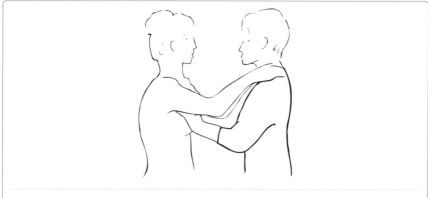

Figure 1F-5: Position while feeling in the armpits for nodes.

Feel in the two armpits at the same time for any lumps. This allows you to compare the two armpits which are shaped like pyramids. You should feel along the inside wall and towards the front (anterior) for lymph nodes. Remember to feel at the top of the armpit also. If you think you feel a lump, examine that armpit very carefully.

J. Palpation of the breasts

Finally lie the woman down flat on her back and examine one breast at a time. Ask her to raise that arm above her head on the bed. This will flatten the breast and make examination easier. It helps to think of the breasts being divided into strips and then examine each strip of breast from the centre of the chest outwards. The breast extends from the clavicle above to the 6th rib below and also towards the axilla. The whole area of the breast must be carefully examined. Always use the tips of your fingers (the most sensitive part of your hand) with the rest of your hand gently resting against the breast. Do not use cold hands.

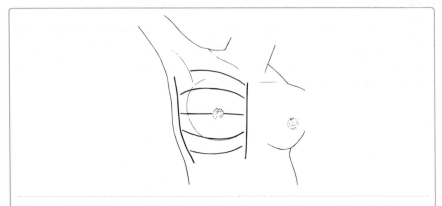

Figure 1F-6: The breast is palpated in strips to make sure the whole breast is examined.

J. Palpate behind the nipples

Never forget to examine behind the nipples and surrounding areolae for any abnormalities such as skin changes, lumps or an inverted nipple. It is best to leave the nipple examination to the end once you have won the woman's trust.

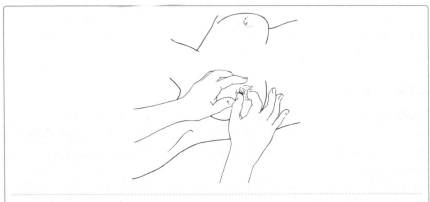

Figure 1F-7: The breast being examined using finger tips with a flat hand.

Examining a woman's breasts provides an excellent opportunity to teach her how to examine her own breasts each month after the end of her period when her breasts are softer. This is something all women should learn and practice regularly as it increases the chance of detecting an early breast cancer which can be cured.

This skills chapter is adapted from the Bettercare book *Breast Care: A health professional's guide to the diagnosis and management of common breast conditions* by Jenny Edge and Dave Woods.

2

Assessment of fetal growth and condition during pregnancy

Take the chapter test before and after you read this chapter.

Objectives

When you have completed this unit you should be able to:

- Assess normal fetal growth.
- List the causes of intra-uterine growth restriction.
- Understand the importance of measuring the symphysis-fundus height.
- Understand the clinical significance of fetal movements.
- Use a fetal-movement chart.
- Manage a patient with decreased fetal movements.
- Understand the value of antenatal fetal heart rate monitoring.

Introduction

During the antenatal period, both maternal and fetal growth must be continually monitored.

Individualised care will improve the accuracy of antenatal observations.

At every antenatal visit from 28 weeks gestation onwards, the wellbeing of the fetus must be assessed.

2-1 How can you assess the condition of the fetus during pregnancy?

The condition of the fetus before delivery is assessed by:

1. Documenting fetal growth.
2. Recording fetal movements.

> When managing a pregnant woman, remember that you are caring for two individuals.

Fetal growth

2-2 What is normal fetal growth?

If the assessed fetal weight is within the expected range for the duration of pregnancy, then the fetal growth is regarded as normal.

> To determine fetal growth you must have an assessment of both the duration of pregnancy and the weight of the fetus.

2-3 When may fetal growth appear to be abnormal?

Fetal growth will appear to be abnormal when the assessed fetal weight is greater or less than that expected for the duration of pregnancy. Remember that incorrect menstrual dates are the commonest cause of an incorrect assessment of fetal growth.

2-4 When is intra-uterine growth restriction suspected?

Intra-uterine growth restriction is suspected when the weight of the fetus is assessed as being less than the normal range for the duration of pregnancy.

2-5 What maternal and fetal factors are associated with intra-uterine growth restriction?

Intra-uterine growth restriction may be associated with either maternal, fetal or placental factors:

1. *Maternal* factors
   - Low maternal weight, especially a low body-mass index resulting from undernutrition.
   - Tobacco smoking.
   - Alcohol intake.
   - Strenuous physical work.
   - Poor socio-economic conditions.
   - Pre-eclampsia and chronic hypertension.

   Poor maternal weight gain is of very little value in diagnosing intra-uterine growth restriction.

2. *Fetal* factors
   - Multiple pregnancy.
   - Chromosomal abnormalities, e.g. trisomy 21.
   - Severe congenital malformations.
   - Chronic intra-uterine infection, e.g. congenital syphilis.

3. *Placental* factors
   - Poor placental function (placental insufficiency) is usually due to a maternal problem such as pre-eclampsia.
   - Smoking. Poor placental function is uncommon in a healthy woman who does not smoke.

If severe intra-uterine growth restriction is present, it is essential to look for a maternal or fetal cause. Usually a cause can be found.

NOTE
True primary placental inadequacy is an uncommon cause of intra-uterine growth restriction as placental causes are almost always secondary to an abnormality of the spiral arteries.

2-6 How can you estimate fetal weight?

The following methods can be used:

1. Measure the size of the uterus on abdominal examination.

2. Palpate the fetal head and body on abdominal examination.
3. Measure the size of the fetus using antenatal ultrasonography (ultrasound).

2-7 How should you measure the size of the uterus?

1. This is done by determining the symphysis-fundus height (SF height), which is measured in centimetres from the upper edge of the symphysis pubis to the top of the fundus of the uterus.
2. The SF height in centimetres should be plotted against the gestational age on the SF growth curve.
3. From 36 weeks onwards, the presenting part may descend into the pelvis and measurement of the SF height will not accurately reflect the size of the fetus. A reduction in the SF height may even be observed.

2-8 What is the symphysis-fundus growth curve?

The symphysis-fundus growth curve compares the SF height to the duration of pregnancy. The growth curve should preferably form part of the antenatal card. The solid line of the growth curve represents the 50th centile, and the upper and lower dotted lines, the 90th and 10th centiles, respectively. If intra-uterine growth is normal, the SF height will fall between the 10th and 90th centiles. The ability to detect abnormalities from the growth curve is much increased if the same person sees the patient at every antenatal visit.

Between 18 and 36 weeks of pregnancy, the SF height normally increases by about 1 cm a week.

2-9 When will the symphysis-fundus height suggest intra-uterine growth restriction?

If any of the following are found:

1. Slow increase in uterine size until one measurement falls under the 10th centile.
2. Three successive measurements 'plateau' (i.e. remain the same) without necessarily crossing below the 10th centile.
3. A measurement which is less than that recorded two visits previously without necessarily crossing below the 10th centile.

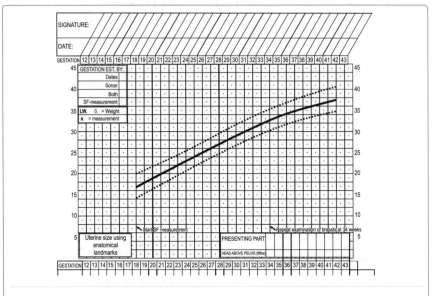

Figure 2-1: The symphysis-fundus growth chart

Note that a measurement that was originally normal, but on subsequent examinations has fallen to below the 10th centile, indicates intra-uterine growth restriction and not incorrect dates.

2-10 How can you identify severe intra-uterine growth restriction?

With *severe* intra-uterine growth restriction, the difference between the actual duration of pregnancy and that suggested by plotting SF height is 4 weeks or more.

2-11 Does descent of the presenting part of the fetus affect your interpretation of the growth curve?

Yes. Descent of the presenting part may occur in the last 4 weeks of pregnancy. Therefore, after 36 weeks the above criteria are no longer valid, if at subsequent antenatal visits progressively less of the fetal head is palpable above the pelvic inlet.

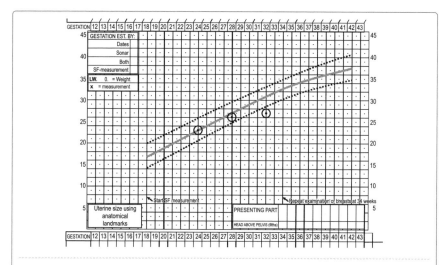

Figure 2-2: One measurement below the 10th centile

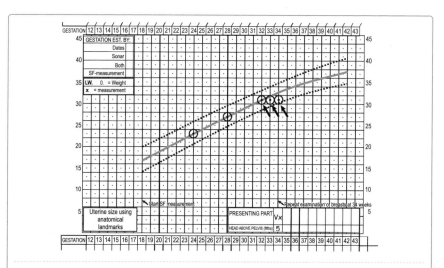

Figure 2-3: Three successive measurements that remain the same

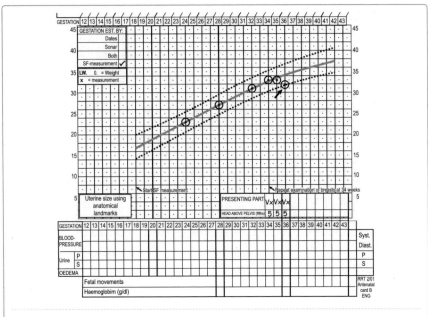

Figure 2-4: A measurement less than that recorded two visits before

2-12 What action would you take if the symphysis-fundus height measurement suggests intra-uterine growth restriction?

1. The patient should stop smoking and rest more, while attention must be given to her diet. It may be necessary to arrange sick leave and social support for the patient.
2. A poor diet which is low in energy (kilojoules) may cause intra-uterine growth restriction, especially in a patient with a low body-mass index. Therefore, ensure that patients with suspected intra-uterine growth restriction receive a high-energy diet. If possible, patients must be given food supplements (food parcels).
3. Exclude pre-eclampsia as a cause.
4. If the gestational age is 28 weeks or more, careful attention must be paid to counting the fetal movements.
5. The patient should be followed up weekly at a level 1 hospital.

2-13 Which special investigation is of great value in the further management of this patient?

The patient must be referred to a fetal evaluation clinic or a level 2 hospital for a Doppler measurement of blood flow in the umbilical arteries:

1. Good flow (low resistance) indicates good placental function. As a result the woman can receive further routine management as a low-risk patient. Spontaneous onset of labour can be allowed. Induction of labour at 38 weeks is not needed.
2. Poor flow (high resistance) indicates poor placental function. Antenatal electronic fetal heart rate monitoring must be done. The further management will depend on the result of the monitoring.

If a Doppler measurement is not available, the patient must be managed as given in 2-14.

2-14 What possibilities must be considered if, after taking the above steps, there is still no improvement in the symphysis-fundus growth?

1. Intra-uterine death must be excluded by the presence of a fetal heartbeat on auscultation.
2. With moderate intra-uterine growth restriction and good fetal movements, the patient must be followed up weekly and delivery at 38 weeks should be considered.
3. If the above patient also has poor social circumstances, an admission to hospital will need to be considered. This should ensure that the patient gets adequate rest, a good diet, and stops smoking.
4. If there are decreased or few fetal movements, the patient should be managed as described in sections 2-25 and 2-26.
5. When there is severe intra-uterine growth restriction, the patient must be referred to a level 2 or 3 hospital for further management.

2-15 What is the management of severe intra-uterine growth restriction?

1. All patients with severe intra-uterine growth restriction must be managed in a level 2 or 3 hospital.

2. An ultrasound examination should be done, if available, to exclude serious congenital abnormalities.
3. If the fetus has reached viability (28 weeks or more, or 1000 g or above), antenatal fetal heart rate monitoring should be done regularly. If this suggests fetal distress, the fetus must be delivered by Caesarean section.
4. In severe intra-uterine growth restriction, the immediate danger is of intra-uterine death, so the delivery of the fetus should be considered at 36 weeks.

Fetal movements

2-16 When are fetal movements first felt?

1. At about 20 weeks in a primigravida.
2. At about 16 weeks in a multigravida.

2-17 Can fetal movements be used to determine the duration of pregnancy accurately?

No, because the gestational age when fetal movements are first felt differs a lot from patient to patient. Therefore, it is only useful as an approximate guide to the duration of pregnancy.

2-18 What is the value of assessing fetal movements?

Fetal movements indicate that the fetus is well. By counting the movements, a patient can monitor the condition of her fetus.

2-19 From what stage of pregnancy will you advise a patient to become aware of fetal movements in order to monitor the fetal condition?

From 28 weeks, because the fetus can now be regarded as potentially viable (i.e. there is a good chance that the infant will survive if delivered). All patients should be encouraged to become aware of the importance of an adequate number of fetal movements.

> Asking the patient if the fetus is moving normally on the day of the visit is an important way of monitoring the fetal wellbeing.

2-20 What is a fetal-movement chart?

A fetal-movement chart records the frequency of fetal movements and thereby assesses the condition of the fetus. The name 'kick chart' is not correct, as all movements must be counted, i.e. rolling and turning movements, as well as kicking.

2-21 Which patients should use a fetal-movement chart?

A fetal-movement chart need not be used routinely by all antenatal patients, but only when:

1. There is concern about the fetal condition.
2. A patient reports decreased fetal movements.

2-22 How should you advise a patient to use the fetal-movement chart?

Fetal movements should be counted and recorded on the chart over a period of an hour per day after breakfast. The patient should preferably rest on her side for this period.

2-23 How accurate is a fetal movement count?

A good fetal movement count always indicates a fetus in good condition. A distressed fetus will never have a good fetal movement count. However, a low count or a decrease in fetal movements may also be the result of periods of rest or sleep in a healthy fetus. The rest and sleep periods can last several hours.

Tests with electronic equipment have shown that mothers can detect fetal movements accurately. With sufficient motivation, the fetal-movement chart can be an accurate record of fetal movements. It is, therefore, not necessary to listen to the fetal heart at antenatal clinics if the patient reports an adequate number of fetal movements, or an adequate number of fetal movements has been recorded for the day.

> A uterus which increases in size normally, and an actively moving fetus, indicate that the fetus is well.

2-24 What is the least number of movements per hour which indicates a good fetal condition?

1. The number of movements during an observation period is less important than a decrease in movements when compared to previous observation periods. If the number of movements is reduced by half, it suggests that the fetus may be at an increased risk of fetal distress.
2. If a fetus normally does not move much, and the count falls to 3 or fewer per hour, the fetus may be in danger.

2-25 What would you advise if the fetal movements suggest that the fetal condition is not good?

1. The mother should lie down on her side for another hour and repeat the count.
2. If the number of fetal movements improves, there is no cause for concern.
3. If the number of fetal movements does not improve, she should report this to her clinic or hospital as soon as possible.

NOTE
A patient who lives far away from her nearest hospital or clinic should continue with bed rest, but if the movements are 3 or fewer over a 6-hour period, then arrangements must be made for her to be moved to the nearest hospital.

2-26 What should you do if a patient with reduced fetal movements arrives at a clinic or hospital without a cardiotocograph (CTG machine)?

1. Listen to the fetal heart with a fetal stethoscope or a doptone to exclude intra-uterine death.
2. The patient should be allowed to rest and count fetal movements over a 6-hour period. With 4 or more movements during the next 6 hours, repeat the fetal movement count the next day, after breakfast. If there are 3 or fewer movements over the next 6 hours, the patient should see the responsible doctor.

The patient should be given a drink containing sugar (e.g. tea) to exclude hypoglycaemia as the cause of the decreased fetal movements.

The management of a patient with confirmed decreased fetal movements in a hospital is demonstrated in Figure 2-6.

2-27 What should the doctor do, in a hospital without fetal heart rate monitoring equipment, if there are decreased fetal movements?

First make sure that the fetus is potentially viable (at least 28 weeks or 1000 g). Further management will then depend on whether or not there are signs of intra-uterine growth restriction:

1. If there *are* clinical signs of intra-uterine growth restriction:
   ○ If the cervix is favourable, the membranes must be ruptured. The fetal heart rate must be very carefully monitored with a stethoscope during labour.
   ○ If the cervix is unfavourable, a Caesarean section must be done.
   ○ If the estimated weight of the fetus is 1500 g or more, the delivery may be managed in a level 1 or 2 hospital. However, if the estimated weight of the fetus is less than 1500 g, then the delivery must take place in a level 2 hospital with a neonatal intensive care unit, or a level 3 hospital.

Intra-uterine growth restriction plus decreased fetal movements is an indication for delivery.

2. If there are *no* clinical signs of intra-uterine growth restriction:
   ○ If the cervix is favourable and the pregnancy is of more than 36 weeks duration, the membranes should be ruptured. The fetal heart rate must be carefully monitored with a stethoscope during labour.
   ○ If the cervix is unfavourable, and the patient is more than 42 weeks pregnant, a Caesarean section must be done.
   ○ If the patient does not fall into either of the above-mentioned categories, she must be observed for a further 6 hours in hospital. If there is no improvement in the number of fetal movements, the

patient must be referred to a hospital which has facilities for electronic fetal heart rate monitoring.

Sections 2-28 to 2-38 need only be studied by nurses and doctors who work in a level 2 or 3 hospital where electronic fetal heart rate monitoring is available. All students must study sections 2-39 and 2-40.

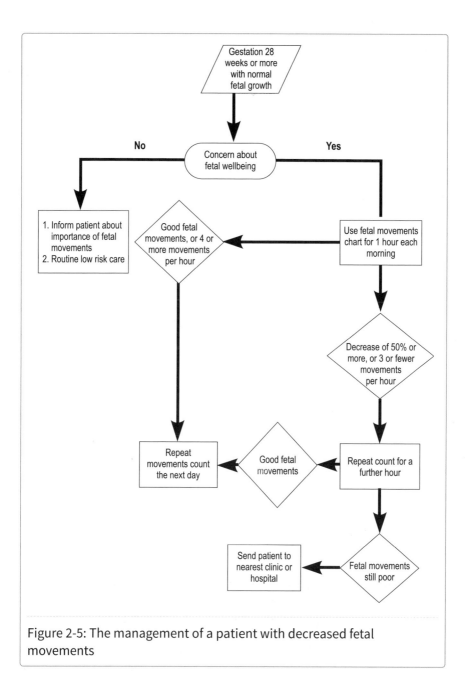

Figure 2-5: The management of a patient with decreased fetal movements

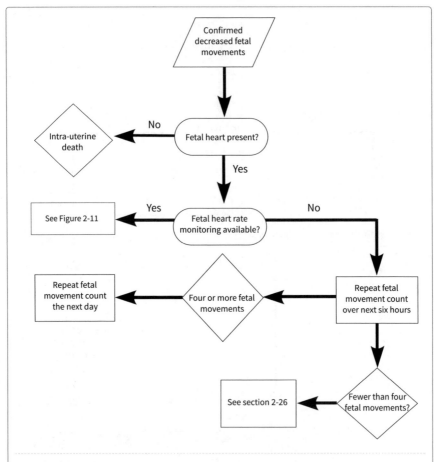

Figure 2-6: The management of a patient with confirmed decreased fetal movements in a hospital

Antenatal fetal heart rate monitoring

2-28 What is antenatal fetal heart rate monitoring?

Antenatal (electronic) fetal heart rate monitoring assesses the condition of the fetus by documenting the pattern of heart rate changes. It is done with a cardiotocograph (the machine) which produces a cardiotocogram (the paper strip showing the uterine contractions and the fetal heart rate pattern).

Antenatal fetal heart rate monitoring is currently regarded as one of the best ways to assess the fetal condition. Fetal heart rate monitoring has the advantage that it can be done reasonably quickly, and that the results are immediately available.

Hospitals which deal with mainly low-risk patients can manage perfectly well without a cardiotocograph. There is also no evidence that antenatal fetal heart monitoring of low-risk patients does anything to improve the outcome of the pregnancy. The interpretation of fetal heart rate patterns needs considerable experience, and should only be done where the necessary expertise is available.

2-29 When is antenatal fetal heart rate monitoring indicated?

1. If a patient with a viable fetus reports a decrease in fetal movements or a poor fetal movement count which does not improve when the count is repeated.
2. If a high-risk patient has a condition for which the value of fetal movement counts has not yet been proven, e.g. insulin-dependent diabetes, preterm rupture of the membranes or severe pre-eclampsia which is being managed conservatively.

2-30 How do you interpret an antenatal fetal heart rate pattern?

1. The fetal condition is good when:
   ◦ There is a reactive (normal) fetal heart rate pattern.
   ◦ There is a normal stress test.

2. No comment can be made about the fetal condition when there is a non-reactive fetal heart rate pattern. In this case there are no contractions and, therefore, one cannot determine whether there is a normal or abnormal stress test. The variability of the heart rate will indicate whether there is fetal wellbeing or possible fetal distress.

3. Fetal distress is present when:
   ◦ There is an abnormal stress test.
   ◦ There are repeated U-shaped decelerations at regular intervals, even though no contractions are observed.

- There is fetal bradycardia, with a fetal heart rate constantly below 100 beats per minute.
- There is a non-reactive fetal heart rate pattern with poor variability (i.e. less than 5 beats).

2-31 What are reactive and non-reactive heart rate patterns?

1. The fetal heart rate pattern is said to be reactive when it has at least 2 accelerations per 10 minutes, each with an amplitude (increase in the number of beats) of 15 or more beats per minute and a duration of at least 15 seconds (Figure 2-5).
2. In a non-reactive fetal heart rate pattern there are no accelerations.

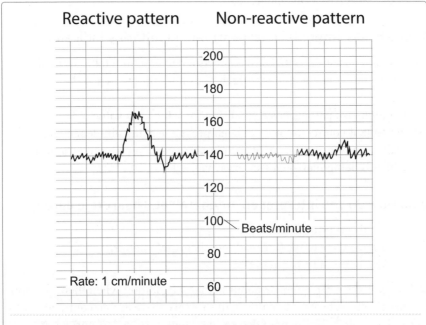

Figure 2-7: Reactive and non-reactive fetal heart rate patterns

2-32 How is the variability in the fetal heart rate used to determine whether a fetal heart rate pattern is non-reactive?

1. With good variability:
   - ○ The variability in the heart rate will be 5 beats or more, in other words, will involve 1 or more blocks in the cardiogram. Each block indicates 5 beats (Figure 2-6).
   - ○ Good variability indicates fetal wellbeing.
2. With poor variability:
   - ○ The variability in the heart rate will be less than 5 beats, in other words, will remain within 1 block (Figure 2-6).
   - ○ The fetal heart monitoring must be repeated after 45 minutes.
   - ○ If the poor variability persists, there is fetal distress.

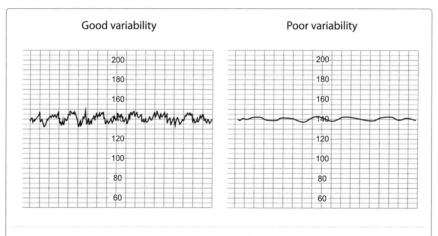

Figure 2-8: Non-reactive fetal heart rate pattern with good and poor variability.

2-33 Why must you repeat the cardiotocogram after 45 minutes in a patient with a non-reactive fetal heart rate pattern and poor variability?

1. Because a sleeping fetus may have a non-reactive fetal heart rate pattern with poor variability.

2. A fetus does not sleep for longer than 45 minutes. In a sleeping fetus the fetal heart rate pattern should, therefore, after 45 minutes have returned to a reactive pattern or a non-reactive pattern with good variability.
3. A persistent non-reactive fetal heart rate pattern with poor variability is abnormal and indicates fetal distress.

2-34 What is a stress test?

If contractions are present during fetal heart rate monitoring in the antenatal period, then the monitoring is called a stress test. The fetal heart rate pattern can now be assessed during the stress of a uterine contraction.

2-35 How is a stress test interpreted?

1. A normal stress test has no fetal heart rate decelerations during or following at least 2 contractions which last at least 30 seconds (Figure 2-7).
2. An abnormal stress test has late decelerations associated with uterine contractions (Figure 2-7). This indicates that the fetus is distressed.

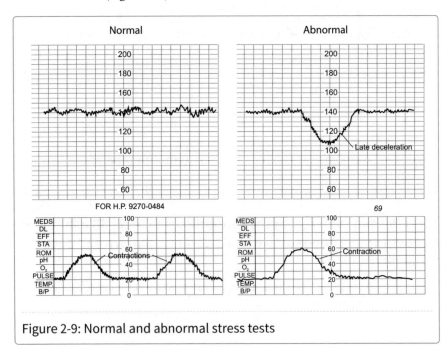

Figure 2-9: Normal and abnormal stress tests

2-36 What are the characteristics of a late deceleration?

On the cardiotocogram the trough of the deceleration occurs 30 seconds or later after the peak of the contraction (Figure 2-8).

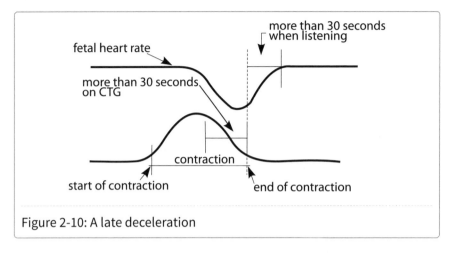

Figure 2-10: A late deceleration

2-37 What should you do in the case of an abnormal stress test, fetal bradycardia, repeated decelerations, or a non-reactive fetal heart rate pattern with persistent poor variability?

1. The patient is managed as an acute emergency as these fetal heart rate patterns indicate fetal distress.
2. However, false-positive abnormal stress tests can be caused by postural hypotension or spontaneous overstimulation of the uterus. Therefore, a stress test must always be performed with the patient on her side in the 15 degrees lateral position.
3. Whenever a fetal heart rate pattern indicates fetal distress, the cardiogram must be repeated immediately. If it is again abnormal, action should be taken as shown in Figure 2-12.
4. A persistent fetal bradycardia is usually a preterminal event and, therefore, an indication for an immediate Caesarean section if the fetus is viable.

The use of antenatal fetal heart rate monitoring is demonstrated in Figure 2-11.

2-38 Why should you not immediately do a Caesarean section if the fetal heart rate pattern indicates fetal distress and the fetus is viable?

Studies have shown that a false-positive abnormal stress test can occur in up to 80% of cases (i.e. an abnormal stress test in a healthy fetus). Therefore, whenever a fetal heart pattern indicates fetal distress, the cardiogram must always be repeated immediately.

2-39 What is the emergency management of proven fetal distress with a viable fetus?

Immediately proceed with fetal resuscitation, as follows:

1. Turn the patient onto her side.
2. Give 40% oxygen through a face mask.
3. Start an intravenous infusion of Ringer's lactate and give 250 µg (0.5 ml) salbutamol slowly intravenously if there are no contraindications. The 0.5 ml salbutamol must first be diluted in 9.5 ml sterile water. Monitor the maternal heart rate for tachycardia.
4. Deliver the infant by the quickest possible route. If the patient's cervix is 9 cm or more dilated and the head is on the pelvic floor, proceed with an assisted delivery. Otherwise, perform a Caesarean section.
5. If the patient cannot be delivered immediately (e.g. she must be transferred to hospital) then a side-infusion of 200 ml saline with 1000 µg salbutamol given at a rate of 30 ml per hour (150 µg per hour) until no further contractions occur, or when the maternal pulse rate reaches 120 beats per minute

It is important that you know how to give fetal resuscitation, as it is a life-saving procedure when fetal distress is present, both during the antepartum period and in labour.

NOTE
Uterine contractions can also be suppressed if 30 mg nifedipine (Adalat) is given my mouth (1 capsule = 10 mg). The 3 capsules must be swallowed and not used sublingually.

2-40 What are the aims of fetal resuscitation?

1. Suppressing uterine contractions and reducing uterine tone, which increases maternal blood flow to the placenta and, thereby, the oxygen supply to the fetus.
2. Giving the mother extra oxygen which will also help the fetus.

It is, therefore, possible to improve the fetal condition temporarily while preparations are being made for the patient to be delivered, or to be transferred to the hospital.

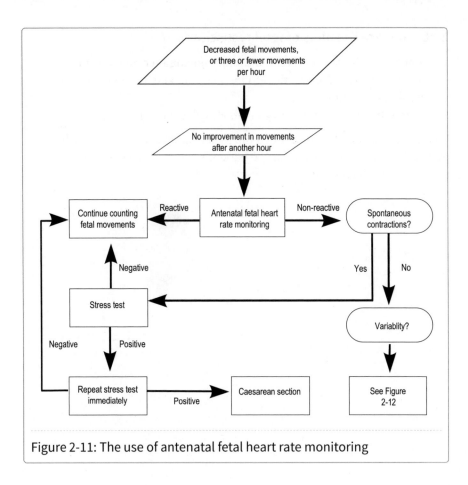

Figure 2-11: The use of antenatal fetal heart rate monitoring

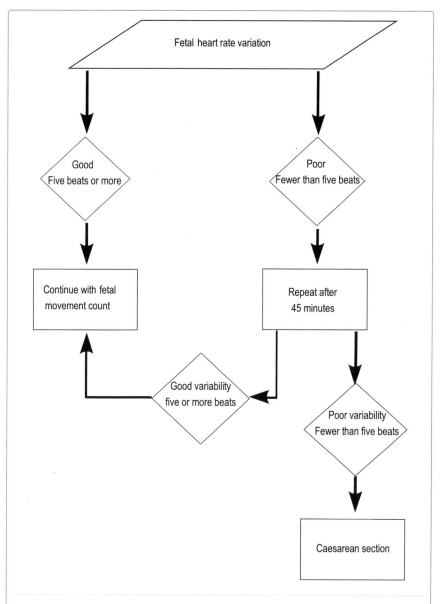

Figure 2-12: The interpretation of variability when the fetal heart rate pattern is nonreactive with no spontaneous uterine contractions

Case study 1

A patient is seen at the antenatal clinic at 37 weeks gestation. She is clinically well and reports normal fetal movements. The SF height was 35 cm the previous week and is now 34 cm. The previous week the fetal head was ballotable above the brim of the pelvis and it is now 3/5 above the brim. The fetal heart rate is 144 beats per minute. The patient is reassured that she and her fetus are healthy, and she is asked to attend the antenatal clinic again in a week's time.

1. Are you worried about the decrease in the SF height since the last antenatal visit?

No, as the fetal head is descending into the pelvis. The head was 5/5 above the brim of the pelvis and is now 3/5 above the brim.

2. What is your assessment of the fetal condition?

The fetus is healthy as the SF height is normal for 37 weeks and the fetus is moving normally.

3. What is the value of a normal fetal heart rate during the antenatal period?

The fetal heart rate is not a useful measure of the fetal condition before the onset of labour. If the fetus moves well during the antenatal period, there is no need to listen to the fetal heart.

4. What is the value of fetal movements during the antenatal period?

Active fetal movements, noted that day, indicate that the fetus is healthy. The patient can therefore monitor the condition of her fetus by taking note of fetal movements.

Case study 2

You examine a 28-year-old gravida 4 para 3 patient who is 34 weeks pregnant. She has no particular problems and mentions that her fetus has moved a lot, as usual, that day. The SF height has not increased over the past three antenatal visits but only the last SF height measurement has fallen to the 10th centile. The patient is a farm labourer and she smokes.

1. What do the SF height measurements indicate?

They indicate that the fetus may have intra-uterine growth restriction, as the last three measurements have remained the same even though the SF height measurement has not fallen below the 10th centile.

2. What are the probable causes of the poor fundal growth?

Hard physical labour and smoking. Both these factors can cause intra-uterine growth restriction.

3. What is the possibility of fetal distress or death in the next few days?

Both these possibilities are most unlikely as the patient has reported normal fetal movements.

4. What can be done to improve fetal growth?

Arrangements should be made, if possible, for the patient to stop working. She must also stop smoking, get enough rest and have a good diet.

5. How should this patient be managed?

She must be given a fetal-movement chart and you must explain clearly to her how to use the chart. She must be placed in the high-risk category and therefore seen at the clinic every week. If the fundal growth does not improve, the patient must be hospitalised and labour should be induced at 38 weeks.

If a Doppler blood flow measurement of the umbilical arteries indicates normal placental function, routine management of a low-risk patient can be given. Induction at 38 weeks is therefore not needed.

Case study 3

A patient, who is 36 weeks pregnant with suspected intra-uterine growth restriction, is asked to record her fetal movements on a fetal-movement chart. She reports to the clinic that her fetus, which usually moves 20 times per hour, only moved five times during an hour that morning.

1. What should the patient have done?

Rather than come to the clinic, she should have counted the number of fetal movements for a further hour.

2. What is the correct management of this patient?

She must not go home unless you are sure that her fetus is healthy. She should lie on her side and count the number of fetal movements during 1 hour. If she has not had breakfast, give her a cold drink or a cup of sweetened tea to make sure that she is not hypoglycaemic.

3. What should you do if the fetus moves more than 10 times during the hour?

If the number of fetal movements returns to more than half the previous count (i.e. more than 10 times per hour), she can go home and return to the clinic in a week. In addition, she must count the fetal movements daily.

4. What should you do if the fetus moves fewer than 10 times during the hour?

If the fetal movement count remains less than half the previous count, the patient should be transferred to a hospital where antenatal electronic fetal heart monitoring can be done. Further management will depend on the result of the monitoring.

5. What is the correct management if electronic fetal heart monitoring is not available?

Fetal movements should be counted for a full 6 hours. If the fetus moves fewer than four times, there is a high chance that the fetus is distressed. A doctor must now examine the patient and decide whether the fetus should be delivered and what would be the safest method of delivery.

Case study 4 need only be attempted by those who have studied the section on antenatal fetal heart rate monitoring.

Case study 4

Antenatal fetal heart rate monitoring is done on a patient who is 36 weeks pregnant and who reports a decrease in the number of fetal movements. She lies flat on her back during the test. A non-reactive fetal heart rate pattern is found.

1. What is wrong with the method used to monitor the fetal heart rate?

The patient should not have been on her back during the test as this can cause postural hypotension resulting in a falsely abnormal fetal heart rate pattern. The patient should lie on her side with a 15 degree lateral tilt while the fetal heart rate is monitored.

2. Does the fetal heart rate pattern indicate fetal distress?

The condition of the fetus cannot be determined if there is a non-reactive antenatal fetal heart rate pattern. The variability must now be examined. If there is good variability (five beats or more), this indicates fetal wellbeing.

3. What must you do if there is poor variability (fewer than 5 beats)?

The test should be repeated after 45 minutes.

4. Why must you repeat the test after 45 minutes if there is a non-reactive pattern with poor variability?

A sleeping fetus may have a fetal heart rate pattern with poor variability. However, a fetus does not sleep for longer than 45 minutes. The fetal heart rate pattern in that case will therefore have reverted to normal when the test is repeated 45 minutes later.

5. What must you do if the test, performed 45 minutes later, continues to show poor variability?

The test now indicates fetal distress. If the fetus is viable, arrangements must be made to deliver it (see Figure 2-12).

Skills: Routine use of the antenatal card

Objectives

When you have completed this skills chapter you should be able to:

- Plot the symphysis-fundus height.
- Use the symphysis-fundus height graph to assess whether the fetus is growing adequately.
- Plot the patient's weight and assess whether the weight gain is normal.

A. Recording information on the antenatal card

The front of the antenatal card is used to record details of the patient's history, examination, special investigations, duration of pregnancy, planned management, and future family planning at the first and second antenatal visits. The back of the antenatal card is used to record the observations made at each antenatal visit throughout pregnancy.

The following items should be recorded on the back of the antenatal card every time the patient attends the antenatal clinic:

1. Date.
2. Blood pressure.
3. Proteinuria or glycosuria.
4. Oedema.
5. Fetal movements from 28 weeks onwards.
6. Presenting part from 34 weeks onwards.
7. Haemoglobin concentration at 28 and 34 weeks.
8. The symphysis-fundus height from 18 weeks.
9. Any additional notes.
10. Signature of the responsible midwife or doctor.

The symphysis-fundus (SF) height is recorded on the antenatal graph while the other information is recorded in the spaces provided (see Figure 2A-1).

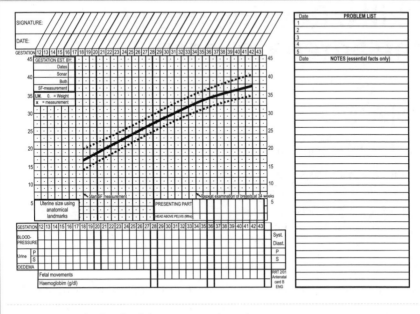

Figure 2A-1: The back of the antenatal card

B. Recording the results of the rapid HIV test on the antenatal card.

1. If the first rapid test is negative, it is accepted that the patient is HIV negative. In the space for special investigations on the front of the antenatal card, 'Yes' must be circled as the test was done (i.e. accepted) and then 'No' must be circled as the result was negative for RVD (i.e. precautions are not needed). RVD is the abbreviation for Retro Viral Disease (see Figure 2A-2).

2. If both the first rapid test and the confirmatory (second) test are positive, it is accepted that the patient is HIV positive. Circle 'Yes' for the test being done and again 'Yes' for the test being positive for RVD. The test was therefore accepted and precautions are needed (see Figure 2A-3). The patient must receive appropriate antiretrovirals to prevent mother-to-child transmission of HIV.

3. If, after counselling, the patient decides not to have an HIV test, 'No' must be circled as the test was not done. As the test was not done, a decision about precautions is not required (see Figure 2A-4).

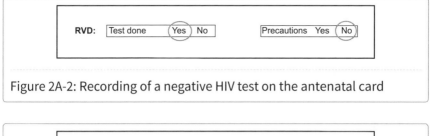

Figure 2A-2: Recording of a negative HIV test on the antenatal card

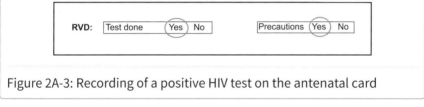

Figure 2A-3: Recording of a positive HIV test on the antenatal card

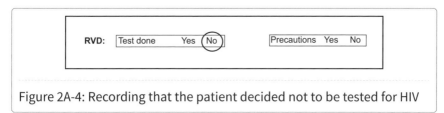

Figure 2A-4: Recording that the patient decided not to be tested for HIV

C. The significance of the lines on the graph

There are three oblique lines on the antenatal graph.

The three lines represent the normal increase in the symphysis-fundus or SF height (i.e. a centile growth chart of fundal height). The solid line in the centre is the 50th centile or average growth line. The dotted lines above and below this represent the 90th and 10th centiles respectively (i.e. the upper and lower limits of normal fundal growth).

D. Plotting the symphysis-fundus height for the first time when the patient is sure of the date of her last menstrual period

1. Calculate the period of gestation in weeks. The gestational age is given along the top and bottom of the graph (the horizontal axis). The patient's gestational age is 24 weeks.
2. Measure the SF height. The SF height in centimetres is given on both sides of the graph (the vertical axis). The patient's SF height measures 21 cm.
3. Knowing the gestational age and the SF height, the SF height for the gestational age can be plotted on the graph and should be recorded by making a dot. A small circle is drawn around the dot to make sure that it is clearly seen (Figure 2A-5).
4. The date of the antenatal visit should be written at the top of the card in the square opposite the gestational age of the patient. The person recording the observations on the antenatal card must also write her or his name next to the date.
5. The method whereby the gestational age was determined must now be ticked in the appropriate block at the top left-hand corner of the chart. In this case 'Dates' should be ticked.
6. Between 18 and 36 weeks the SF height in centimetres should be plotted on the SF curve to determine the gestational age in weeks. If the fundal height is at the level of the umbilicus or higher, and the SF height differs from the gestational age by 4 weeks or more, the SF height should be plotted.

E. Plotting the SF height for the first time when the patient does not know the date of her last menstrual period

1. The patient's SF height measures 27 cm. Plot the measurement on the 50th centile opposite the 27 cm on the vertical axis (figure 2A-6).
2. By plotting the SF height measurement on the 50th centile you are *assuming* that the fetus is growing normally and that the measurement on the horizontal axis represents the approximate gestational age. In this case the approximate gestational age is 28 weeks.

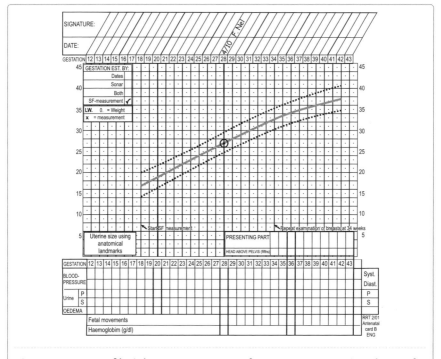

Figure 2A-5: An s-f height measurement of 21 cm at a gestational age of 24 weeks is plotted on July 27th

3. The method whereby the gestational age was determined must now be ticked in the appropriate block at the top left-hand corner of the chart. In this case 'SF-measurement' should be ticked.

4. The fundal growth must be carefully recorded at the following visits. If little or no growth occurs in the next 4 weeks, the diagnosis of intra-uterine growth restriction must be made. If excessive growth occurs, multiple pregnancy must be excluded. Normal growth with the SF height between the 90th and 10th centiles confirms a normal growing singleton pregnancy.

F. The first recording of the SF height when the duration of pregnancy, as determined by her last normal menstrual period,

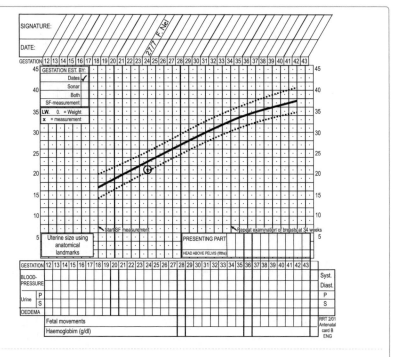

Figure 2A-6: Recording the s-f height of 27 cm on the 50th centile when a patient could not remember the date of her last menstrual period. The patient attended the antenatal clinic on 4 October.

differs from that determined by the SF height by four or more weeks.

1. According to the patient's last menstrual period, she is 31 weeks pregnant. The SF height measurement is 25 cm which indicates a gestational age of 26 weeks if plotted on the 50th centile of the SF curve (Figure 2A-7).
2. In this case the fundal height is above the umbilicus, and the gestational age estimated from the mother's last menstrual period and the SF height differ by 5 weeks. The SF height probably indicates the true gestational age. Make a mark on the 50th centile opposite 25 cm. This indicates an estimated gestational age of 26 weeks.

3. The method by which the gestational age is estimated must be recorded in the box at the top left-hand corner of the growth chart. In this case a tick should be made opposite 'SF measurement'.

4. The fundal growth must be carefully recorded at the following visits. If little or no growth occurs in the next 4 weeks, a diagnosis of intra-uterine growth restriction must be made. If excessive growth occurs, multiple pregnancy must be excluded. Normal growth with the SF height between the 90th and 10th centiles confirms a normal growing singleton pregnancy. This information also confirms that using the SF height to determine gestational age was correct.

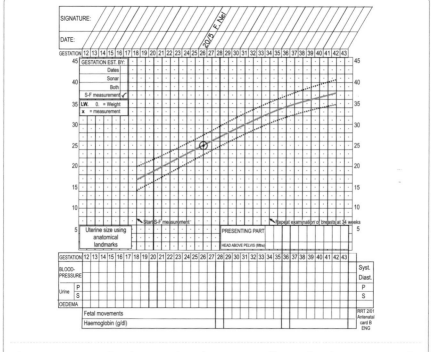

Figure 2A-7: A patient's gestational age, according to her last menstrual period, is 31 weeks and the s-f height measurement is 25 cm.

G. Plotting the symphysis-fundus height at subsequent antenatal visits

The symphysis-fundus height must be plotted on the graph at every subsequent antenatal clinic visit. As before, the symphysis-fundus height measurement and the gestational age are used to determine where the dot should be made on the graph. For example, if the patient's present visit is 4 weeks after she last attended the antenatal clinic, the SF height measurement must be plotted 4 weeks later on the graph (Figure 2A-8).

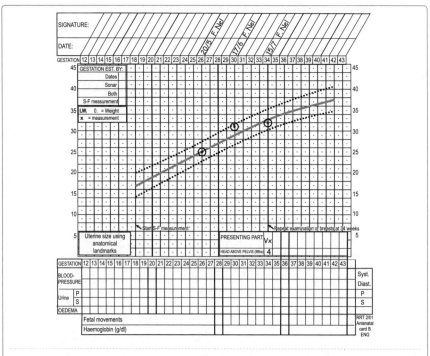

Figure 2A-8: A patient's SF height measurement is 25 cm at 26 weeks and then 31 cm at 30 weeks. Four weeks after her last visit the SF height is 32 cm.

H. Recording the presenting part and the amount of fetal head palpable above the brim of the pelvis

From 34 weeks gestation onwards the lie and the presenting part must be determined at every visit. The presenting part may be a vertex or breech. If the presenting part is a fetal head, then the amount of head above the pelvic brim must be determined.

I. Writing notes on the antenatal record card

A space for brief notes is provided on the antenatal card. A block is also provided for a problem list. Few notes are needed and usually there are no notes for patients that are assessed as being low risk with normal pregnancies (Figure 2A-9).

Date	PROBLEM LIST
1 20/5	Grande multipara
2 20/5	Gestational diabetes
3 23/6	Pre-eclamsia
4	
5	

Date	NOTES (essential facts only)
20/5	Diabetes to be managed with diet
23/6	Good diabetic control
	Admit to ward for PET assessment
	and management
	Requests tubal ligation

Figure 2A-9: A problem list with short notes

3

Hypertensive disorders of pregnancy

Take the chapter test before and after you read this chapter.

Objectives

When you have completed this unit you should be able to:

- Define hypertension in pregnancy.
- Give a simple classification of the hypertensive disorders of pregnancy.
- Diagnose pre-eclampsia and chronic hypertension.
- Explain why the hypertensive disorders of pregnancy must always be regarded as serious.
- List which patients are at risk of developing pre-eclampsia.
- List the complications of pre-eclampsia.
- Differentiate pre-eclampsia from severe pre-eclampsia.
- Give a practical guide to the management of pre-eclampsia.
- Provide emergency management for eclampsia.
- Manage gestational hypertension and chronic hypertension during pregnancy.

The hypertensive disorders of pregnancy

3-1 What is the normal blood pressure during pregnancy?

The normal systolic blood pressure is less than 140 mm Hg and the diastolic blood pressure is less than 90 mm Hg. During the second trimester both the systolic and diastolic blood pressures usually fall and then rise again toward the end of pregnancy. A mild rise in blood pressure early in the third trimester can therefore be normal.

3-2 What is hypertension during pregnancy?

Hypertension during pregnancy is defined as a diastolic blood pressure of 90 mm Hg or more and/or a systolic blood pressure of 140 mm Hg or more.

A diastolic blood pressure of 90 mm Hg or more or a systolic blood pressure of 140 mm hg or more during pregnancy is abnormal.

An abnormally high blood pressure during pregnancy is often accompanied by proteinuria.

3-3 What is proteinuria?

Proteinuria is defined as an excessive amount of protein in the urine. Normally the urine contains no protein or only a trace of protein. Therefore, just a trace of protein in the urine is not regarded as abnormal.

Proteinuria during pregnancy is diagnosed when either of the following is present:

1. 0.3 g or more of protein in a 24-hour urine specimen.
2. 1+ or more protein as measured with a reagent strip (e.g. Albustix, Labstix, Uristix, Multistix, Lenstrip, etc.).

Proteinuria during pregnancy may also be caused by:

1. A urinary tract infection or renal disease.
2. Contamination of the urine by a vaginal discharge or leucorrhoea.

Patients with proteinuria must be asked to collect a second sample, as a midstream specimen of urine (MSU). The correct method of collecting an MSU must be carefully explained to the patient. The amount of proteinuria present in the MSU will be the correct one and must, therefore, be recorded in the notes. The further management will be dictated by the amount of proteinuria in the MSU.

1+ or more protein in the urine is abnormal.

The classification of hypertension during pregnancy

3-4 How is hypertension during pregnancy classified?

The classification of hypertension during pregnancy depends on:

1. Whether the hypertension started before or after the 20th week of pregnancy.
2. Whether or not proteinuria is also present.

> The classification of hypertension during pregnancy depends on the time of onset of the hypertension and the presence or absence of proteinuria.

Classifying hypertension is important, as the cause of the hypertension and the risk to the mother and fetus vary between the different groups.

The common forms of hypertension during pregnancy that will be discussed in this unit are:

1. Pre-eclampsia (gestational proteinuric hypertension).
2. Gestational hypertension.
3. Chronic hypertension.
4. Chronic hypertension with superimposed pre-eclampsia.
5. Eclampsia.

NOTE
> Based on the above criteria, hypertension during pregnancy is at present divided into the following conditions:
> • Gestational proteinuric hypertension (or pre-eclampsia).
> • Gestational hypertension.
> • Chronic hypertension and chronic renal disease with hypertension.
> • Chronic hypertension with superimposed gestational proteinuric hypertension (or pre-eclampsia).
> • Unclassified hypertension and unclassified proteinuric hypertension (if the patient is seen for the first time in the second half of pregnancy, with hypertension and/or proteinuria).
> • Eclampsia.

3-5 What is pre-eclampsia?

Pre-eclampsia presents with hypertension and proteinuria which develop in the second half of pregnancy. Pre-eclampsia may present during pregnancy, labour, or the puerperium.

Pre-eclampsia is also called gestational (pregnancy-induced) proteinuric hypertension.

3-6 What is gestational hypertension?

In contrast to pre-eclampsia, gestational hypertension is not accompanied by proteinuria but also presents in the second half of pregnancy. Should proteinuria develop in a patient with gestational hypertension, the diagnosis must be changed to pre-eclampsia.

> Pre-eclampsia presents with hypertension and proteinuria in the second half of pregnancy.

NOTE
The term pre-eclampsia (rather than gestational proteinuric hypertension) will be used, as it is still widely known as such.

3-7 What is chronic hypertension?

Chronic hypertension is hypertension, with or without proteinuria, that presents during the first half of pregnancy. There is usually a history of hypertension before the start of the pregnancy.

NOTE
Chronic hypertension without proteinuria is usually due to essential hypertension. If the chronic hypertension is accompanied by proteinuria during the first half of pregnancy, then the hypertension is usually due to chronic renal disease.

3-8 What is chronic hypertension with superimposed pre-eclampsia?

This is hypertension presenting during the first half of pregnancy that is complicated by the appearance of proteinuria during the second half of pregnancy. In other words it is chronic hypertension that is complicated by the development of pre-eclampsia.

NOTE
Patients who book in the second half of pregnancy cannot be classified into any of the above types of hypertension, as it is not known whether the hypertension started in the first or second half of pregnancy. If a patient has hypertension without proteinuria when she books during the second half of pregnancy, she is said to have unclassified hypertension. However, if she has both hypertension and proteinuria when she books during the second half of pregnancy, she is said to have unclassified proteinuric hypertension. Most patients with unclassified hypertension probably have chronic hypertension, while most patients with unclassified proteinuric hypertension probably have pre-eclampsia.

3-9 What is eclampsia?

Eclampsia is a serious complication of pre-eclampsia that presents with convulsions during pregnancy, labour, or the first 7 days of the puerperium. Convulsions could also be the result of other causes such as epilepsy, but the possibility of eclampsia must be carefully ruled out whenever convulsions occur.

Pre-eclampsia

Pre-eclampsia is the hypertensive disorder of pregnancy which occurs most commonly and also causes the most problems for the mother and fetus.

Gestational proteinuric hypertension and chronic hypertension with superimposed pre-eclampsia will subsequently be discussed under the heading 'pre-eclampsia' because the management is similar.

3-10 How frequently does pre-eclampsia occur?

In the Western Cape 5–6% of all pregnant women develop pre-eclampsia.

3-11 Is pre-eclampsia a danger to the mother?

Yes, it is one of the most important causes of maternal death in most parts of southern Africa.

3-12 What are the maternal complications of pre-eclampsia?

The two most important complications of pre-eclampsia are also important causes of maternal death during pregnancy:

1. Intracerebral haemorrhage.
2. Eclampsia.

NOTE
Other, less common, complications of pre-eclampsia are pulmonary oedema and the HELLP (Haemolysis, Elevated Liver enzymes, and a Low Platelet count) syndrome. Rupture of the liver, renal failure, the adult respiratory distress syndrome, and a generalised disorder of blood coagulation may also occur, but fortunately, those are rare complications.

3-13 Which patients are at an increased risk of intracerebral haemorrhage?

The risk of intracerebral haemorrhage is especially high if the diastolic blood pressure is 110 mm Hg or more and/or a systolic blood pressure of 160 mm Hg or more.

3-14 Does eclampsia only occur at a very high diastolic blood pressure?

No, eclampsia can occur at a much lower blood pressure, especially in young patients.

3-15 Why is pre-eclampsia a danger to the fetus and newborn infant?

Pre-eclampsia is an important cause of perinatal death because:

1. Preterm delivery is often necessary because of a deterioration in the maternal condition or the development of fetal distress.
2. Abruptio placentae is more common in patients with pre-eclampsia and often results in an intra-uterine death.
3. Pre-eclampsia is associated with decreased placental blood flow. As a result of decreased placental blood flow the fetus may suffer from:
   ○ Intra-uterine growth restriction or wasting.
   ○ Fetal distress.

> Pre-eclampsia may result in intra-uterine growth restriction, fetal distress, preterm delivery and intra-uterine death.

3-16 How can the severity of pre-eclampsia be graded?

The severity of pre-eclampsia can be graded by:

1. The diastolic and/or systolic blood pressure.
2. The amount of proteinuria.
3. Signs and symptoms of imminent eclampsia.
4. The presence of convulsions.

Patients with pre-eclampsia can be divided into four grades of severity:

1. *Pre-eclampsia*: A diastolic blood pressure of 90–109 mm Hg and/or a systolic blood pressure of 140–159 mm Hg and proteinuria.
2. *Severe pre-eclampsia*: Any of the following:
   ◦ A diastolic blood pressure of 110 mm Hg or more and/or a systolic blood pressure of 160 mm Hg or more on two occasions, 4 hours apart.
   ◦ A diastolic blood pressure of 120 mm Hg or more, and/or a systolic blood pressure of 170 mm Hg or more, on one occasion, and proteinuria.
3. *Imminent eclampsia*: These patients have symptoms and/or signs that indicate that they are at extremely high risk of developing eclampsia at any moment. The diagnosis does *not* depend on the degree of hypertension or the amount of proteinuria present.
4. *Eclampsia*: Eclampsia is diagnosed when a patient with any of the grades of pre-eclampsia has a convulsion.

> If there is any doubt about the grade of pre-eclampsia, the patient should always be placed in the more severe grade.

Patients who improve on bed rest should be kept in the grade of pre-eclampsia which they were given at the initial evaluation on admission. Further management should be in accordance with this grade.

3-17 What are the symptoms and signs of imminent eclampsia?

The *symptoms* are:

1. Headache.
2. Visual disturbances or flashes of light seen in front of the eyes.
3. Upper abdominal pain, in the epigastrium and/or over the liver.

The *signs* are:

1. Tenderness over the liver.
2. Increased tendon reflexes, e.g. knee reflexes.

> The diagnosis of imminent eclampsia is made even if only one of the symptoms or signs is present, irrespective of the blood pressure or the amount of proteinuria.

3-18 How common is eclampsia?

In the Western Cape, the incidence of eclampsia is 1 per 1000 pregnancies.

Patients at increased risk of pre-eclampsia

3-19 Which patients are at an increased risk of pre-eclampsia?

1. Primigravidas.
2. Patients with chronic hypertension.
3. Patients over 34 years of age.
4. Patients with a multiple pregnancy.
5. Diabetics.
6. Patients with a past history of a pregnancy complicated by pre-eclampsia, especially if the pre-eclampsia developed during the late 2nd or early 3rd trimester.
7. Patients who develop generalised oedema, especially facial oedema.

3-20 What advice should be given to patients at an increased risk of pre-eclampsia?

They must be told about the symptoms of imminent eclampsia, and advised to contact the clinic or hospital immediately, if these symptoms appear.

3-21 What special care should be given to patients at an increased risk of pre-eclampsia?

In the second half of pregnancy, the following must be carefully watched for:

1. A rise in diastolic blood pressure.
2. Proteinuria.
3. Symptoms and signs of imminent eclampsia.

Patients with an obstetric history of pre-eclampsia that developed late in the second trimester or early in the third trimester, must receive 75 mg aspirin (a quarter Disprin) daily from a gestational age of 14 weeks. This will reduce the risk that pre-eclampsia may develop.

3-22 What should you do if a patient develops generalised oedema, but remains normotensive and does not have proteinuria?

1. She should rest as much as possible.
2. She should be followed up weekly at the antenatal clinic and carefully checked for the development of hypertension and proteinuria.
3. She should carefully monitor the fetal movements.

The management of pre-eclampsia

3-23 What should you do if a patient develops pre-eclampsia?

1. A patient with pre-eclampsia must be admitted to hospital. Such a patient may be safely cared for in a level 1 hospital.
2. Methyldopa (Aldomet) must be prescribed to control the blood pressure.

All patients with pre-eclampsia must be admitted to hospital, irrespective of the level of their blood pressure.

3-24 How should you monitor the fetus to ensure fetal wellbeing?

Patients with pre-eclampsia often have placental insufficiency, associated with intra-uterine growth restriction. Fetal distress, therefore, occurs commonly. If this is not diagnosed, and the fetus is not delivered soon, intra-uterine death will result. These patients are also at high risk of abruptio placentae, followed by fetal distress and frequently also intra-uterine death. The fetal condition must, therefore, be carefully monitored in all patients with pre-eclampsia.

Fetal movements must be counted and recorded by the patient twice a day.

NOTE
In level 2 and 3 hospitals antenatal fetal heart rate monitoring (CTG) for fetal distress must be done at least daily.

Patients with pre-eclampsia are at high risk of developing fetal distress. They must, therefore, be carefully monitored for fetal distress.

3-25 When should you deliver a patient with pre-eclampsia?

Patients who have a gestational age of 36 weeks or more should have their labour induced on the day that the diagnosis is made. If the patient has a favourable ('ripe')cervix, a surgical induction can be done.

A patient with an unfavourable ('unripe') cervix must be referred to a level 2 hospital. There, labour is induced by first 'ripening' the cervix with a very low dose of oral misoprostol (Cytotec) or prostaglandin E2, after which the membranes are ruptured. A patient must always be carefully monitored for an hour after oral misoprostol or the insertion of the prostaglandin, because overstimulation of the uterus may cause fetal distress.

Patients with a gestation of less than 36 weeks must be managed as described in sections 3-23 and 3-24.

3-26 What should you do if a patient with pre-eclampsia develops severe pre-eclampsia?

1. If the patient is 34 weeks pregnant or more, labour must be induced.
2. If she is less than 34 weeks pregnant, she must be managed as indicated in section 3-37.

The management of pre-eclampsia is bed rest and careful monitoring, to detect a worsening of the pre-eclampsia or the development of fetal distress.

3-27 What special investigations are indicated in pre-eclampsia?

1. An MSU must be examined microscopically for a urinary tract infection, or sent to the laboratory for culture, as a urinary tract infection may be responsible for the proteinuria.
2. A platelet count must be done, if a laboratory is available. A platelet count of less than 100 000 is an indication for referral of the patient to a level 2 hospital.

A urinary tract infection must be excluded in all patients with proteinuria in pregnancy.

The emergency management of severe pre-eclampsia and imminent eclampsia

The management of patients with severe pre-eclampsia and imminent eclampsia is the same and consists of stabilising the patient, followed by referral to a level 2 or 3 hospital.

3-28 What are the greatest dangers to a patient with severe pre-eclampsia?

The two greatest dangers which are a threat to the patient's life are eclampsia and an intracerebral haemorrhage.

3-29 How should you manage a patient with severe pre-eclampsia or imminent eclampsia?

The main aims of management are to:

1. Prevent eclampsia by giving magnesium sulphate.
2. Prevent intracerebral haemorrhage by decreasing the blood pressure with parenteral dihydralazine (Nepresol) or oral nifedipine capsules (Adalat).

> The initial management of severe pre-eclampsia and imminent eclampsia is aimed at the prevention of eclampsia and intracerebral haemorrhage.

The steps in the management of severe pre-eclampsia are:

Step 1: An intravenous infusion is started (Plasmalyte B or Ringer's lactate) and magnesium sulphate is administered as follows:

1. Give 4 g slowly intravenously over 10 minutes. Prepare the 4 g by adding 8 ml 50% magnesium sulphate (i.e. 2 ampoules) to 12 ml sterile water.
2. Then give 5 g (i.e. 10 ml 50% magnesium sulphate) by deep intramuscular injection into each buttock.

A total of 14 g of magnesium sulphate is given.

NOTE
300 ml of the intravenous infusion is given rapidly over half an hour. Thereafter, the infusion is given slowly, at a rate of 80 ml per hour.

Step 2: After the magnesium sulphate has been administered, a Foley catheter is inserted into the patient's bladder to monitor the urinary output.

Step 3: After giving the magnesium sulphate, the blood pressure must be measured again. If the diastolic blood pressure is still 110 mg Hg or more and/or the systolic blood pressure 160 mm Hg or more, oral nifedipine (Adalat) or dihydralazine (Nepresol) is given as follows:

- Give 10 mg (1 capsule) nifedipine orally or 6.25 mg dihydralazine by intramuscular injection.
- The patient's blood pressure is taken every 5 minutes for the next 30 minutes.
- If the blood pressure drops too much, intravenous Balsol or Ringer's lactate is administered rapidly, until the blood pressure returns to normal.
- If the diastolic blood pressure remains 110 mm Hg and/or the systolic blood pressure 160 mm Hg or more after 30 minutes, patients who received 10 mg nifedipine orally can be given a second dose of 10 mg nifedipine orally. If necessary, 10 mg of nifedipine can be repeated half-hourly up to a maximum dose of 50 mg.

Or

- If dihydralazine was used, an ampoule of dihydralazine (25 mg) should be mixed with 20 ml of sterile water. Bolus doses of 2 ml (2.5 mg) are given slowly intravenously, at 20-minute intervals, until the diastolic blood pressure drops to below 110 mm Hg and/or the systolic blood pressure below 160 mm Hg.

Nifedipine 10 mg capsules must always be given orally and not given sublingually (under the tongue). The 10 mg capsules must not be confused with Adalat XL tablets which are slowly dissolved and not suitable for rapidly lowering blood pressure.

Step 4: When the blood pressure is controlled, the patient is transferred to a level 2 or 3 hospital.

> Patients with severe pre-eclampsia or imminent eclampsia must always be stabilised before they are transferred, or until further management is decided upon.

3-30 What can be done to ensure maximal safety for the patient during her transfer to hospital?

1. A doctor or registered nurse or midwife should accompany the patient.

2. Resuscitation equipment, together with magnesium sulphate, calcium gluconate and dihydralazine or nifedipine, must be available in the ambulance. Respiration may be depressed if a large dose of magnesium sulphate is given too rapidly. Calcium gluconate is the antidote to be given in the event of an overdose of magnesium sulphate.
3. Convulsions must be watched for and the patient's blood pressure must also be carefully observed.
4. If the patient begins to convulse in the ambulance, she must be given a further 2 g of magnesium sulphate intravenously. The dose may, if required, be repeated once. (Make up the solution beforehand and keep it ready in a 20 ml syringe). Further maintenance doses of magnesium sulphate must be given if more than 4 hours pass after the loading dose.
5. If the blood pressure again rises to 110 mm Hg and/or the systolic blood pressure 160 mm Hg or more while the patient is being transported, you should give a second dose of 10 mg nifedipine orally or 6.25 mg dihydralazine intramuscularly. Remember that with every administration of dihydralazine there is a danger that the patient may become hypotensive. Another side effect is tachycardia, and if the pulse rate rises to 120 beats per minute or above, further administration of dihydralazine must be stopped.

3-31 How and when should you give maintenance doses of magnesium sulphate?

After the initial loading dose of magnesium sulphate, the patient will need regular maintenance doses until 24 hours after delivery. Magnesium sulphate 5 g is given every 4 hours by deep intramuscular injection into alternate buttocks. The injections are less painful if the magnesium sulphate is injected together with 1 ml 1% lignocaine.

3-32 What are the adverse effects of an overdose of magnesium sulphate and how can they be prevented?

An overdose of magnesium sulphate causes respiratory and cardiac depression. Here, the patellar reflex acts as a convenient warning. If the reflex is present, the drug may safely be given, as there is no danger of overdosage. If the reflex is absent or very reduced, there is a danger of overdosage and the next dose must not be given.

Magnesium sulphate is excreted by the kidneys. If the urinary output is less than 30 ml per hour, follow-up doses must only be given if there is a definite patellar reflex present.

3-33 What should you do if the patient develops the effects of an overdose of magnesium sulphate?

This is a life-threatening emergency and the following steps must be taken immediately:

1. The patient must be intubated and ventilated or else temporarily ventilated with a bag and face mask. External cardiac massage may also be needed.
2. Give 10 ml of 10% calcium gluconate slowly intravenously. This is an antidote for magnesium sulphate poisoning.

The management of eclampsia

3-34 What is your immediate management if a patient convulses?

The management of eclampsia is as follows:

Step 1: Prevent aspiration of the stomach contents by:

- Turning the patient immediately onto her side.
- Keeping the airway open by suctioning (if necessary) and inserting an airway.
- Administering oxygen.

Step 2: Stop the convulsion and prevent further convulsions by putting up an intravenous infusion of Balsol or Ringer's lactate and giving magnesium sulphate as described in 3-30.

Step 3: After the magnesium sulphate has been given, insert a Foley catheter to monitor the urinary output.

Step 4: If the diastolic blood pressure is 110 mm Hg and/or the systolic blood pressure 160 mm Hg or more, it must be reduced with dihydralazine (Nepresol). Oral nifedipine can be used if the patient is fully conscious after the convulsion, as described in 3-29.

Step 5: The patient must now be urgently transferred to a level 2 or 3 hospital.

> **Eclampsia is a life-threatening condition for both the mother and the fetus. Immediate management is therefore needed.**

3-35 What should you do if the patient convulses again?

If the patient convulses again, after the initial loading dose of 14 g of magnesium sulphate has controlled the first convulsion, a further 2 g of magnesium sulphate should be administered intravenously. This dose can be repeated once more in the unlikely event of the patient having yet another convulsion.

The following management is not essential knowledge, but should be read by medical and nursing staff working in level 2 or 3 hospitals.

The further management of severe pre-eclampsia and imminent eclampsia at the referral hospital

3-36 How should you manage the patient further in a level 2 or 3 hospital?

Further management consists of either delivery or conservative treatment, depending on:

1. The degree to which the patient's condition stabilises, i.e. the diastolic blood pressure remains below 110 mm Hg and/or the systolic blood pressure below 160 mm Hg, and there are no symptoms or signs of imminent eclampsia. (Oral anti-hypertensive drugs must be given to control the blood pressure, if it is decided to continue conservative management).
2. The duration of the pregnancy.
3. The condition of the fetus.

The patient must be delivered if any of the following apply:

1. The patient's condition does not stabilise.
2. The fetus is not nearing viability (it is less than 26 weeks).
3. The duration of pregnancy is 34 or more weeks.
4. There is fetal distress.

If none of the above apply then the patient can be managed conservatively until 34 weeks gestation or until the maternal condition deteriorates or fetal distress develops.

> The maternal condition must always be stabilised first. Thereafter, the condition of the fetus and the duration of the pregnancy must be taken into consideration in planning the further management of the patient.

3-37 What is the conservative management of severe pre-eclampsia?

1. Magnesium sulphate must be stopped.
2. The patient must be hospitalised for bed rest in a level 2 or 3 hospital.
3. The fetal movements must be monitored daily.
4. Antenatal cardiotocography (CTG) is very useful and if possible must be done twice or more daily. This is because of the risk of fetal distress, as a result of placental insufficiency or abruptio placentae.
5. Urinary tract infection must be excluded.
6. A platelet count and renal function tests (urea and creatinine) must be done twice a week. If the platelet count is less than 100 000, liver function tests should be done. Poor renal function, raised liver enzymes or a platelet count that falls further are indications for delivery.
7. An ultrasound examination is of value to assess fetal weight, and to assess fetal viability. Remember that a patient with a viable, growth-restricted fetus can present with a fundal height of 24, or even 22 weeks gestation. Fetal growth must also be monitored.
8. Because of the danger of hyaline membrane disease in a newborn infant who, though viable, has a gestational age of less than 34 weeks, steroids (betamethasone 12 mg, Celestone-Soluspan) must be given

intramuscularly to the patient, to enhance fetal lung maturity. A second dose must be repeated 24 hours later.

9. If the duration of the pregnancy is unknown, and the clinical assessment or ultrasound size suggests a pregnancy of 34 weeks or more, the fetus must be delivered.
10. If there is no fetal distress and the presentation is cephalic, a medical or surgical induction of labour must be done at 34 weeks gestation.
11. If fetal distress is present, or the presentation is abnormal, a Caesarean section must be done.
12. A patient whose condition becomes well stabilised, must be placed on an oral antihypertensive drug. Alpha methyldopa is the drug of choice. A high dosage (such as 500 mg 8-hourly that can be increased to 750 mg 8-hourly) must be used. If the diastolic blood pressure remains at 110 mm Hg and/or the systolic blood pressure 160 mm Hg or higher, a second or even a third antihypertensive drug is added.

NOTE

Nifedipine (Adalat) is the drug of choice, if a second antihypertensive drug is required. Prazosin (Minipress) or labetalol (Trandate) may be added, if a third drug is required. This form of management must take place in a level 3 hospital.

If the decision is taken to manage the patient conservatively, the danger of prematurity (if the fetus is delivered) must continually be weighed against the danger of fetal distress or abruptio placentae (which could result in an intra-uterine death).

Gestational hypertension

3-38 What should you do if a patient develops gestational hypertension?

A patient with a slightly elevated blood pressure (a diastolic blood pressure of 90 to 95 mm Hg), which develops in the second half of pregnancy, in the absence of proteinuria, may be managed in a level 1 hospital or clinic. If the home circumstances are poor, she must be admitted to hospital for bed rest. Where the home circumstances are good, the patient is allowed bed rest at home, under the following conditions:

1. The patient must be told about the symptoms of imminent eclampsia. Should any of these occur, she must contact or attend the hospital or clinic immediately.
2. The patient must be seen weekly at a high-risk antenatal clinic. In addition, she must be seen once between visits, to check her blood pressure and test her urine for protein.
3. If the patient cannot be seen more frequently, she must be given urinary reagent strips to take home. She must then test her urine daily and go to the clinic, should there be 1+ proteinuria or more.
4. No special investigations are indicated.
5. Alpha methyldopa (Aldomet) must be prescribed to control her blood pressure. The initial dosage of alpha methyldopa (Aldomet) is 500 mg 8-hourly.

Patients with a diastolic blood pressure of 100 mm Hg and/or a systolic blood pressure 150 mm Hg or higher must be admitted to hospital and alpha methyldopa (Aldomet) must be prescribed. Once the diastolic blood pressure has dropped below 100 mm Hg and the systolic blood pressure to below 150 mm Hg, they are managed as indicated above.

3-39 How should you monitor the fetus in order to ensure fetal wellbeing?

Fetal movements must be counted and recorded twice daily.

3-40 When should you deliver a patient with gestational hypertension?

If the blood pressure remains well controlled, no proteinuria develops, and the fetal condition remains good, the pregnancy must be allowed to continue until 40 weeks when labour must be induced.

Chronic hypertension

These patients have hypertension in the first half of pregnancy, or are known to have had hypertension before the start of pregnancy.

3-41 Which patients with chronic hypertension should be referred to a level 2 or 3 hospital?

A good prognosis can be expected if:

1. Renal function is normal (there is a normal serum creatinine concentration).
2. Pre-eclampsia is not superimposed on the chronic hypertension.
3. The blood pressure is well controlled (a diastolic blood pressure of 90 mm Hg and/or the systolic blood pressure 140 mm Hg or less) from early in pregnancy.

These women can be managed at a level 1 hospital. However, women with chronic hypertension should be referred to a level 2 or 3 hospital for further management if:

1. Renal function is abnormal (serum creatinine more than 120 mmol/l).
2. Proteinuria develops.
3. The diastolic blood pressure is 110 mm Hg and/or the systolic blood pressure 160 mm Hg or higher.
4. There is intra-uterine growth restriction.
5. More than 1 drug is required to control the blood pressure.

3-42 Will you adjust the medication of a patient with chronic hypertension when she becomes pregnant?

Yes, she must change to alpha methyldopa (Aldomet) 500 mg 8-hourly. Other antihypertensives (i.e. diuretics, beta blockers and ACE inhibitors) must be stopped.

NOTE
> In pregnancy, beta-blockers are not completely safe for the fetus, while diuretics reduce the intravascular fluid compartment, with adverse effects on placental and renal perfusion. An ACE inhibitor, such as captopril (Capoten and enalapril (Renitec)), is completely contraindicated in pregnancy, as intra-uterine deaths have occurred in patients on this drug.

3-43 What special care is needed for a patient with chronic hypertension during pregnancy?

1. Any rise in the blood pressure or the development of proteinuria must be carefully looked for, as they indicate an urgent need for referral.
2. A Doppler measurement of the blood flow in the umbilical artery should be done to determine placental function.
3. Postpartum sterilisation must be discussed with the patient, and is recommended when the patient is a multigravida.

3-44 When should you deliver a patient with chronic hypertension?

The management is the same as that for gestational hypertension.

Case study 1

A 21-year-old primigravida patient is attending the antenatal clinic. Her pregnancy progresses normally to 33 weeks. At the next visit at 35 weeks, the patient complains that her hands and feet have started to swell over the past week. On examining her, you notice that her face is also slightly swollen. Her blood pressure at present is 120/80, which is the same as at her previous visit, and she has no proteinuria. She reports that her fetus moves frequently.

1. Why is this patient at high risk of developing pre-eclampsia?

Because she is a primigravida and has developed generalised oedema over the past week.

2. How should this patient be managed further?

She should rest a lot. She should also be seen at the antenatal clinic again in a week when she must be carefully examined for a rise in blood pressure or the presence of proteinuria.

3. What advice should this patient be given?

She should be told about the symptoms of imminent eclampsia, i.e. headache, flashes of light before the eyes, and upper abdominal pain. She should also be asked to count and record fetal movements twice a day. If any of the above-mentioned symptoms are experienced, or if fetal movements decrease, she must immediately report to the clinic or hospital.

4. When you see the patient a week later she has a diastolic blood pressure of 90 mm Hg, but there is still no proteinuria. How should she be managed further?

The patient has pregnancy-induced hypertension. If the home conditions are satisfactory, she can be managed with bed rest at home. The hypertension must be controlled with alpha methyldopa (Aldomet). She must be seen twice a week and carefully monitored to detect a rise in her blood pressure and the possible development of proteinuria. If her blood pressure rises and/ or proteinuria develops, she must be admitted to hospital. If the home conditions are poor, she should be admitted to hospital for bed rest.

Case study 2

At an antenatal clinic you see a patient who is 39 weeks pregnant. Up until now she has had a normal pregnancy. On examination, you find that her diastolic blood pressure is 95 mm Hg and that she has 2+ proteinuria.

1. How should this patient be managed?

She should be admitted to hospital as all patients with 2+ proteinuria must be hospitalised. She should also be delivered, as she is more than 38 weeks pregnant.

2. On examining this patient you observe that she has increased patellar reflexes i.e. brisk knee jerks. How should this observation alter her management?

Increased tendon reflexes are a sign of imminent eclampsia. The diagnosis must be made, irrespective of the degree of hypertension or the amount of proteinuria. To prevent the development of eclampsia, the patient must be given magnesium sulphate.

3. What is the danger to this patient's health?

The patient has severe pre-eclampsia. Therefore, the immediate danger to her life is the development of eclampsia or an intracerebral haemorrhage.

4. How should this patient be managed?

Her clinical condition must first be stabilised. An intravenous infusion should be started and a loading dose of 14 g magnesium sulphate must be given. This should prevent the development of eclampsia. A Foley catheter must be inserted in her bladder.

5. Is a loading dose of magnesium sulphate also adequate to control the high blood pressure?

No. Sometimes with severe pre-eclampsia, the blood pressure will drop to below 160/110 mm Hg after the loading dose of magnesium sulphate has been given. In that case, no further management is needed for the hypertension. However, if the patient's blood pressure does not drop after administering the magnesium sulphate, 10 mg (1 capsule) oral nifedipine (Adalat) or intramuscular dihydralazine (Nepresol) 6.25 mg should be given.

Case study 3

While working at a level 1 hospital you admit a patient with a blood pressure of 170/120 mm Hg and 3+ proteinuria. She is 32 weeks pregnant. On further questioning and examination, she has no symptoms or signs of imminent eclampsia.

1. What is the danger to this patient's health?

The patient has severe pre-eclampsia. Therefore, the immediate danger to her life is the development of eclampsia or an intracerebral haemorrhage.

2. How should this patient be managed?

Her clinical condition must first be stabilised. An intravenous infusion should be started and a loading dose of 14 g magnesium sulphate must be given. This should prevent the development of eclampsia. A Foley catheter must be inserted in her bladder.

3. Following the administration of magnesium sulphate, the blood pressure is 160/110 mm Hg. What should the further management be?

Her blood pressure needs to be lowered. 10 mg (1 capsule) oral nifedipine (Adalat) or intramuscular dihydralazine (Nepresol) 6.25 mg should be given. If the diastolic blood pressure remains 110 mm Hg and/or the systolic blood pressure 160 mm Hg or more after 30 minutes, patients who received 10 mg nifedipine orally can be given a second dose of 10 mg nifedipine orally. If dihydralazine was used, an ampoule of dihydralazine (25 mg) should be mixed with 20 ml of sterile water. A bolus doses of 2 ml (2.5 mg) should be given slowly intravenously.

4. Should you continue to manage this patient at a level 1 hospital?

No. The patient should be transferred to a level 2 or 3 hospital for further management.

Case study 4

A 37-year-old gravida 4, para 3 patient books for antenatal care. She has chronic hypertension and is managed with a diuretic. By dates and examination she is 14 weeks pregnant.

1. Should the management of the patient's hypertension be changed during the pregnancy?

Yes. The diuretic should be stopped, as these drugs are not completely safe during pregnancy. Instead, the patient should be treated with alpha methyldopa (Aldomet).

2. What factors indicate a good prognosis for a patient with chronic hypertension during pregnancy?

Normal renal function, no superimposed pre-eclampsia and good control of the blood pressure during pregnancy.

3. How can superimposed pre-eclampsia be diagnosed during pregnancy?

The patient will develop proteinuria and/or a rise in blood pressure during the second half of pregnancy.

4. Why is it important to detect superimposed pre-eclampsia in a patient with chronic hypertension?

Because the risk of complications increases and as a result, a preterm delivery may be necessary. The patient should, therefore, be transferred to a level 2 or 3 hospital if superimposed pre-eclampsia develops.

5. What should be seriously recommended during the puerperium in this patient?

A postpartum sterilisation. Postpartum sterilisation should be discussed with the patient during the pregnancy. Postpartum sterilisation is particularly important as the patient is a 37-year-old multipara.

Skills: Measuring blood pressure and proteinuria

Objectives

When you have completed this skills chapter you should be able to:

- Measure blood pressure.
- Measure the amount of protein in the urine.

Measuring blood pressure

A. The standardised method of measuring blood pressure

The following are important if you want to measure the blood pressure accurately:

1. The right upper arm is used.
2. The arm must be taken out of the sleeve.
3. The patient should lie on her right side with a 30 degree lateral tilt or sit in a chair.
4. Take the blood pressure after a five-minute period of rest.
5. The cuff must be applied correctly. If the patient is sitting in a chair, the blood pressure apparatus must be at the same level as her upper arm.
6. The systolic blood pressure is taken at Korotkoff phase 1.
7. The diastolic blood pressure is taken at Korotkoff phase 5.

> The patient should lie on her right side or sit when her blood pressure is measured.

B. Use the right arm

The examination couches in most clinics stand with their left side against a wall as it is most convenient for a right-handed person to examine from the right side of the patient. The lower arm (i.e. the right arm if she is lying on her right side) should be used, as the upper arm will give false low readings as it is above the level of the heart. The arm must be fully undressed so that the cuff can be correctly applied.

C. The patient must not lie on her back

The patient should lie down on her side or sit. She should always lie slightly turned onto her side. Lying on her back may cause the uterus to press on the inferior vena cava resulting in a decreased return of blood to the heart and a drop in blood pressure. A false low blood pressure may, therefore, be recorded.

D. Allow the patient to rest for 5 minutes before measuring the blood pressure

Anxiety and the effort of climbing onto the couch often increases the blood pressure. This will usually return to a resting value if the patient can lie down and relax for 5 minutes.

E. How to apply the cuff

A standard-size cuff (width of 14.5 cm) is usually used. If the mid-upper arm circumference is more than 33 cm, then use a wide cuff (17.5 cm) to get a correct reading. The cuff must be applied firmly around the arm, not allowing more than 1 finger between the cuff and the patient's arm.

F. Listening to the pulse

The cuff should be pumped up with a finger feeling the brachial or radial pulse. Only when the pulse can no longer be felt, should the stethoscope be put over the brachial pulse and the pressure released slowly.

G. Recognising the Korotkoff phases 1 and 5

The Korotkoff phases are times when the sound of the pulse changes during the measurement of the blood pressure:

Phase 1 is the first sound which you hear after the cuff pressure is released. This indicates the systolic pressure.

Phase 5 is the time when the sound of the pulse disappears. Usually the sound gets softer before it disappears, but sometimes it disappears without first becoming softer. However, in all cases the diastolic blood pressure must be read when the sound of the pulse disappears.

Measuring proteinuria

H. Measuring the amount of proteinuria

The amount of protein in a sample of urine is simply and easily measured with a plastic reagent strip.

I. Grading the amount of proteinuria

Using a reagent strip the amount of proteinuria is graded as follows:

1+ = 0.3 g/l

2+ = 1.0 g/l

3+ = 3.0 g/l

4+ = 10 g/l

Remember that a trace (0.1g/l) of protein is not regarded as significant proteinuria and may occur normally.

J. The use of a reagent strip to measure the amount of proteinuria

1. Collect a fresh specimen of urine.
2. Remove a reagent strip from the bottle and replace the cap.
3. Dip the strip into the urine so that all the test areas are completely covered, then immediately remove the strip.

4. Wait 60 seconds.
5. Hold the strip horizontally and compare with the colour blocks on the side of the bottle. Hold the strip close to the bottle to match the colours but do not rest it on the bottle as the urine will damage the colour chart. The darker the colour of the reagent strip, the greater is the amount of proteinuria.

K. Reagent strips can give a false reading

Reagent strips may incorrectly assess the degree of proteinuria if the urine is very concentrated or very dilute. Do not use the first urine passed in the morning as it may be concentrated and, therefore, give a falsely high reading.

Antepartum haemorrhage

Take the chapter test before and after you read this chapter.

Objectives

When you have completed this unit you should be able to:

- Understand why an antepartum haemorrhage should always be regarded as serious.
- Provide the initial management of a patient presenting with an antepartum haemorrhage.
- Understand that it is sometimes necessary to deliver the fetus as soon as possible, in order to save the life of the mother or infant.
- Diagnose the cause of the bleeding from the history and examination of the patient.
- Correctly manage each of the causes of antepartum haemorrhage.
- Diagnose the cause of a blood-stained vaginal discharge and administer appropriate treatment.

Antepartum haemorrhage

4-1 What is an antepartum haemorrhage?

An antepartum haemorrhage is any vaginal bleeding which occurs at or after 24 weeks (estimated fetal weight at 24 weeks = 500 g) and before the birth of the infant. A bleed before 24 weeks is regarded as a threatened miscarriage.

NOTE
A fetus is viable from 28 weeks, or an estimated weight of 1000 g, if the duration of pregnancy is uncertain. Antepartum haemorrhage before the fetus is viable has the same serious complications as that with a viable fetus. In both cases, the management is the same except for fetal monitoring, which is only done from 28 weeks (or 1000 g).

4-2 Why is an antepartum haemorrhage such a serious condition?

1. The bleeding can be so severe that it can endanger the life of both the mother and fetus.
2. Abruptio placentae is a common cause of antepartum haemorrhage and an important cause of perinatal death in many communities.

Therefore, all patients who present with an antepartum haemorrhage must be regarded as serious emergencies until a diagnosis has been made. Further management will depend on the cause of the haemorrhage.

Any vaginal bleeding during pregnancy may be an important danger sign that must be reported immediately.

4-3 What advice about vaginal bleeding should you give to all patients?

Every patient must be advised that any vaginal bleeding is potentially serious and told that this complication must be reported immediately.

4-4 What is the management of an antepartum haemorrhage?

The management consists of four important steps that should be carried out in the following order:

1. The maternal condition must be evaluated and stabilised, if necessary.
2. The condition of the fetus must then be assessed.
3. The cause of the haemorrhage must be diagnosed.
4. Finally, the definitive management of an antepartum haemorrhage, depending on the cause, must be given.

It must also be decided whether the patient should be transferred for further treatment.

The initial emergency management of antepartum haemorrhage

The management must always be provided in the following order:

1. Assess the condition of the patient. If the patient is shocked, she must be resuscitated immediately.
2. Assess the condition of the fetus. If the fetus is viable but distressed, an emergency delivery is needed.
3. Diagnose the cause of the bleeding, taking the clinical findings into account and, if necessary, the results of special investigations.

The initial management and diagnosis of a patient with vaginal bleeding is summarised in Figure 4-1.

4-5 What symptoms and signs indicate that the patient is shocked due to blood loss?

1. Dizziness is the commonest symptom of shock.
2. On general examination the patient is sweating, her skin and mucous membranes are pale, and she feels cold and clammy to the touch.
3. The blood pressure is low and the pulse rate fast.

4-6 How should you manage a shocked patient with an antepartum haemorrhage?

When there are symptoms and signs to indicate that the patient is shocked, you must:

1. Put up *2* intravenous infusions ('drips') with Balsol or Ringer's lactate, to run in quickly in order to actively resuscitate the patient.
2. Insert a Foley catheter into the patient's bladder to measure the urinary volume and to monitor further urine output.

3. If blood is available, take blood for cross-matching at the time of putting up the intravenous infusion and order 2 or more units of blood urgently.
4. Listen to the fetal heart:
   ○ If fetal distress is present and the fetus is assessed to be viable (28 weeks or an estimated weight of 1000 g or more), then deliver by the quickest possible method, usually by Caesarean section.
   ○ If fetal distress is excluded, if the fetus is too preterm to be viable, or if there is an intra-uterine death, then more attention can be given to the history and examination of the patient in order to make a diagnosis of the cause of the bleeding.

4-7 What must you do if a patient presents with a life-threatening haemorrhage?

The maternal condition takes preference over that of the fetus. The patient, therefore, is actively resuscitated while arrangements are made to terminate the pregnancy by Caesarean section.

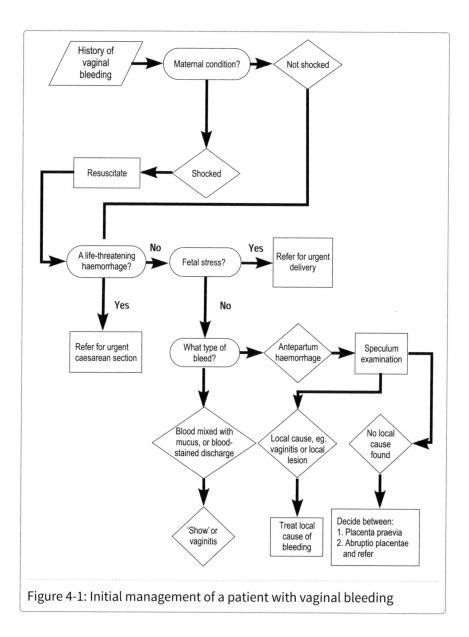

Figure 4-1: Initial management of a patient with vaginal bleeding

Diagnosing the cause of the bleeding

4-8 Should you treat all patients with antepartum haemorrhage in the same way, irrespective of the amount and character of the bleed?

No. The management differs depending on whether the vaginal bleeding is diagnosed as a 'haemorrhage' on the one hand, or a blood-stained vaginal discharge or a 'show' on the other hand. A careful assessment of the amount and type of bleeding is, therefore, very important.

1. Any vaginal bleeding at or after 24 weeks must be diagnosed as an *antepartum haemorrhage* if any of the following are present:
   - A sanitary pad is at least partially soaked with blood.
   - Blood runs down the patient's legs.
   - A clot of blood has been passed.

   A diagnosis of a haemorrhage always suggests a serious complication.

2. *A blood-stained vaginal discharge* will consist of a discharge mixed with a small amount of blood.
3. A 'show' will consist of a small amount of blood mixed with mucus. The blood-stained vaginal discharge or 'show' will be present on the surface of the sanitary pad but will not soak it.

If the maternal and fetal conditions are satisfactory, then a careful speculum examination should be done to exclude a local cause of the bleeding. Do *not* perform a digital vaginal examination, as this may cause a massive haemorrhage if the patient has a placenta praevia.

> Do not do a digital vaginal examination until placenta praevia has been excluded.

4-9 How does a speculum examination help you determine the cause of the bleeding?

1. Bleeding through a closed cervical os confirms the diagnosis of a haemorrhage.

2. If the cervix is a few centimetres dilated with bulging membranes, or the presenting part of the fetus is visible, this suggests that the bleed was a 'show'.
3. A blood-stained discharge in the vagina, with no bleeding through the cervical os, suggests a vaginitis.
4. Bleeding from the surface of the cervix caused by contact with the speculum (i.e. contact bleeding) may indicate a cervicitis or cervical intra-epithelial neoplasia (CIN).
5. Bleeding from a cervical tumour or an ulcer may indicate an infiltrating carcinoma.

4-10 Can you rely on clinical findings to determine the cause of a haemorrhage?

In many cases the history and examination of the abdomen will enable the patient to be put into one of two groups:

1. Abruptio placentae.
2. Placenta praevia.

There are some patients in whom no reason for the haemorrhage can be found. Such a haemorrhage is classified as an antepartum haemorrhage of unknown cause.

4-11 What is the most likely cause of an antepartum haemorrhage with fetal distress?

Abruptio placentae is the commonest cause of antepartum haemorrhage leading to fetal distress. However, sometimes there may be very little or no bleeding even with a severe abruptio placentae.

An antepartum haemorrhage with fetal distress or fetal death is almost always due to abruptio placentae.

4-12 What is the most likely cause of a life-threatening antepartum haemorrhage?

A placenta praevia is the most likely cause of a massive antepartum haemorrhage that threatens the patient's life.

Antepartum bleeding caused by abruptio placentae

4-13 What is abruptio placentae?

Abruptio placentae (placental abruption) means that part or all of the normally implanted placenta has separated from the uterus before delivery of the fetus. The cause of abruptio placentae remains unknown.

4-14 Which patients are at increased risk of abruptio placentae?

Patients with:

1. A history of an abruptio placentae in a previous pregnancy. (There is a 10% chance of recurrence after an abruptio placentae in a previous pregnancy and a 25% chance after two previous pregnancies with an abruptio placentae.)
2. Pre-eclampsia (gestational proteinuric hypertension) and, to a lesser extent, any of the other hypertensive disorders of pregnancy.
3. Intra-uterine growth restriction.
4. Cigarette smoking.
5. Poor socio-economic conditions.
6. A history of abdominal trauma, e.g. a fall or kick on the abdomen.

4-15 What symptoms point to a diagnosis of abruptio placentae?

1. An antepartum haemorrhage which is associated with continuous severe abdominal pain.
2. A history that the blood is dark red with clots.
3. Absence of fetal movements following the bleeding.

4-16 What do you expect to find on examination of the patient?

1. The general examination and observations show that the patient is shocked, often out of proportion to the amount of visible blood loss.
2. The patient usually has severe abdominal pain.

3. The abdominal examination shows the following:
   - The uterus is tonically contracted, hard and tender, so much so that the whole abdomen may be rigid.
   - Fetal parts cannot be palpated.
   - The uterus is bigger than the patient's dates suggest.
   - The haemoglobin concentration is low, indicating severe blood loss.
4. The fetal heartbeat is almost always absent in a severe abruptio placentae.

These symptoms and signs are typical of a severe abruptio placentae. However, abruptio placentae may present with symptoms and signs which are less obvious, making the diagnosis difficult.

The management of abruptio placentae is summarised in Figure 4-2.

> The diagnosis of severe abruptio placentae can usually be made from the history and physical examination.

4-17 What would you do if the fetal heartbeat was still present?

If the fetal heartbeat is still present with an abruptio placentae, there will usually be signs of fetal distress. The infant will die in utero if not delivered immediately.

4-18 How should you decide on the method of delivery if the fetal heartbeat is still present?

1. If the symptoms and signs are typical of an abruptio placentae, a vaginal examination should be done.
2. If the cervix is at least 9 cm dilated, and the presenting part is well down in the pelvis, then the membranes should be ruptured and the infant delivered vaginally. If these conditions are not present, an emergency Caesarean section should be done.
3. If the fetus is not viable, it should be delivered vaginally if the diagnosis is abruptio placentae.
4. While preparations for delivery are being made, the mother must be resuscitated and intra-uterine resuscitation of the fetus started.

However, salbutamol or nifedipine must *not* be given to a patient who shows any evidence of shock.

5. When there is doubt about the diagnosis, specifically when placenta praevia cannot be excluded on history and examination, then a digital vaginal examination should *not* be done. If fetal distress is present and the fetus is viable, a Caesarean section must be done. If there is neither fetal distress nor severe vaginal bleeding, the possibility of a placenta praevia must be investigated. An ultrasound examination or vaginal examination in theatre must then be done.

4-19 What should you do if the fetal heartbeat is absent?

1. Active resuscitation of the mother is a priority and should have been started as part of the initial emergency management:
   o 2 intravenous infusion lines are usually needed, one of which can be a central venous pressure line inserted in the antecubital fossa.
   o 2 units of fresh frozen plasma, and at least 4 units of whole blood are usually needed for effective resuscitation.

2. A Foley catheter is inserted into the bladder.

3. The pulse rate and blood pressure must be checked every 15 minutes until the patient's condition stabilises, and half-hourly thereafter. The urinary output must be recorded hourly.

4. The membranes are then ruptured, following which cervical dilatation and delivery of the fetus usually occur quickly.

5. Pain relief in the form of pethidine or morphine and promethazine (Phenergan) or hydroxyzine (Aterax) should be given once the patient is adequately resuscitated.

4-20 Why is it important to remember that many patients with abruptio placentae have underlying pre-eclampsia?

1. Signs of shock may be present even with a normal blood pressure. These patients, nevertheless, need active resuscitation.

2. After resuscitation a hypotensive patient may become hypertensive, so much so that dihydralazine (Nepresol) may have to be given parenterally or nifedipine (Adalat) orally.

3. Magnesium sulphate must be given if the patient develops imminent eclampsia.

These patients are haemodynamically very unstable. Although initially they also require active resuscitation, they quickly become fluid overloaded, resulting in pulmonary oedema. Renal complications, such as acute tubular necrosis, commonly occur.

Abruptio placentae with pre-eclampsia is a serious condition with a high risk of maternal death.

4-21 At your initial assessment of the patient, how would you know whether or not there is underlying pre-eclampsia present?

By finding protein in the patient's urine.

4-22 What complication should you watch for after delivery?

Postpartum haemorrhage, as this is common after abruptio placentae.

4-23 What action should you take to prevent postpartum haemorrhage?

1. Syntometrine 1 ampoule should be given intramuscularly, if the patient is not hypertensive. Only oxytocin is used in a hypertensive patient.
2. In addition, 20 units of oxytocin are put in the intravenous infusion bottle.
3. The uterus is rubbed up well.
4. The patient is carefully observed for bleeding.

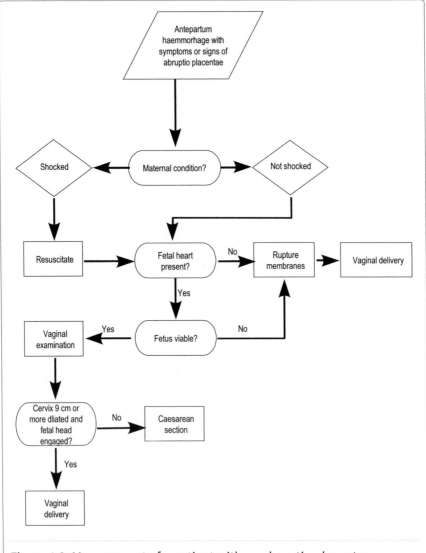

Figure 4-2: Management of a patient with an abruptio placentae

Antepartum bleeding caused by placenta praevia

4-24 What is placenta praevia?

Placenta praevia means that the placenta is implanted either wholly or partially in the lower segment of the uterus. It may extend down to, or cover the internal os of the cervix. When the lower segment starts to form or the cervix begins to dilate, the placenta becomes partially separated and this causes maternal bleeding.

4-25 Which patients have the highest risk of placenta praevia?

1. With regard to their previous obstetric history, patients who:
   - Are grande multiparas, i.e. who are para 5 or higher.
   - Have had a previous Caesarean section.

2. With regard to their present obstetric history, patients who:
   - Have a multiple pregnancy.
   - Have had a threatened abortion, especially in the second trimester.
   - Have an abnormal presentation.

4-26 What in the history of the bleeding suggests the diagnosis of placenta praevia?

1. The bleeding is painless and bright red in colour.
2. Fetal movements are still present after the bleed.

4-27 What are the typical findings on physical examination in a patient with placenta praevia?

1. General examination may show signs that the patient is shocked, and the amount of bleeding corresponds to the degree of shock. The patient's haemoglobin concentration is normal or low depending on the amount of blood loss and the time interval between the haemorrhage and the haemoglobin measurement. However, the first bleed is usually not severe.
2. Examination of the abdomen shows that:
   ○ The uterus is soft and not tender to palpation.
   ○ The uterus is not bigger than it should be for the patient's dates.
   ○ The fetal parts can be easily palpated, and the fetal heart is present.
   ○ There may be an abnormal presentation. Breech presentation or oblique or transverse lies are commonly present.
   ○ In cephalic presentations, the head is not engaged and is easily ballotable above the pelvis.

The diagnosis of placenta praevia can usually be made from the history and physical examination.

4-28 Do you think that engagement of the head can occur if there is a placenta praevia present?

No. If there is 2/5 or less of the fetal head palpable above the pelvic brim on abdominal examination, then placenta praevia can be excluded and a digital vaginal examination can be done safely. The first vaginal examination must always be done carefully.

2/5 or less of the fetal head palpable above the pelvic brim excludes the possibility of placenta praevia.

4-29 What do you understand by a 'warning bleed'?

This is the first bleeding that occurs from a placenta praevia, when the lower segment begins to form at about 34 weeks, or even earlier.

4-30 Are there any investigations that can confirm the diagnosis of placenta praevia?

1. If the patient is less than 38 weeks pregnant and *not bleeding actively*, an ultrasound examination must be done in order to localise the placenta.
2. If the patient is 38 or more weeks pregnant, and *not bleeding actively*:
   ○ If ultrasonology is available, an ultrasound examination can be done in order to localise the placenta.
   ○ If ultrasonology is not available, a digital vaginal examination can be done in theatre with everything ready for a Caesarean section.

4-31 What action should you take if a routine ultrasound examination early in pregnancy shows a placenta praevia?

In most cases, the position of the placenta moves away from the internal os of the cervix as pregnancy continues. A follow-up ultrasound examination must be arranged at a gestational age of 32 weeks.

4-32 What is the further management after making the diagnosis of placenta praevia?

1. If the patient is not bleeding actively, further management depends on the gestational age:
   ○ With a gestational age of less than 38 weeks, the patient is hospitalised and managed conservatively until 38 weeks or until active bleeding starts.
   ○ If the fetus is viable (28 weeks or more) but the gestational age is less than 34 weeks, steroids must be given to stimulate fetal lung maturity as delivery may become necessary within a few days.
   ○ With a gestational age of 38 weeks or more, the fetus should be delivered.

   The further management of a patient when her pregnancy has reached 36 weeks depends on the grade of placenta praevia.

2. A patient who is actively bleeding must be delivered irrespective of the gestational age, because this is a life-threatening condition for the patient. An emergency Caesarean section or hysterotomy must be done.

The management of a patient with a placenta praevia is summarised in Figures 4-3 and 4-4.

4-33 When a patient with placenta praevia is less than 38 weeks pregnant and is being managed conservatively, what amount of bleeding would indicate that you should deliver the fetus?

1. Any sudden, severe haemorrhage.
2. Any continuous, moderate bleeding, such that the drop in the patient's haemoglobin concentration requires a blood transfusion.

4-34 How will you further manage a patient who has been treated conservatively?

1. With a grade 3 or 4 placenta praevia, a Caesarean section should be done at 36 weeks.
2. With a grade 2 placenta praevia, a Caesarean section should be done at 38 weeks.
3. With a grade 1 placenta praevia which bleeds now, and a presenting part that remains high above the pelvis, a Caesarean section should be done at 38 weeks.
4. With a grade 1 placenta praevia, which does not bleed and where the fetal head is engaged (2/5 or less palpable above the brim), you can wait for the spontaneous onset of labour. The first vaginal examination must be done very carefully.

4-35 How do you go about doing a vaginal examination in theatre?

1. The theatre sister must be scrubbed up with her trolley ready.
2. The anaesthetist must be ready with his drugs drawn up so that, if necessary, he can proceed immediately with the induction of anaesthesia.
3. A careful digital examination must be done. First feel in all four vaginal fornices:
   - If there is soft tissue between the examining finger and the fetal skull, then placenta praevia is diagnosed.

- If the fetal skull is easily felt in all four fornices, then a careful examination is done through the cervix.
- If placental tissue is felt, then a Caesarean section should be done. If not, the membranes can be ruptured with the aim of allowing a vaginal delivery.

4-36 If the fetus is alive, why is urgent delivery of less importance in placenta praevia than in abruptio placentae?

Compared with abruptio placentae, intra-uterine death is uncommon in placenta praevia. However, a serious vaginal bleed due to placenta praevia may still necessitate an immediate delivery to save the mother's life.

4-37 Why do patients with a placenta praevia have an increased risk of postpartum haemorrhage?

The placenta was implanted in the lower segment which does not have the same ability as the upper segment to contract and retract after delivery. Therefore, the same measures taken with abruptio placentae must be taken to prevent postpartum haemorrhage.

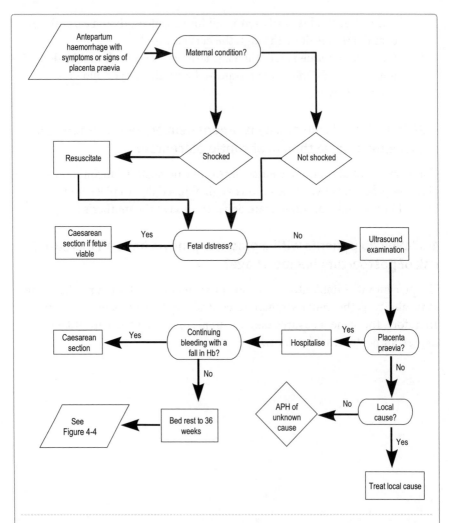

Figure 4-3: Management of a patient with a placenta praevia before 36 weeks

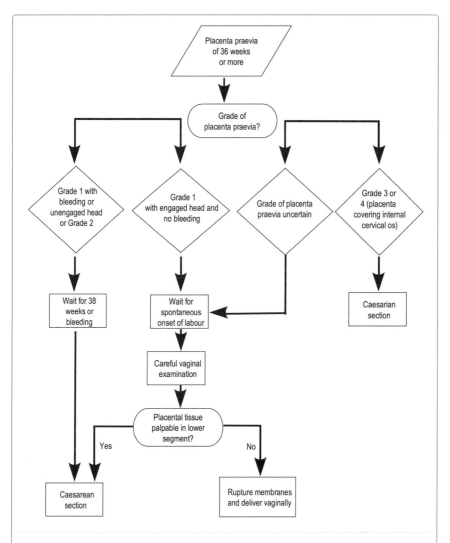

Figure 4-4: Management of a patient with a placenta praevia at 36 weeks or more

Antepartum haemorrhage of unknown cause

4-38 When would you suspect an antepartum haemorrhage of unknown cause?

In patients who fulfill *all* the following requirements:

1. Less severe antepartum bleeding, without signs of shock, and when the fetal condition is good.
2. When the history and examination do not suggest a severe abruptio placentae.
3. When local causes have been excluded on speculum examination.
4. When placenta praevia has been excluded by an ultrasound examination.

4-39 What should you do to exclude other causes of bleeding if you do not have ultrasound facilities ?

1. Abruptio placentae can usually be excluded on history and examination.
2. Local causes are excluded on speculum examination.
3. With a gestational age of 38 weeks or more, a vaginal examination is done in theatre to confirm or exclude placenta praevia.
4. If the gestational age is less than 38 weeks, the patient must be admitted to hospital and close attention paid to fetal movements, especially in the first 24 hours.

NOTE
  If available, antenatal fetal heart rate monitoring should be done on admission to hospital and every 6 hours during the first 24 hours.

4-40 What is the most likely cause of an antepartum haemorrhage of unknown cause?

A small abruptio placentae that does not cause any other signs or symptoms. If the placental separation is going to extend, it will usually happen within the first 24 hours following the bleed. Therefore, the patient must be hospitalised and closely observed during this period for signs of fetal distress.

4-41 How should you manage a patient with an antepartum haemorrhage of unknown cause?

1. The patient must be hospitalised.
2. Careful attention must be given to fetal movements, especially during the first 24 hours.

   NOTE
   If available, a cardiotocogram must be recorded on admission and then every 6 hours during the first 24 hours.

3. If there is no further bleeding in the next 48 hours, the patient can be discharged. She must abstain from coitus for the rest of her pregnancy.
4. As a high-risk pregnancy, the patient must have weekly follow-ups and is advised to report immediately if there is any decrease in fetal movements, or further bleeding. No digital vaginal examination must be done.
5. The patient must be allowed to go into spontaneous labour at term.

> A patient with an antepartum haemorrhage of unknown cause must be closely observed for fetal distress during the first 24 hours after the bleed.

4-42 Why is an antepartum haemorrhage of unknown cause always regarded in a serious light?

There is the possibility that abruptio placentae may be present. If the abruptio placentae is going to extend, intra-uterine death may result. The risk of such an event is greatest during the 24 hours following the bleed.

NOTE
Antepartum haemorrhage could also be due to vasa praevia. This rare cause of antepartum haemorrhage occurs when the vessels of the umbilical cord cross the membranes near to the internal os. When the membranes rupture, a small amount of continuous bright red bleeding occurs. The blood is from the fetal circulation and, therefore, the fetus can bleed to death. If the cervix is almost fully dilated, the fetus can be delivered vaginally. If not, a Caesarean section

must be done. The presence of fetal blood is confirmed by performing the sodium hydroxide (Apt) test: Add 1 drop of blood to 9 drops of 1% sodium hydroxide in a glass test tube. Read at 1 minute. If the blood is fetal, the mixture remains pink. However, if the blood is maternal, the mixture becomes brown.

Referral of a patient with an antepartum haemorrhage

4-43 How should you decide whether a patient can be managed locally or whether she should be transferred?

1. Clinics and level 1 hospitals which do not have blood available must refer all patients with an antepartum haemorrhage.
2. Level 1 hospitals which have blood available, and level 2 hospitals, must manage patients with the following problems:
   o A life-threatening bleed from placenta praevia.
   o Fetal distress present with a viable fetus.
   o Abruptio placentae with a live, viable fetus.
3. Abruptio placentae with a dead fetus must be managed in at least a level 2 hospital, because of the risk of clotting defects.
4. A patient with abruptio placentae and pre-eclampsia must be referred to a level 3 hospital as this patient is at high risk of pulmonary oedema and acute tubular necrosis.
5. A patient with a grade 3 or 4 placenta praevia and a viable fetus of less than 34 weeks, who is going to be managed conservatively, should be managed in at least a level 2 hospital with a neonatal intensive care unit, or a level 3 hospital.

4-44 When you refer a patient, what precautions should you take to ensure the safety of the patient in transit?

1. A shocked patient should have 2 intravenous infusion lines with Plasmalyte B or Ringer's lactate running in fast. A doctor should accompany the patient if possible. If not possible, a registered nurse should accompany her.
2. A patient who is no longer bleeding should also have an intravenous infusion and be accompanied by a registered nurse whenever possible.

A blood-stained vaginal discharge

4-45 How would a patient generally describe a blood-stained vaginal discharge?

A patient would probably describe a blood-stained vaginal discharge as a vaginal discharge mixed with a small amount of blood.

4-46 How would a patient generally describe a 'show'?

A patient would probably describe a 'show' as a slight vaginal bleed consisting of blood mixed with mucus.

4-47 How should you manage a patient with a history of a blood-stained vaginal discharge or a 'show'?

1. After getting a good history and ensuring that the condition of the fetus is satisfactory, a careful speculum examination should be done.
2. The speculum is only inserted for 5 cm, carefully opened, and then introduced further until the cervix can be seen.
3. Any bleeding through a closed cervical os indicates an antepartum haemorrhage.
4. A 'show' is the most likely cause of the discharge if the cervix is a few centimetres dilated with bulging membranes, or if the presenting part of the fetus is visible.
5. A vaginitis is the most likely cause, if a blood-stained discharge is seen in the vagina.

4-48 How should you treat a blood-stained discharge due to vaginitis in pregnancy?

1. If a microscope is available, make a wet smear of the discharge. The specific organism causing the vaginitis can then be identified and treated.

   NOTE
   A wet smear of the discharge is made, in both saline and 2% potassium hydroxide and examined.

2. If a microscope is not available:

   o Organisms identified on the cervical cytology smear are the most likely cause of the vaginitis.
   o If no organisms are identified on the cytology smear, or a smear was not done, then *Trichomonas vaginalis* is most probably present.

To treat a Trichomonal vaginitis, both the patient and her partner should receive a single dose of 2 g metronidazole (Flagyl) orally.

4-49 Should metronidazole be used during pregnancy?

Metronidazole should not be used in the first trimester of pregnancy, unless absolutely necessary, as it may cause congenital abnormalities in the fetus. The patient and her partner must be warned that metronidazole causes severe nausea and vomiting if it is taken with alcohol. The risk of congenital abnormalities caused by alcohol may also be increased by metronidazole.

4-50 How do you manage a patient with contact bleeding?

1. When there is normal cervical cytology (Papanicolaou smear), the contact bleeding is probably due to a cervicitis. If it is troublesome, the patient should be given a course of oral erythromycin 500 mg 6-hourly for seven days.
2. With abnormal cervical cytology, the patient should be managed correctly. Cervical intra-epithelial neoplasia causes contact bleeding.

4-51 What action should you take when the bleeding is from a cervical ulcer or tumour?

The patient most probably has an infiltrating cervical carcinoma and should be correctly managed.

NOTE

When there is doubt about the diagnosis, a cytology smear and biopsy of the lesion must be taken. The results should be obtained as soon as possible.

Case study 1

A patient who is 35 weeks pregnant presents with a history of vaginal bleeding.

1. Why does this patient need to be assessed urgently?

Because an antepartum haemorrhage should always be regarded as an emergency, until a cause for the bleeding is found. Thereafter, the correct management can be given.

2. What is the first step in the management of a patient with an antepartum haemorrhage?

The clinical condition of the patient must be assessed. Special attention must be paid to signs of shock. If shock is present, resuscitation must be started urgently.

3. What is the next step in the management of a patient with an antepartum haemorrhage?

The condition of the fetus must be assessed. The presence of fetal distress will influence the choice of management.

4. What should be done once the condition of the patient and her fetus have been assessed, and the patient resuscitated, if necessary?

The cause of the antepartum haemorrhage must be sought and managed.

Case study 2

A patient who is 32 weeks pregnant, according to her antenatal card, presents with a history of severe vaginal bleeding and abdominal pain. The blood contains dark clots. Since the haemorrhage, the patient has not felt her fetus move. The patient's blood pressure is 80/60 mm Hg and the pulse rate 120 beats per minute.

1. What is your clinical diagnosis?

The history is typical of an abruptio placentae.

2. If the clinical examination confirms the diagnosis, what should be the first step in the management of this patient?

The patient's blood pressure and pulse rate indicate that she is shocked. Therefore, she must first be resuscitated.

3. What is the next step that requires urgent attention in the management of the patient?

As the fetus is viable, it is of great importance to establish whether the fetus is still alive. Therefore, it must be urgently established whether the fetal heartbeat is present or not.

4. How should you manage the patient if a fetal heartbeat is heard?

A vaginal examination must be done. If the cervix is 9 cm or more dilated and the fetal head is on the pelvic floor, then the membranes should be ruptured and the fetus delivered vaginally as quickly as possible. Otherwise, an emergency Caesarean section must be done as soon as the patient has been resuscitated. Immediately before starting the Caesarean section, make sure that the fetal heartbeat is still present.

5. Should the above patient be transferred to a level 2 or 3 hospital for delivery, if the fetus is still alive?

The patient should be delivered in any hospital which has facilities for doing a Caesarean section. Moving the patient because the fetus is regarded as preterm may result in an intra-uterine death during transport. If necessary, the newborn infant can be transported to a level 2 hospital with a neonatal intensive care unit. The risk of a clotting defect is low if the fetus is still alive.

6. How should you manage this patient if a fetal heartbeat is not heard?

The membranes should be ruptured and the fetus delivered vaginally, if possible.

Case study 3

A patient is seen at the antenatal clinic at 35 weeks gestation with a breech presentation. The patient is referred to see the doctor the following week, for an external cephalic version. That evening she has a painless, bright red vaginal bleed.

1. What is your diagnosis?

The history and the presence of an abnormal lie suggest that the bleeding is the result of a placenta praevia.

2. What should the initial management of the patient be?

The condition of the mother should first be assessed and the patient resuscitated, if necessary. Then the fetal condition must be assessed. The patient's abdomen should also be examined, to determine whether the clinical signs support the diagnosis of placenta praevia.

3. How should the patient be managed if she should have a severe bleed?

An emergency Caesarean section must be done, as soon as the patient has been adequately resuscitated.

4. What investigations should be done if the patient is not bleeding actively during your initial clinical examination?

A ultrasound examination must be done to confirm the clinical diagnosis. After placenta praevia has been excluded, a careful speculum examination should be done to exclude any local cause for the bleeding.

5. How should the patient be managed if she has had no further severe bleeding after the initial bleed?

She should be hospitalised and managed conservatively until 36 or 38 weeks gestation, or until she starts to bleed actively again. Depending on the degree of placenta praevia, a Caesarean section should be done at 36 or 38 weeks or spontaneous labour can be awaited.

Case study 4

A patient books for antenatal care at 30 weeks gestation. When you inform her of the danger signs during pregnancy, she says that she has had a vaginal discharge for the past 2 weeks. At times the discharge has been blood stained.

1. Has this patient had a antepartum haemorrhage?

The history suggests a blood-stained vaginal discharge rather than an antepartum haemorrhage.

2. What is the most probable cause of the blood-stained vaginal discharge?

A vaginitis. This can usually be confirmed by a speculum examination.

3. How can the cause of the vaginitis be determined?

During the speculum examination, a sample of the discharge should be taken and a wet smear made. Organisms seen on the wet smear are probably the cause of the vaginitis.

4. What is the most likely cause of a vaginitis with a blood-stained discharge?

Trichomonas vaginalis. Therefore, if a microscope is not available, Trichomonas vaginalis is presumed to be the cause of the vaginitis.

5. How should you treat a patient with Trichomonal vaginitis?

A single dose of 2 g metronidazole (Flagyl) is given orally to both the patient and her partner. Both must be warned against drinking alcohol for a few days after taking metronidazole.

5

Preterm labour and preterm rupture of the membranes

Take the chapter test before and after you read this chapter.

Objectives

When you have completed this unit you should be able to:

- Define preterm labour and preterm rupture of the membranes.
- Understand why these conditions are very important.
- Understand the role of infection in causing preterm labour and preterm rupture of the membranes.
- List which patients are at increased risk of these conditions.
- Understand what preventive measures should be taken.
- Diagnose preterm labour and preterm rupture of the membranes.
- Manage these conditions.

Preterm labour and preterm rupture of the membranes

5-1 What is preterm labour?

Preterm labour is diagnosed when there are regular uterine contractions before 37 weeks of pregnancy, together with either of the following:

1. Cervical effacement and/or dilatation.
2. Rupture of the membranes.

5-2 What is preterm rupture of the membranes?

Preterm rupture of the membranes is diagnosed when the membranes rupture before 37 weeks, in the absence of uterine contractions.

NOTE
Preterm rupture of the membranes (as defined above) is sometimes called preterm, prelabour rupture of the membranes in literature.

5-3 What is prelabour rupture of the membranes?

Prelabour rupture of the membranes is defined as rupture of the membranes for at least 1 hour before the onset of labour in a term pregnancy.

5-4 How should you diagnose preterm labour if the gestational age is unknown?

Preterm labour is diagnosed if the estimated fetal weight is below 2500 g. The symphysis-fundus height will be less than 35 cm.

5-5 Why are preterm labour and preterm rupture of the membranes important?

Preterm labour and preterm rupture of the membranes are major causes of perinatal death because:

1. Preterm delivery, especially before 34 weeks, commonly results in the birth of an infant who develops hyaline membrane disease and other complications of prematurity.
2. Preterm labour and preterm rupture of the membranes are often accompanied by bacterial infection of the membranes and placenta that may cause complications for both the mother and the fetus. The mother and fetus may develop severe infection, which is life threatening

5-6 What is the commonest known cause of preterm labour and preterm rupture of the membranes?

In many cases the cause is unknown, but increasing evidence points to infection of the membranes and placenta as the commonest known cause of both preterm labour and preterm rupture of the membranes.

> Infection of the membranes and placenta is the commonest recognised cause of preterm labour and preterm rupture of the membranes.

5-7 What is infection of the membranes and placenta?

Infection of the membranes and placenta causes an acute inflammation of the placenta, membranes and decidua. This condition is called *chorioamnionitis*. It may occur with intact or ruptured membranes.

Bacteria from the cervix and vagina spread through the endocervical canal to infect the membranes and placenta. Later these bacteria may colonise the liquor, from where they may infect the fetus.

Chorioamnionitis may cause the release of prostaglandins which in turn stimulate uterine contractions and cause the onset of labour. Chorioamnionitis may also weaken the membranes and lead to their rupture. If the membranes have already been ruptured due to other causes, such as polyhydramnios, vaginal bacteria can spread directly into the liquor. The longer the duration of ruptured membranes, the greater the risk of chorioamnionitis. The risk of infection is also increased by digital vaginal examinations after rupture of the membranes.

NOTE
 After delivery, the diagnosis of chorioamnionitis can be confirmed by:
 • Noting that the infant and placenta have an offensive smell.
 • Noting that the membranes are cloudy.
 • Finding pus cells and bacteria on microscopic examination of the infant's gastric aspirate immediately after birth.
 • Finding acute inflammation in the membranes and placenta on histology after delivery.

> Infection of the membranes and placenta (chorioamnionitis) may occur with either intact or ruptured membranes.

5-8 What is the clinical presentation of chorioamnionitis?

Usually chorioamnionitis is asymptomatic (subclinical chorioamnionitis) and, therefore, the clinical diagnosis is often not made. However, the following signs may be present:

1. Fetal tachycardia.
2. Maternal pyrexia and/or tachycardia.
3. Tenderness of the uterus.
4. Drainage of offensive liquor, if the membranes have ruptured.

If any of the above signs are present, a diagnosis of clinical chorioamnionitis must be made.

NOTE
There is no proof that daily white cell counts or determination of C-reactive protein (CRP) are of any greater diagnostic value in making an early diagnosis of chorioamnionitis.

5-9 What factors may predispose a woman to chorioamnionitis?

1. Rupture of the membranes.
2. Exposure of the membranes due to dilatation of the cervix.
3. Coitus during the second half of pregnancy.

However, in many cases, the factors that result in chorioamnionitis are not known.

5-10 Can chorioamnionitis cause complications during the puerperium?

Yes. Chorioamnionitis may cause infection of the genital tract (puerperal sepsis) which, if not treated correctly, may result in septicaemia, the need for hysterectomy, and possibly in maternal death. These complications can usually be prevented by starting a course of broad spectrum antibiotics (e.g. ampicillin plus metronidazole), as soon as the diagnosis of clinical chorioamnionitis is made.

Bacteria that have colonised the amniotic fluid may infect the fetus, and the infant may present with signs of infection at, or soon after, birth.

5-11 What factors other than chorioamnionitis can lead to preterm labour and preterm rupture of the membranes?

The following maternal, fetal and placental factors may be associated with preterm labour and/or preterm rupture of the membranes:

1. Maternal factors:
   ○ Pyrexia, as the result of an acute infection other than chorioamnionitis, e.g. acute pyelonephritis or malaria.
   ○ Uterine abnormalities, such as congenital uterine malformations (e.g. septate or bicornuate uterus) and uterine myomas (fibroids).
   ○ Incompetence of the internal cervical os ('cervical incompetence').

2. Fetal factors:
   ○ A multiple pregnancy.
   ○ Polyhydramnios (both cause overdistension of the uterus.)
   ○ Congenital malformations of the fetus.
   ○ Syphilis.

3. Placental factors:
   ○ Placenta praevia.
   ○ Abruptio placentae.

NOTE
Polyhydramnios, multiple pregnancy and cervical incompetence cause preterm dilatation of the cervix with exposure of the membranes to the vaginal bacteria. This may predispose to chorioamnionitis. Polyhydramnios has several causes, but it is important to remember that oesophageal atresia is one of the causes which need to be excluded after delivery.

5-12 Which patients are at an increased risk of preterm labour or preterm rupture of the membranes?

Both preterm labour and preterm rupture of membranes are more common in patients who:

1. Have a past history of preterm labour.
2. Have no antenatal care.
3. Live in poor socio-economic circumstances.
4. Smoke, use alcohol or abuse habit-forming drugs.
5. Are underweight due to undernutrition.

6. Have coitus in the second half of pregnancy, when they are at an increased risk of preterm labour
7. Have any of the maternal, fetal or placental factors listed in 5-11.

> **The most important risk factor for preterm labour is a previous history of preterm delivery.**

5-13 What can be done to decrease the incidence of these complications?

1. Take measures to ensure that all pregnant women receive antenatal care.
2. Identify patients with a past history of preterm labour.
3. Give advice about the dangers of smoking, alcohol and the use of habit-forming drugs.
4. Advise against coitus during the late second and in the third trimester in pregnancies at high risk for preterm labour or preterm rupture of the membranes. If coitus occurs during pregnancy in these patients, the use of condoms must be recommended as this may reduce the risk of chorioamnionitis.
5. At 14–16 weeks, insert a McDonald suture in patients with a proven incompetent internal cervical os.
6. Prevent teenage pregnancies.
7. Improve the socio-economic and nutritional status of poor communities.
8. Arrange that the workload of women, who have to do heavy manual labour, is decreased when they are pregnant and that an opportunity to rest during working hours is allowed.

5-14 How should you manage a patient at increased risk of preterm labour or preterm rupture of the membranes?

1. Patients at increased risk must have two weekly vaginal examinations from 24 weeks, in order to make an early diagnosis of preterm cervical effacement and/or dilatation.
2. In all women with cervical effacement or dilatation before 34 weeks, the following preventive measures can then be taken:
   - Bed rest. This can be at home, except when the home circumstances are poor, in which case the patient should be admitted to hospital.

- Sick leave must be arranged for working patients.
- Coitus must be forbidden.
- Patients must immediately report if contractions or rupture of the membranes occur.
- Women with preterm labour or preterm rupture of the membranes must be seen as soon as possible, and the correct measures taken to prevent the delivery of a severely preterm infant.

> All patients should be told to immediately report preterm labour or preterm rupture of the membranes.

5-15 What should you do if a patient threatens to deliver a preterm infant?

1. Infants born between 34 and 36 weeks can usually be cared for in a level 1 hospital.
2. However, women who deliver between 28 and 33 weeks, should be referred to a level 2 or 3 hospital with a neonatal intensive care unit.
3. If the birth of a preterm baby cannot be prevented, it must be remembered that the best incubator for transporting an infant is the mother's uterus. Even if the delivery is inevitable, an attempt to suppress labour should be made, so that the patient can be transferred before the infant is born.
4. The better the condition of the infant on arrival at the neonatal intensive care unit, the better the prognosis.

Diagnosis of preterm labour and preterm rupture of the membranes

5-16 How should you distinguish between Braxton Hicks contractions and the contractions of preterm labour?

Braxton Hicks contractions:

1. Are irregular.
2. May cause discomfort but are not painful.

3. Do not increase in duration or frequency.
4. Do not cause cervical effacement or dilatation.

The duration of contractions cannot be used as a distinguishing factor, as Braxton Hicks contractions may last up to 60 seconds.

In contrast, the contractions of preterm or early labour:

1. Are regular, at least 1 per 10 minutes.
2. Are painful.
3. Increase in frequency and duration.
4. Cause effacement and dilatation of the cervix.

5-17 How should you confirm the diagnosis of preterm labour?

Both of the following will be present in a patient of less than 37 weeks gestation:

1. Regular uterine contractions, palpable on abdominal examination, of at least 1 per 10 minutes.
2. A history of rupture of the membranes, or cervical effacement and/or dilatation, on vaginal examination.

5-18 How can you diagnose preterm rupture of the membranes?

1. A patient of less than 37 weeks gestation will give a history of sudden drainage of liquor followed by a continual leak of smaller amounts, without associated uterine contractions.
2. A sterile speculum examination will confirm the diagnosis of ruptured membranes.
3. *A digital vaginal examination must not be done* as it is of little value in diagnosing rupture of the membranes and may increase the risk of infection.

A digital vaginal examination must not be done if there is preterm rupture of the membranes.

5-19 What is the value of a sterile speculum examination when preterm rupture of the membranes is suspected?

1. The danger of ascending infection is not increased by this procedure.
2. Observing drainage of liquor from the cervical os confirms the diagnosis of ruptured membranes.
3. If no drainage of liquor is observed, drainage can sometimes be seen if the patient is asked to cough.
4. If no drainage of liquor is seen, a smear should be taken from the posterior vaginal fornix with a wooden spatula to determine the pH and to test for ferning.
5. The possibility of cord prolapse can be excluded or confirmed.
6. It is also important to see whether the cervix is long and closed, or whether there is already clear evidence of cervical effacement and/or dilatation.
7. A patient with a profuse vaginal discharge or stress incontinence (leaking urine when coughing or laughing) may think that she is draining liquor. A speculum examination will help to confirm or rule out this possibility.

NOTE
If the facilities are available, and preterm rupture of the membranes has been confirmed, an endocervical swab could be taken to culture for Group B Streptococcus and Gonococcus.

5-20 How should you test the vaginal pH?

1. The pH of the vagina is acidic but the pH of liquor is alkaline.
2. Red litmus paper is pressed against the moist spatula. If the red litmus changes to blue, then liquor is present in the vagina, indicating that the membranes have ruptured. If blue litmus is used, it will remain blue with rupture of membranes or change to red if the membranes are intact.

5-21 How will you test for ferning?

1. The vaginal fluid on the wooden spatula is spread on a microscope slide and allowed to dry.
2. The slide is then examined under the low power lens of a microscope. An unmistakable pattern of a fern leaf will be observed if the specimen is liquor.

Management of preterm labour

5-22 How will you manage a patient in preterm labour?

Step 1: Listen to the fetal heart to rule out fetal distress and determine the duration of pregnancy as accurately as possible:

1. If fetal distress is present and the fetus is assessed to be viable (28 weeks or more), then the infant must be delivered as soon as possible.
2. If the pregnancy is 34 weeks or more, labour should be allowed to continue.
3. If the infant is assessed to be 24 weeks or more but less than 34 weeks, other contraindications for the suppression of preterm labour must be excluded. Subsequently the contractions should be suppressed with a calcium channel blocker, e.g. nifedipine (Adalat), or a beta2 stimulant, e.g. salbutamol (Ventolin). The further management of these patients must take place in a level 2 or 3 hospital.
4. The administration of steroids to enhance fetal lung maturity prior to transfer should be discussed with the referral hospital.

Step 2: Look for treatable causes of preterm labour, such as urinary tract infection or malaria.

The management of a patient with preterm labour is summarised in Figure 5-1.

5-23 What are the contraindications to the suppression of preterm labour?

1. Fetal distress.
2. A pregnancy where the duration is 34 weeks or more, or 24 weeks or less.
3. Chorioamnionitis.
4. Intra-uterine death.
5. Congenital abnormalities incompatible with life.
6. Pre-eclampsia.
7. Antepartum haemorrhage of unknown cause.

8. Cervical dilatation of more than 6 cm. (However, contractions should be temporarily suppressed while the patient is being transferred to a hospital where preterm infants can be managed.)
9. Severe intra-uterine growth restriction.

NOTE

Antepartum haemorrhage of unknown cause may be due to a small abruptio placentae. It is, therefore, advisable not to suppress labour should it occur.

5-24 How will you decide that a patient is less than 36 weeks pregnant if the duration of the pregnancy is unknown?

This is done by measuring the symphysis-fundus height and by doing a complete abdominal examination.

Labour must be suppressed if the estimated fetal weight is less than 2000 g or the estimated gestational age less than 34 weeks. The symphysis-fundus height measurement will be less than 33 cm.

5-25 How should you give nifedipine for the suppression of preterm labour?

1. Three nifedipine (Adalat) 10 mg capsules (total 30 mg) should be taken by mouth. If there are no further contractions and no continuing cervical dilatation and effacement, 20 mg should be given 8-hourly.
2. If there are still contractions with cervical dilatation and effacement 3 hours after the initial dose, a second dose of 20 mg should be given, followed by 8-hourly doses.

Nifedipine (Adalat) has fewer side effects than salbutamol for the mother. Following the latest research, nifedipine (Adalat) has been recommended as the drug of choice in suppressing uterine contractions.

5-26 What are the contraindications to the use of nifedipine in suppressing labour?

1. Nifedipine (Adalat) cannot be used for the suppression of preterm labour if patients have hypertension, or are suffering from any of the hypertensive disorders of pregnancy.
2. Hypovolaemia or surgical shock due to any reason.
3. Any condition that impairs the function of the myocardium.

5-27 How should you use salbutamol for the suppression of preterm labour?

1. Start an intravenous infusion of Ringer's lactate and give 250 µg (0.5 ml) salbutamol slowly intravenously, after ensuring that there is no contraindication to its use. The 0.5 ml salbutamol is diluted with 9.5 ml sterile water and given slowly intravenously over 5 minutes while the maternal heart rate is carefully monitored for tachycardia.
2. The initial dose is followed by a side-infusion of 200 ml saline with 1000 µg salbutamol given at a rate of 30 ml per hour (150 µg per hour) until no further contractions occur, or when the maternal pulse rate reaches 120 beats per minute. If contractions persist, after 2 hours the dose is doubled to 60 ml per hour (300 µg per hour) until no further contractions occur, or when the maternal pulse rate reaches 120 beats per minute. The administration of the salbutamol infusion is continued until there are no further contractions, effacement, and/or dilatation of the cervix for at least 6 hours.
3. The patient must be warned that salbutamol causes tachycardia (palpitations).
4. Patients should be monitored with an ECG monitor while receiving intravenous salbutamol. This should ideally occur within a high-care unit.

If the contractions are still occurring, and there is progressive effacement and dilatation of the cervix in spite of an adequate rate of administration, alternative measures must be taken to suppress labour. Otherwise, administration of the drug should be stopped and preparation made for the delivery of a preterm infant.

5-28 What are the contraindications to the use of beta2 stimulants in suppressing labour?

1. Heart valve disease. The use of beta2 stimulants, such as salbutamol, can endanger the patient's life, especially if she has a narrowed heart valve, e.g. mitral stenosis.
2. A shocked patient.
3. A patient with tachycardia, e.g. as the result of an acute infection.

5-29 What additional action must you take to suppress labour?

Prostaglandin antagonists, e.g. indomethacin (Indocid), are prescribed. 1 indomethacin 100 mg rectal suppository is administered 12-hourly. 2 doses are usually sufficient. The total dose should not exceed 4 doses (i.e. it shouldn't be taken for more than 48 hours).

The following side effects make indomethacin potentially dangerous:

1. Gastrointestinal irritation.
2. Suppression of platelet function.
3. Fluid retention.
4. Premature closure of the ductus arteriosus in the fetus.
5. Renal failure in a patient with poor renal function.

Indomethacin is also a useful drug to use if there is a contraindication to giving a beta2 stimulant, e.g. maternal tachycardia due to pyrexia. The risk of fetal death due to closure of the ductus arteriosus by indomethacin is much greater after 31 weeks. Therefore, indomethacin should not be used from 32 weeks gestation.

Successful suppression of preterm labour with nifedipine (Adalat) or salbutamol together with indomethacin is more likely if antibiotics (ampicillin and metronidazole) are given in addition. Possible asymptomatic chorioamnionitis will then be treated as well.

5-30 How should you manage the patient further, after labour has been successfully suppressed?

1. If there is a treatable cause, e.g. a urinary tract infection, then no further suppression of labour is necessary after the cause has been treated.
2. If nothing can be done about the cause of the preterm labour, e.g. in the case of a multiple pregnancy or polyhydramnios, nifedipine (Adalat) 20 mg may be given orally every 6 hours.

5-31 What other action can be taken to improve the fetal outcome?

1. Steroids administered parenterally to the mother cross the placenta and hasten the onset of fetal lung maturity. Betamethasone (Celestone-Soluspan) 12 mg (2 ml) intramuscularly is the drug of choice.

2. 2 doses of 12 mg each are given 24 hours apart. Fetal lung maturity is usually, but not always, achieved 24 hours after the second dose. Suppression of labour for 48 hours in order to give betamethasone is, therefore, of value.
3. If the infant is not delivered and there is still a risk of preterm delivery, a single dose of 12 mg can be given after a week. The dose should not be repeated weekly until a gestational age of 33 weeks is reached.

NOTE
Fetuses that are exposed to repeated doses of steroids in pregnancy are born with a smaller head circumference and length. As the long-term neurological outcome is uncertain, the maximum dose described here should not be exceeded.

5-32 What are the dangers of using steroids to promote fetal lung maturity?

1. Steroids must not be given if a clinically detectable infection is the cause of the preterm labour, because they may make the infection worse.
2. Steroids cause fluid retention. Consequently, the amount of intravenous fluid which is used to administer the salbutamol must be restricted.
3. The patient must continually be observed for signs of fluid overload, the first sign of which is the presence of crepitations in the lungs as a result of pulmonary oedema.

5-33 If the delivery of a preterm infant cannot be prevented, what action should you take in order to make the delivery as safe as possible?

1. The mother must be transferred before delivery to a hospital where preterm infants can be managed.
2. Entonox (50% nitrous oxide and 50% oxygen) or an epidural anaesthetic are the preferred methods of providing analgesia.
3. The membranes should not be ruptured as they form a better cervical dilator than the small fetal head. If they rupture spontaneously, a sterile vaginal examination must be done to exclude an umbilical cord prolapse.
4. A spontaneous vertex delivery, with an episiotomy if necessary, is the best method of delivery. A well-controlled delivery of the fetal head

reduces the risk of intracranial haemorrhage. There is no evidence that the routine use of forceps has any advantage for the preterm infant.

5. Before the delivery, you must make sure that the equipment you need for the resuscitation and management of the preterm infant is available and in working order.

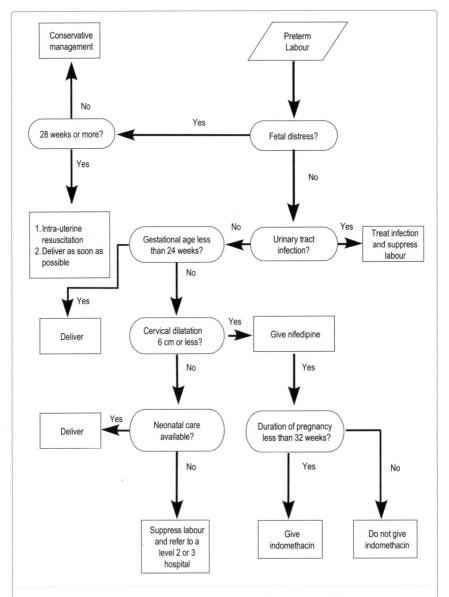

Figure 5-1: The management of a patient with preterm labour when the duration of pregnancy is less than 34 weeks

Management of preterm rupture of the membranes

5-34 How should you manage preterm rupture of the membranes?

There are two possible ways of managing preterm rupture of the membranes:

1. Labour can be induced.
2. The pregnancy can be allowed to continue.

The management of a patient with preterm rupture of the membranes is summarised in Figure 5-2.

5-35 How should you decide which method of management to use?

The danger of prematurity if the fetus is delivered must be weighed against the risk of infection in both the mother and the fetus if the pregnancy is allowed to continue.

5-36 What is the reason for allowing the pregnancy to continue with preterm rupture of the membranes?

To provide time for the fetal lungs to mature and, thereby, to reduce the danger of hyaline membrane disease after delivery.

Prematurity remains the commonest cause of neonatal death resulting from preterm rupture of the membranes.

5-37 Which patients with preterm rupture of the membranes are at an increased risk of chorioamnionitis?

Patients with preterm rupture of the membranes plus one or more of the following factors are at a particularly high risk of chorioamnionitis:

1. HIV-positive patients with immune suppression, either:
   - A CD4 count of less than 350 cells/mm³.
   - An AIDS-defining infection that indicates clinical immune suppression.
2. Rupture of the membranes during or following coitus.
3. A digital vaginal examination following rupture of the membranes.
4. No antenatal care.

5-38 What should you do once preterm rupture of the membranes has occurred?

1. Check whether the fetus is still alive, and exclude fetal distress by assessing fetal movements. Antenatal fetal heart rate monitoring is of great value.
2. Determine the duration of the pregnancy as accurately as possible. Remember, with preterm rupture of the membranes, both clinical and ultrasound examinations tend to underestimate the duration of pregnancy.
3. Look for signs of clinical chorioamnionitis.

If the history and clinical examination indicate a pregnancy of less than 34 weeks duration, an ultrasound examination is of value in determining fetal size and possible gross congenital abnormalities.

5-39 What are the indications for induction of labour when preterm rupture of the membranes has occurred?

1. An HIV-positive patient.
2. A duration of pregnancy of 34 weeks or more.
3. A duration of pregnancy less than 26 weeks.
4. Intra-uterine death or severe fetal congenital abnormalities.
5. Signs of clinical chorioamnionitis.
6. Maternal illness such as pre-eclampsia or diabetes mellitus.

7. Severe intra-uterine growth restriction.
8. Antepartum haemorrhage of unknown cause.

5-40 What method of induction should you use?

The method of choice is to stimulate uterine contractions with oxytocin. If there are contraindications to stimulating labour or to a vaginal delivery, then a Caesarean section is done.

5-41 What should the daily care of a patient include if pregnancy is allowed to continue?

1. The patient must be kept on bed rest, being allowed up to the toilet. She must not sit in a bath, but should use a shower.
2. Digital vaginal examinations must *not* be done.
3. The condition of the fetus must be monitored daily, preferably with a cardiotocograph. If this is not available, fetal movements must be counted and recorded.
4. Observations for signs of clinical chorioamnionitis must be done:
   - The maternal pulse rate and temperature and the fetal heart rate must be checked 4-hourly.
   - An abdominal examination is done twice a day to check for uterine tenderness.
   - At the same time it is noted whether or not the liquor is offensive.

The first digital vaginal examination in a patient with preterm rupture of the membranes is done only when she is in established labour.

5-42 How long should you allow the pregnancy to continue?

1. If complications, such as chorioamnionitis and fetal distress, do not develop, the pregnancy is allowed to continue until the patient goes into labour. However, if the pregnancy reaches 34 weeks duration and the patient is still draining liquor, an oxytocin induction is done.
2. A patient who has stopped draining liquor completely and where liquor is present on abdominal examination, with no signs of chorioamnionitis, may be allowed to continue her pregnancy until the spontaneous onset

of labour. The patient may be allowed home if no liquor has drained for two days. However, she is not allowed to sit in a bath or to have coitus. The patient must be followed up weekly at a high-risk clinic.

5-43 Which physical signs will be present if a patient develops severe infection (septic shock) and what will the initial management be?

1. The signs of clinical chorioamnionitis already mentioned will be present. In addition, there will be a drop in the blood pressure and cold clammy extremities, if severe infection (septic shock) develops.
2. The patient must be actively resuscitated and treated with ampicillin, metronidazole (Flagyl) and gentamicin. The patient must then be referred to a level 2 or 3 hospital.

5-44 What advice should you give to a woman who has delivered a preterm infant?

1. She should be seen before her next pregnancy to be assessed for possible causes, e.g. cervical incompetence.
2. She must book early in any future pregnancy.

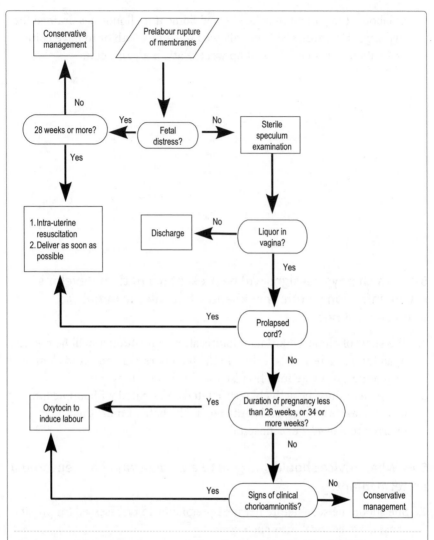

Figure 5-2: The management of a patient with preterm prelabour rupture of the membranes

Prelabour rupture of the membranes

5-45 How should you manage a patient with prelabour rupture of the membranes?

1. If a patient has prelabour ruptured membranes and there are signs of chorioamnionitis, then labour should be induced without delay.
2. HIV-positive patients should be started on a course of antibiotics and labour should be induced:
   - The longer the interval between rupture of the membranes and delivery, the greater the risk of mother-to-child transmission of HIV.
   - The patient has a higher risk of chorioamnionitis.
3. However, if the patient is at low risk of chorioamnionitis and both fetal and maternal conditions are good, you can wait for 24 hours after the membranes have ruptured before inducing labour. About 80% of patients will go into labour spontaneously within this period. A digital vaginal examination should not be done until the patient is in labour.

NOTE
In busy hospitals with a high bed occupancy rate, patients with prelabour rupture of the membranes can have their labour induced with oxytocin after the diagnosis is confirmed. Induction of labour in these circumstances does not result in a higher Caesarean section rate but reduces hospital stay by 24 hours.

Case study 1

A patient, 32 weeks pregnant, presents with regular painful uterine contractions. She is apyrexial and appears clinically well. On vaginal examination, the cervix is 4 cm dilated. The fetal heart rate is 138 beats per minute with no decelerations.

1. Is the patient in true or false labour? Give the reasons for your diagnosis.

She is in true labour because she is getting regular painful contractions and her cervix is 4 cm dilated.

2. What signs exclude a diagnosis of clinical chorioamnionitis?

The patient is apyrexial, clinically well and has a normal fetal heart rate.

3. Why could chorioamnionitis still be the cause of her preterm labour?

Because chorioamnionitis is often asymptomatic.

4. Would you allow labour to continue or would you suppress labour?

Labour should be suppressed because the pregnancy is of less than 34 weeks duration, the fetus is viable, and there are no signs of clinical chorioamnionitis or fetal distress.

5. How should labour be suppressed?

Labour must be suppressed using nifedipine (Adalat) or salbutamol (Ventolin).

6. Which other drugs would increase the chance of successful suppression of preterm labour?

Antibiotics, such as ampicillin and metronidazole (Flagyl), increase the likelihood of successful suppression of preterm labour if the labour is caused by asymptomatic chorioamnionitis.

7. Must indomethacin (Indocid) also be given?

No, as the patient is already 32 weeks pregnant. The risk of closing the ductus arteriosus and causing intra-uterine deaths increases from 32 weeks.

8. Which drugs can be used to hasten fetal lung maturity, and would you give one of these drugs to this patient?

Steroids, such as betamethasone, can be given to the patient to hasten lung maturity in the fetus. As this patient's pregnancy is less than 34 weeks and there are no signs of clinical chorioamnionitis, steroids must be given.

Case study 2

A patient, who is 36 weeks pregnant, reports that she has been draining liquor since earlier that day. The patient appears well, with normal observations, no uterine contractions and the fetal heart rate is normal.

1. Would you diagnose rupture of the membranes on the history given by the patient?

No, other causes of fluid draining from the vagina may cause confusion, e.g. a vaginitis or stress incontinence.

2. How would you confirm rupture of the membranes?

A sterile speculum examination should be done. If there is no clear evidence of liquor draining, the vaginal pH using litmus paper and microscopy for ferning can be used to identify liquor.

3. Why should you not perform a digital vaginal examination to assess whether the cervix is dilated or effaced?

A digital vaginal examination is contraindicated in the presence of rupture of the membranes if the patient is not already in labour, because of the risk of introducing infection.

4. Is this patient at high risk of having or developing chorioamnionitis?

Yes. The preterm prelabour rupture of the membranes may have been caused by chorioamnionitis. In addition, all patients with ruptured membranes are at an increased risk of developing chorioamnionitis.

5. Should you induce labour? Give your reasons.

Yes. As she is more than 34 weeks pregnant, one should induce labour. As the patient does not fall into a high-risk group for infection, a waiting period of 24 hours from the time of rupture can be allowed before inducing labour. Most patients will go into labour spontaneously during this period.

6. Should you prescribe antibiotics? Give your reasons.

There is no indication for giving antibiotics as there are no signs of clinical chorioamnionitis. However, a careful watch must be kept for early signs of maternal infection or fetal tachycardia.

Case study 3

An unbooked patient presents with a five-day history of ruptured membranes. She is pyrexial with lower abdominal tenderness and is draining offensive liquor. She is uncertain of her dates but abdominal examination suggests that she is at term. Treatment has been started with oral amoxicillin.

1. What signs of clinical chorioamnionitis does the patient have?

She is pyrexial, with lower abdominal tenderness and she has offensive liquor.

2. Would you induce labour in this patient? Give your reasons.

Yes, because there is danger of spreading infection in both the mother and fetus if the infant is not delivered. The patient is in grave danger of developing septic shock. Labour should be induced with oxytocin, if there is no indication for an immediate delivery, e.g. fetal distress. With signs of septic shock, the patient must be actively resuscitated and treated with broad-spectrum antibiotics, followed by delivery of the fetus. The earliest sign of septic shock will be a fall in the blood pressure, followed by the patient developing cold, clammy extremities.

3. Should you continue to treat the patient with oral amoxicillin? Give your reasons.

She should be treated with appropriate broad-spectrum antibiotics, given in adequate dosages until her pyrexia has subsided. As it is not clear how long the infection has been present, gentamicin must be added to the ampicillin and metronidazole (Flagyl) until the patient has been apyrexial for 24 hours.

The gentamicin and ampicillin must initially be given intravenously and the metronidazole as a rectal suppository.

4. Why is the infant at increased risk for neonatal complications?

The chorioamnionitis has already spread to the liquor as this is offensive. Therefore, the fetus may also be infected and may present with congenital pneumonia or septicaemia at birth.

6

Monitoring the condition of the mother during the first stage of labour

Take the chapter test before and after you read this chapter.

Objectives

When you have completed this unit you should be able to:

- Monitor the condition of the mother during the first stage of labour.
- Record the clinical observations on the partogram.
- Explain the clinical significance of the observations.
- Manage any abnormalities which are detected.

Monitoring labour

6-1 What is labour?

Labour is the process whereby the fetus and the placenta are delivered. The uterine contractions cause the cervix to dilate and eventually push the fetus and placenta through and out of the vagina.

6-2 What are the stages of labour?

Labour is divided into three stages:

1. The first stage of labour.

2. The second stage of labour.
3. The third stage of labour.

Each stage of labour is important as it must be correctly diagnosed and managed. There are dangers to the mother in each of the three stages of labour.

Labour is divided into three stages.

6-3 What is the first stage of labour?

The first stage of labour starts with the onset of regular uterine contractions and ends when the cervix is fully dilated.

6-4 What must be monitored in the first stage of labour?

1. The condition of the mother.
2. The condition of the fetus.
3. The progress of labour.

6-5 What four questions should be asked about each of these observations?

1. How often must the observations be done?
2. How are the findings recorded?
3. What is the clinical significance of the findings?
4. What should be done if an observation is abnormal?

6-6 What is the partogram?

The partogram is a chart which shows the progress of labour over time. It also displays observations reflecting the maternal and fetal condition. The observations of every patient in the first stage of labour must be charted on a partogram.

All the observations of every patient in the first stage of labour must be recorded on a partogram.

6-7 What maternal observations are recorded on the partogram?

Notes on the general condition of the patient, as well as observations of the temperature, pulse rate, blood pressure, urine volume and chemistry are recorded on the partogram.

6-8 How should each observation be assessed?

At the completion of any set of observations, you must ask yourself the following questions:

1. *Is everything normal?* If the answer is *no*, then you must ask:
   ◦ *What* is not normal and *why* is it not normal?
2. Finally you must ask the question: *What must I do about the problem?*

6-9 How is the condition of the patient monitored?

By regular observations of the following:

1. The general condition of the patient.
2. Temperature.
3. Pulse rate.
4. Blood pressure.
5. Urine output and urinalysis for protein and ketones.

Assessing the general condition of the patient

6-10 Why is it important to observe the general condition of the patient during the first stage of labour?

If the general condition of the patient is not normal, there will usually be further abnormal findings when the other observations are made.

6-11 When can the general condition of the patient be regarded as normal?

A patient in the first stage of labour will normally appear calm and relaxed between contractions and does not look pale. During contractions, her respiratory rate will increase and she will experience pain. However, she should not have pain between contractions. When a patient's cervix is fully dilated, or almost fully dilated, she becomes restless, may vomit, and has an uncontrollable urge to bear down with contractions.

6-12 How often should the general condition of the patient be observed?

The general condition of the patient should be observed continuously, but noted specially when other observations are made.

6-13 When is the general condition of the patient abnormal?

When any of the following are present:

1. Excessive anxiety.
2. Severe, continuous pain.
3. Severe exhaustion.
4. Dehydration.
5. Marked pallor of the face and mucous membranes.

6-14 What causes severe anxiety?

Anxiety is usually seen in primigravidas who:

1. Are not prepared for the process of labour and the labour ward.
2. Are not accompanied by a friend or family member in the labour ward.
3. Cannot communicate due to language differences.

6-15 What should you do if the patient is very anxious and is experiencing very painful contractions?

1. The patient must be comforted and reassured. If possible, someone she knows should stay with her.
2. The patient must be offered appropriate pain relief.

6-16 What causes severe, continuous pain in the first stage of labour?

Severe, continuous pain always indicates that a complication is present, such as:

1. Abruptio placentae.
2. Rupture of the uterus.
3. An infection, such as acute pyelonephritis and chorioamnionitis.

6-17 When may severe exhaustion or dehydration occur?

With a prolonged labour, e.g. with cephalopelvic disproportion.

6-18 What may cause a pale face and mucous membranes?

This is usually due to either of the following:

1. Chronic anaemia, e.g. iron deficiency, malaria, etc.
2. Blood loss, e.g. placenta praevia, abruptio placentae or rupture of the uterus.

6-19 Where must abnormalities in the patient's general condition be recorded?

If the general condition of the patient becomes abnormal, this must be noted in the appropriate space at the bottom of the partogram as shown in figure 6-1.

Assessing the temperature

6-20 What is a normal temperature?

The normal range of oral temperature is 36.0 to 37.0 °C. Therefore, a temperature higher than 37.0 °C is abnormal and is regarded as pyrexia.

6-21 How often should you monitor the temperature?

4-hourly, unless there is a particular reason to do so more frequently.

6-22 How is the temperature recorded?

The temperature is recorded in the appropriate space on the partogram as shown in figure 6-1.

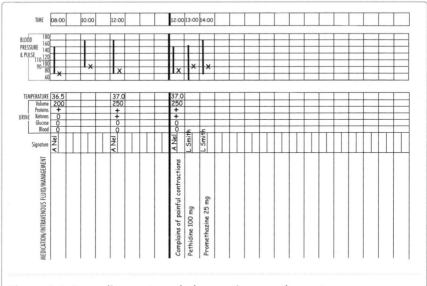

Figure 6-1: Recording maternal observations on the partogram

6-23 What are the causes of pyrexia during labour?

There are two main causes of a high maternal temperature:

1. Infection: This will most probably be in the urogenital tract, e.g. acute pyelonephritis or chorioamnionitis. However, it must be remembered that any other infection may be present during labour.
2. Maternal exhaustion: Dehydration causes pyrexia.

6-24 How should you manage a patient with pyrexia?

1. The cause of the high temperature must be found and treated. It is particularly important to look for acute pyelonephritis, chorioamnionitis, and evidence of maternal exhaustion. A high temperature may also be due to an infection unrelated to the pregnancy, e.g. pneumonia, viral infections, malaria, etc.
2. The temperature may be brought down with paracetamol (e.g. Panado).

6-25 What are the dangers of pyrexia?

1. To the mother: The temperature on its own does not constitute a risk. However, if the pyrexia is caused by an infection, the infection may be dangerous to the mother. Fever may cause a patient to go into labour.
2. To the fetus: A high temperature can cause fetal tachycardia. Preterm delivery with complications of immaturity in the newborn infant may also result. If the pyrexia is due to chorioamnionitis, the fetus is at high risk of becoming infected and may present with pneumonia or septicaemia.

Assessing the pulse rate

6-26 What is the normal maternal pulse rate?

The normal range of the maternal pulse rate is 80 to 100 beats per minute.

6-27 How often should you monitor the pulse rate?

The pulse rate is monitored 2-hourly during the latent phase of labour, and hourly during the active phase of the first stage of labour.

6-28 How is the pulse rate recorded?

The pulse rate is recorded in the appropriate space on the partogram as shown in figure 6-1.

6-29 What are the causes of a rapid pulse rate?

The commonest causes of a rapid pulse rate (tachycardia) are:

1. Anxiety.
2. Pain.
3. Pyrexia.
4. Exhaustion.
5. Shock.

6-30 What action should be taken if the patient has tachycardia?

The cause of the tachycardia should be determined and treated.

Assessing the blood pressure

6-31 What is a normal blood pressure?

The normal range of blood pressure during the first stage of labour is 100/60 mm Hg or above, but less than 140/90 mm Hg.

6-32 How often should you monitor the blood pressure?

Blood pressure should be monitored 2-hourly during the latent phase of labour, and hourly during the active phase of labour.

6-33 How is the blood pressure recorded?

The blood pressure is recorded in the appropriate space on the partogram as shown in figure 6-1.

6-34 What are the causes of hypertension (high blood pressure)?

1. Anxiety.
2. Pain.
3. Any one of the hypertensive disorders of pregnancy.

6-35 What are the causes of hypotension (low blood pressure)?

1. Some patients may normally have a low blood pressure. Therefore, the blood pressure during labour must be compared with that recorded during the antenatal visits.
2. Pressure of the uterus on the inferior vena cava when the patient lies on her back may decrease the venous return to the heart and, thereby, cause the blood pressure to fall. This is called supine hypotension.
3. Shock. This is usually due to blood loss.

6-36 What are the risks of hypotension?

1. To the mother: If hypotension is due to shock, the mother may suffer kidney damage. Severe and uncorrected hypotension may result in maternal death.
2. To the fetus: A fall in blood pressure results in decreased blood flow to the placenta, reducing the supply of oxygen to the fetus. This may cause fetal distress.

6-37 What should you do for a patient with hypotension?

1. Establish the cause of the hypotension.
2. If the hypotension is due to the patient lying on her back, she should be turned onto her side. The blood pressure usually returns to normal within 1 or 2 minutes. The fetal heart rate should then be checked again.
3. If the hypotension is due to haemorrhage, the patient must be resuscitated urgently and be managed according to the cause of the bleeding.

6-38 How do you recognise shock?

Shock presents with one or more of the following features:

1. Tachycardia.
2. Hypotension.
3. Cold, sweaty skin.

6-39 What are the common causes of shock in the first stage of labour?

1. Shock during the first stage of labour is almost always due to haemorrhage, for example:
   - Abruptio placentae.
   - Placenta praevia.
   - A ruptured uterus.

2. Infection as a cause of shock must always be considered.

Assessing the urine

6-40 What urine tests should be done during labour?

1. Volume.
2. Protein.
3. Ketones.

The presence and degree of proteinuria and ketonuria is measured and graded with a reagent strip, such as Dipstix.

6-41 How often should you test the urine?

1. Every 4 hours during the latent phase of labour.
2. Every 2 hours during the active phase of labour.
3. Each time the patient passes urine, if more frequently than above.

6-42 How are the urinary observations recorded?

The observations are recorded on the partogram:

1. Volume in ml.
2. Protein and ketones are recorded as 0 if absent and 1+ to 4+ if present.

The urinary observations should be recorded on the partogram as shown in figure 6-1.

6-43 What volume of urine passed indicates oliguria (decreased urine output)?

An amount of less than 20 ml per hour.

6-44 What are the causes of oliguria?

1. Dehydration.
2. Severe pre-eclampsia.
3. Shock.

Patients suffering from any of these conditions must have their urinary output accurately monitored. An indwelling urinary catheter must, therefore, be passed.

NOTE
The antidiuretic effect of oxytocin may also cause oliguria.

The cause of the oliguria must be diagnosed and treated.

6-45 How can normal hydration during labour be ensured?

1. If a vaginal delivery is expected, the patient should be encouraged to eat and drink during the latent phase of the first stage of labour.
2. If a Caesarean section is expected, the patient must be kept nil per mouth while in labour in preparation for surgery.
3. Low-risk patients must continue taking fluids, while patients with risk factors should be kept nil per mouth, during the active phase of the first stage of labour. Intravenous fluids must be given to patients with risk factors as well as to patients with long labours.

Always ensure that a patient in labour has an adequate fluid intake. Fluids should be given intravenously if necessary.

6-46 What is the significance of proteinuria?

Proteinuria of more than a trace is never normal. It is an important sign of:

1. Pre-eclampsia.
2. Urinary tract infection.
3. Renal disease.

When there is proteinuria, the urine must always be examined for evidence of infection. However, infection alone will not cause more than 1+ proteinuria. Proteinuria of 2+ or more should always be regarded as indicating pre-eclampsia or chronic renal disease.

6-47 What is the management of a patient with proteinuria?

The cause of the proteinuria must be determined, and the appropriate management given.

6-48 What is the clinical significance of ketonuria?

Ketonuria is common in labour and may be normal. However, if a woman has ketonuria, it is important to look for signs of maternal exhaustion.

Maternal exhaustion

Maternal exhaustion is a term used to describe a clinical condition consisting of dehydration and exhaustion during prolonged labour. It should not be confused with pain, anxiety or shock.

6-49 How do you recognise maternal exhaustion?

The following physical signs may be present:

1. Tachycardia.
2. Pyrexia.
3. A dry mouth.
4. Oliguria.
5. Ketonuria.

6-50 What causes maternal exhaustion?

A long labour with an insufficient supply of fluid and energy to the patient.

6-51 What are the effects of maternal exhaustion?

1. On the mother: Inadequate progress of labour due to poor uterine action in the first stage, and poor maternal effort in bearing down during the second stage of labour.
2. On the fetus: Fetal distress due to hypoxia. This often results from incorrectly managed cephalopelvic disproportion.

6-52 How can you prevent maternal exhaustion?

1. Make sure that the patient gets an adequate intake of fluid and energy during labour. It may be necessary to give fluid intravenously. Ringer's lactate with 5% dextrose will also ensure an adequate energy supply to the patient.
2. Ensure that the patient gets adequate analgesia during labour.
3. Ensure that labour does not become prolonged.

6-53 How do you treat a patient with maternal exhaustion?

If a patient has signs of maternal exhaustion then she should receive:

1. An intravenous infusion, giving 2 litres of Ringer's lactate with 5% dextrose. The first litre must be given quickly and the second litre given over 2 hours. It is contra-indicated to give a patient in labour 50 ml of 50% dextrose intravenously as this may be harmful to the fetus.
2. Adequate analgesia.

> Maternal exhaustion may result in poor progress of labour, while poor progress of labour may result in maternal exhaustion.

6-54 Is it necessary for every patient to receive intravenous fluid during labour?

No. Low-risk patients who are progressing well in labour do not need intravenous fluid, even if 1+ or 2+ ketonuria is present. If there are no contraindications, patients should be encouraged to take oral fluids during labour.

Case study 1

A patient is admitted at 32 weeks gestation. She complains of lower abdominal pain and fever. On general examination her temperature is 38 °C.

1. Does this patient have a normal temperature?

No. She is pyrexial as her temperature is higher than 37 °C.

2. Where should her temperature be recorded?

In the appropriate space on the partogram.

3. What are the most likely causes of her pyrexia?

An acute pyelonephritis or chorioamnionitis as she has pyrexia with lower abdominal pain.

4. How should you manage this patient's pyrexia?

Diagnose and treat the cause of the high temperature. The temperature should be brought down with paracetamol.

5. What are the dangers of maternal pyrexia to the fetus?

Pyrexia may cause preterm labour, resulting in the delivery of a preterm infant with all the complications of immaturity. If the pyrexia is due to chorioamnionitis a preterm infant will be born with a high risk of congenital pneumonia.

Case study 2

A patient is admitted to hospital with a history of labour for 24 hours. On admission she appears anxious, has a dry mouth and a pulse rate of 120 beats per minute. She is able to pass only 30 ml of urine which is dark in colour. She has not passed any urine for the previous few hours.

1. What is the probable diagnosis?

Maternal exhaustion due to a long labour with an inadequate fluid and energy intake. The diagnosis is confirmed by the presence of maternal tachycardia and a dry mouth.

2. What other findings would help confirm this diagnosis?

Pyrexia and ketonuria.

3. Does this patient have oliguria?

Yes, as she obviously has passed less than 20 ml per hour during the past number of hours.

4. Is ketonuria always abnormal?

No, ketonuria on its own may be normal.

5. How could maternal exhaustion be avoided?

By making sure that every patient receives an adequate intake of fluid and energy during labour. If a vaginal delivery is expected and no high-risk factors are present, a patient should continue to take fluids orally during the active phase of the first stage of labour. Any patient with prolonged labour should receive fluids intravenously.

6. How should the patient's exhaustion be treated?

She should be given 2 litres of Ringer's lactate with 5% dextrose intravenously. The first litre must be given quickly and the second litre over 2 hours. In addition, adequate analgesia should be given if needed.

7

Monitoring the condition of the fetus during the first stage of labour

Take the chapter test before and after you read this chapter.

Objectives

When you have completed this unit you should be able to:

- Monitor the condition of the fetus during labour.
- Record the findings on the partogram.
- Understand the significance of the findings.
- Understand the causes and signs of fetal distress.
- Interpret the significance of different fetal heart rate patterns and meconium-stained liquor.
- Manage any abnormalities which are detected.

Monitoring the fetus

7-1 Why should you monitor the fetus during labour?

It is essential to monitor the fetus during labour in order to assess how it responds to the stresses of labour. The stress of a normal labour usually has no effect on a healthy fetus.

7-2 What may stress the fetus during labour?

1. Compression of the fetal head during contractions.
2. A decrease in the supply of oxygen to the fetus.

7-3 How does head compression stress the fetus?

During uterine contractions compression of the fetal skull causes vagal stimulation which slows the fetal heart rate. Head compression usually does not harm the fetus. However, with a long labour due to cephalopelvic disproportion, the fetal head may be severely compressed. This may result in fetal distress.

7-4 What may reduce the supply of oxygen to the fetus?

1. Uterine contractions: Uterine contractions are the commonest cause of a decrease in the oxygen supply to the fetus during labour.
2. Reduced blood flow through the placenta: The placenta may fail to provide the fetus with enough oxygen and nutrition due to a decrease in the blood flow through the placenta, i.e. placental insufficiency. Patients with pre-eclampsia have poorly formed spiral arteries that provide maternal blood to the placenta. This can also be caused by narrowing of the uterine blood vessels due to maternal smoking.
3. Abruptio placentae: Part or all of the placenta stops functioning because it is separated from the uterine wall by a retroplacental haemorrhage. As a result, the fetus does not receive enough oxygen.
4. Cord prolapse or compression: This stops the transport of oxygen from the placenta to the fetus.

Uterine contractions are the commonest cause of a decreased oxygen supply to the fetus during labour.

7-5 How do contractions reduce the supply of oxygen to the fetus?

Uterine contractions may:

1. Reduce the maternal blood flow to the placenta due to the increase in intra-uterine pressure.
2. Compress the umbilical cord.

7-6 When do uterine contractions reduce the supply of oxygen to the fetus?

Usually uterine contractions do not reduce the supply of oxygen to the fetus, as there is an adequate store of oxygen in the placental blood to meet the fetal needs during the contraction. Normal contractions in labour do not affect the healthy fetus with a normally functioning placenta, and, therefore, are not dangerous.

However, contractions may reduce the oxygen supply to the fetus when:

1. There is placental insufficiency.
2. The contractions are prolonged or very frequent.
3. There is compression of the umbilical cord.

7-7 How does the fetus respond to a lack of oxygen?

A reduction in the normal supply of oxygen to the fetus causes fetal hypoxia. This is a lack of oxygen in the cells of the fetus. If the hypoxia is mild the fetus will be able to compensate and, therefore, show no response. However, severe fetal hypoxia will result in fetal distress. Severe, prolonged hypoxia will eventually result in fetal death.

7-8 How is fetal distress recognised during labour?

Fetal distress caused by a lack of oxygen results in a decrease in the fetal heart rate.

NOTE
The fetus responds to hypoxia with a bradycardia to conserve oxygen. In addition, blood is shunted away from less important organs, such as the gut and kidney, to essential organs, such as the brain and the heart. This may cause ischaemic damage to the gut and kidneys, and intraventricular haemorrhage in the brain. Severe hypoxia will eventually cause a decreased cardiac output leading to myocardial and cerebral ischaemia. Hypoxia also results in anaerobic metabolism which causes fetal acidosis (a low blood pH).

7-9 How do you assess the condition of the fetus during labour?

Two observations are used:

1. The fetal heart rate pattern.
2. The presence or absence of meconium in the liquor.

Fetal heart rate patterns

7-10 What devices can be used to monitor the fetal heart rate?

Any one of the following three pieces of equipment:

1. A fetal stethoscope.
2. A 'doptone' (Doppler ultrasound fetal heart rate monitor).
3. A cardiotocograph (CTG machine).

In most low-risk labours the fetal heart rate can be determined adequately using a fetal stethoscope. However, a doptone is helpful if there is difficulty hearing the fetal heart, especially if intra-uterine death is suspected. If available, a doptone is the preferred method in primary-care clinics and hospitals. Cardiotocograph is not needed in most labours but is an important and accurate method of monitoring the fetal heart in high-risk pregnancies.

> A doptone is the preferred method in primary-care clinics and hospitals.

7-11 How should you monitor the fetal heart rate?

Because uterine contractions may decrease the maternal blood flow to the placenta, and thereby cause a reduced supply of oxygen to the fetus, it is essential that the fetal heart rate should be monitored during a contraction. In practice, this means that the fetal heart pattern must be checked before, during and after the contraction. A comment on the fetal heart rate, without knowing what happens *during* and *after* a contraction, is almost valueless.

> The fetal heart rate must be assessed before, during, and after a contraction.

7-12 How often should you monitor the fetal heart rate?

1. For low-risk patients who have had normal observations on admission:
   - 2-hourly during the latent phase of labour.
   - Half-hourly during the active phase of labour.

   Patients with a high risk of fetal distress should have their observations done more frequently.

2. Intermediate-risk patients, high-risk patients, patients with abnormal observations on admission, and patients with meconium-stained liquor need more frequent recording of the fetal heart rate:
   - Hourly during the latent phase of labour.
   - Half-hourly during the active phase of labour.
   - At least every 15 minutes if fetal distress is suspected.

7-13 What features of the fetal heart rate pattern should you always assess during labour?

There are two features that should always be assessed:

1. *The baseline fetal heart rate*: This is the heart rate between contractions.
2. *The presence or absence of decelerations*: If present, the relation of the deceleration to the contraction must be determined:
   - Decelerations that occur only *during* a contraction (i.e. early decelerations).
   - Decelerations that occur *during and after* a contraction (i.e. late decelerations).
   - Decelerations that have *no fixed relation* to contractions (i.e. variable decelerations).

NOTE
In addition, the variability of the fetal heart rate can also be evaluated if a cardiotocograph is available. Good variability gives a spiky trace while poor variability gives a flat trace.

7-14 What fetal heart rate patterns can be recognised with a fetal stethoscope?

1. Normal.
2. Early deceleration.
3. Late deceleration.

4. Variable deceleration.
5. Baseline tachycardia.
6. Baseline bradycardia.

These fetal heart rate patterns (with the exception of variable decelerations) can be easily recognised with a stethoscope or doptone. However, cardiotocograph recordings (figures 7-1, 7-2 and 7-3) are useful in learning to recognise the differences between the three types of deceleration.

It is common to get a combination of patterns, e.g. a baseline bradycardia with late decelerations. It is also common to get one pattern changing to another pattern with time, e.g. early decelerations becoming late decelerations.

NOTE
    Variability is assessed with a CTG. The variation in the fetal heart normally exceeds 5 beats or more per minute, giving the baseline a spiky appearance on a CTG trace. A loss or reduction in variability to below 5 beats per minute gives a flat baseline (a flat trace), which suggest fetal distress. However, a flat baseline may also occur if the fetus is asleep or as a result of the administration of analgesics (pethidine, morphine) or sedatives (phenobarbitone).

7-15 What is a normal fetal heart rate pattern?

1. No decelerations during or after contractions.
2. A baseline rate of 100–160 beats per minute.

7-16 What are early decelerations?

Early decelerations are characterised by a slowing of the fetal heart rate starting at the beginning of the contraction, and returning to normal by the end of the contraction. Early decelerations are usually due to compression of the fetal head with a resultant increase in vagal stimulation, which causes the heart rate to slow during the contraction.

7-17 What is the significance of early decelerations?

Early decelerations do not indicate the presence of fetal distress. However, these fetuses must be carefully monitored as they are at an increased risk of fetal distress.

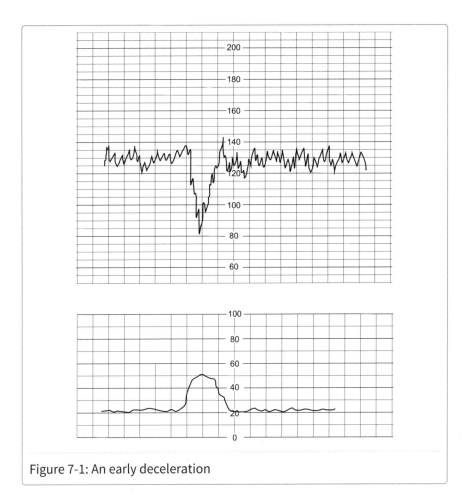

Figure 7-1: An early deceleration

NOTE
When early decelerations occur, normal variability of the fetal heart rate is reassuring that the fetus is not hypoxic.

7-18 What are late decelerations?

A late deceleration is a slowing of the fetal heart rate during a contraction, with the rate only returning to the baseline 30 seconds or more after the contraction has ended.

> **With a late deceleration the fetal heart rate only returns to the baseline 30 seconds or more after the contraction has ended.**

NOTE

When using a cardiotocograph, a late deceleration is diagnosed when the lowest point of the deceleration occurs 30 seconds or more after the peak of the contraction.

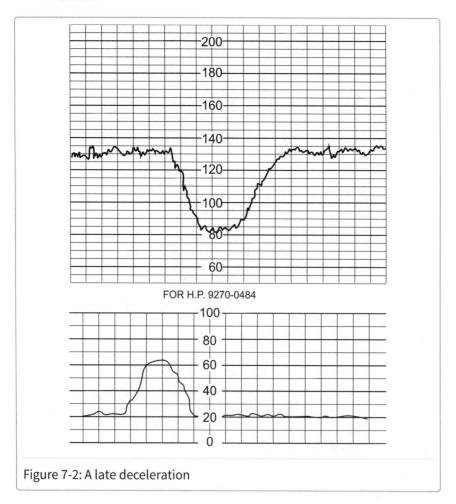

FOR H.P. 9270-0484

Figure 7-2: A late deceleration

7-19 What is the significance of late decelerations?

Late decelerations are a sign of fetal distress and are caused by fetal hypoxia. The degree to which the heart rate slows is not important. It is the timing of the deceleration that is important.

> **Late decelerations indicate fetal distress.**

7-20 What are variable decelerations?

Variable decelerations have no fixed relationship to uterine contractions. Therefore, the pattern of decelerations changes from 1 contraction to another. Variable decelerations are usually caused by compression of the umbilical cord and do not indicate the presence of fetal distress. However, these fetuses must be carefully monitored as they are at an increased risk of fetal distress.

Variable decelerations are not easy to recognise with a fetal stethoscope or doptone. They are best detected with a cardiotocograph.

NOTE
Variable decelerations accompanied by loss of variability may indicate fetal distress. Variable decelerations with good variability is reassuring.

7-21 What is a baseline tachycardia?

A baseline fetal heart rate of more than 160 beats per minute.

7-22 What are the causes of a baseline tachycardia?

1. Maternal pyrexia.
2. Maternal exhaustion.
3. Salbutamol (Ventolin) administration.
4. Chorioamnionitis (infection of the placenta and membranes).
5. Fetal haemorrhage or anaemia.

7-23 What is a baseline bradycardia?

A baseline fetal heart rate of less than 100 beats per minute.

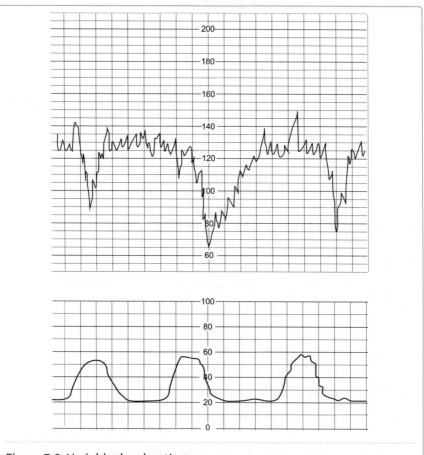

Figure 7-3: Variable decelerations

7-24 What is the cause of a baseline bradycardia?

A baseline bradycardia of less than 100 beats per minute usually indicates fetal distress which is caused by severe fetal hypoxia. If decelerations are also present, a baseline bradycardia indicates that the fetus is at great risk of dying.

7-25 How should you assess the condition of the fetus on the basis of the fetal heart rate pattern?

1. The fetal condition is *normal* if a normal fetal heart rate pattern is present.
2. The fetal condition is *uncertain* if the fetal heart rate pattern indicates that there is an increased risk of fetal distress.
3. The fetal condition is *abnormal* if the fetal heart rate pattern indicates fetal distress.

7-26 What is a normal fetal heart rate pattern during labour?

A normal baseline fetal heart rate without any decelerations.

7-27 Which fetal heart rate patterns indicate an increased risk of fetal distress during labour?

1. Early decelerations.
2. Variable decelerations.
3. A baseline tachycardia.

These fetal heart rate patterns do not indicate fetal distress but warn that the patient must be closely observed as fetal distress may develop.

NOTE
If electronic monitoring is available, the fetal heart rate pattern must be monitored electronically.

7-28 What fetal heart rate patterns indicate fetal distress during labour?

1. Late decelerations.
2. A baseline bradycardia.

NOTE
On cardiotocography, loss of variability of beat-to-beat variation lasting more than 60 minutes also suggests fetal distress.

7-29 How should the fetal heart rate pattern be observed during labour?

The fetal heart rate must be observed before, during and after a contraction. The following questions must be answered and recorded on the partogram:

1. What is the baseline fetal heart rate?
2. Are there any decelerations?
3. If decelerations are observed, what is their relation to the uterine contractions?
4. If the fetal heart rate pattern is abnormal, how must the patient be managed?

7-30 Which fetal heart rate pattern indicates that the fetal condition is good?

1. The baseline fetal heart rate is normal.
2. There are *no* decelerations.

7-31 What must be done if decelerations are observed?

First the relation of the decelerations to the uterine contractions must be observed to determine the type of deceleration. Then manage the patient as follows:

1. If the decelerations are early or variable, the fetal heart rate pattern warns that there is an increased risk of fetal distress and, therefore, the fetal heart rate must be checked every 15 minutes.
2. If late decelerations are present, the management will be the same as that for fetal bradycardia.

The observations of the fetal heart rate must be recorded on the partogram as shown in figure 7-4. A note of the management decided upon must also be made under the heading 'Management' at the bottom of the partogram.

7-32 What must be done if a fetal bradycardia is observed?

Fetal distress due to severe hypoxia is present. Therefore, you should immediately do the following:

1. Exclude other possible causes of bradycardia by turning the patient onto her side to correct supine hypotension, and stopping the oxytocin infusion to prevent uterine overstimulation.
2. If the fetal bradycardia persists, intra-uterine resuscitation of the fetus must be continued and the fetus delivered as quickly as possible.

7-33 How is intra-uterine resuscitation of the fetus given?

1. Turn the patient onto her side.
2. Give her 40% oxygen through a face mask.
3. Start an intravenous infusion of Ringer's lactate and give 250 µg (0.5 ml) salbutamol (Ventolin) slowly intravenously, after ensuring that there is no contraindication to its use. (Contraindications to salbutamol are heart valve disease, a shocked patient or patient with tachycardia). The 0.5 ml salbutamol is diluted with 9.5 ml sterile water and given slowly intravenously over 5 minutes.
4. Deliver the infant by the quickest possible route. If the patient's cervix is 9 cm or more dilated and the head is on the pelvic floor, proceed with an assisted delivery (forceps or vacuum). Otherwise, perform a Caesarean section.
5. If the patient cannot be delivered immediately (i.e. there is another patient in theatre) the dose of salbutamol can be repeated if contractions start again, but not within 30 minutes of the first dose or if the maternal pulse is 120 or more beats per minute.

It is important that you know how to give fetal resuscitation, as it is a lifesaving procedure when fetal distress is present, both during the antepartum period and in labour.

Always prepare to resuscitate the infant after birth if fetal distress is diagnosed during labour.

NOTE
Salbutamol (a beta2 stimulant) can also be given from an inhaler, but this method is less effective than the parenteral administration. Give four puffs from a salbutamol inhaler. This can be repeated every 10 minutes until the uterine

contractions are reduced in frequency and duration, or the maternal pulse reaches 120 beats per minute. Uterine contractions can also be suppressed with nifedipine (Adalat). Nifedipine 30 mg is given by mouth (1 capsule = 10 mg). The three capsules must be swallowed and not used sublingually. This method is slower than using intravenous salbutamol and the uterine contractions will only be reduced after 20 minutes.

The liquor

7-34 Is the liquor commonly meconium stained?

Yes, in 10–20% of patients, the liquor is yellow or green due to meconium staining. The incidence of meconium-stained liquor is increased in the group of patients that go into labour after 42 weeks gestation.

7-35 Is it important to distinguish between thick and thin, or yellow and green meconium?

Although fetal and neonatal complications are more common with thick meconium, all cases of meconium-stained liquor should be managed the same during the first stage of labour. The presence of meconium is important and the management does not depend on the consistency of the meconium.

7-36 What is the importance of meconium in the liquor?

1. Meconium-stained liquor usually indicates the presence of fetal hypoxia or an episode of fetal hypoxia in the past. Therefore, fetal distress may be present. If not, the fetus is at high risk of distress.
2. There is a danger of meconium aspiration at delivery.

> Meconium-stained liquor warns that either fetal distress is present or that there is a high risk of fetal distress.

7-37 How should you monitor the fetus during the first stage of labour if the liquor is meconium stained?

1. Listen carefully for late decelerations. If present, then fetal distress must be diagnosed.
2. If late decelerations are absent, then observe the fetus carefully during labour for fetal distress, as about a third of fetuses with meconium-stained liquor will develop fetal distress.
3. If electronic monitoring is available, the fetal heart rate pattern must be monitored.

7-38 How must the delivery be managed if there is meconium in the liquor?

1. The infant's mouth and pharynx must be thoroughly suctioned after delivery of the head, but before the shoulders and chest are delivered, i.e. before the infant breathes. This must be done irrespective of whether a vaginal delivery or Caesarean section is done.
2. Anticipate that the infant may need to be resuscitated at delivery. If the infant has asphyxia and needs intubation, suction the airways via the endotracheal tube before starting ventilation.

7-39 How and when are the liquor findings recorded?

Three symbols are used to record the liquor findings on the partogram:

I = Intact membranes (i.e. no liquor draining).

C = Clear liquor draining.

M = Meconium-stained liquor draining.

The findings are recorded in the appropriate space on the partogram as shown in figure 7-4.

The liquor findings should be recorded when:

1. The membranes rupture.
2. A vaginal examination is done.
3. A change in the liquor findings is noticed, e.g. if the liquor becomes meconium stained.

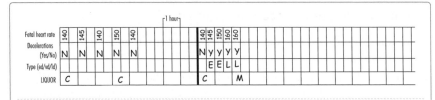

Figure 7-4: Recording fetal observations on the partogram

Case study 1

A primigravida with inadequate uterine contractions during labour is being treated with an oxytocin infusion. She now has frequent contractions, each lasting more than 40 seconds. With the patient in the lateral position, listening to the fetal heart rate reveals late decelerations.

1. What worries you most about this patient?

The late decelerations indicate that fetal distress is present.

2. Should the fetus be delivered immediately?

No. Correctable causes of poor oxygenation of the fetus must first be ruled out, e.g. postural hypotension and overstimulation of the uterus with oxytocin. The oxytocin infusion must be stopped and oxygen administered to the patient. Then the fetal heart rate should be checked again.

3. After stopping the oxytocin, the uterine contractions are less frequent. No further decelerations of the fetal heart rate are observed. What further management does this patient need?

As overstimulation of the uterus with oxytocin was the most likely cause of the late decelerations, labour may be allowed to continue. However, very careful observation of the fetal heart rate pattern is essential, especially if oxytocin is to be restarted. The fetal heart should be listened to every 15 minutes or fetal heart rate monitoring with a cardiotocograph should be started.

Case study 2

A patient who is 38 weeks pregnant presents with an antepartum haemorrhage in labour. On examination, her temperature is 36.8 ℃, her pulse rate 116 beats per minute, her blood pressure 120/80 mm Hg, and there is tenderness over the uterus. The baseline fetal heart rate is 166 beats per minute. The fetal heart rate drops to 130 beats per minute during contractions and then returns to the baseline 35 seconds after the contraction has ended.

1. Which of the maternal observations are abnormal and what is the probable cause of these abnormal findings?

A maternal tachycardia is present and there is uterine tenderness. These findings suggest an abruptio placentae.

2. Which fetal observations are abnormal?

Both the baseline tachycardia and the late decelerations.

3. How can you be certain that these are late decelerations?

Because the deceleration continues for more than 30 seconds after the end of the contraction. This observation indicates fetal distress. The number of beats by which the fetal heart slows during a deceleration is not important.

4. Why should an abruptio placentae cause fetal distress?

Part of the placenta has been separated from the wall of the uterus by a retroplacental clot. As a result, the fetus has become hypoxic.

Case study 3

During the first stage of labour a patient's liquor is noticed to have become stained with thin green meconium. The fetal heart rate pattern is normal and labour is progressing well.

1. What is the importance of the change in the colour of the liquor?

Meconium in the liquor indicates an episode of fetal hypoxia and suggests that there may be fetal distress or that the fetus is at high risk of fetal distress.

2. Can thin meconium be a sign of fetal distress?

Yes. All meconium in the liquor indicates either fetal distress or that the fetus is at high risk of fetal distress. The management does not depend on whether the meconium is thick or thin.

3. How would you decide whether this fetus is distressed?

By listening to the fetal heart rate. Late decelerations or a baseline bradycardia will indicate fetal distress.

4. How should the fetus be monitored during the remainder of the labour?

The fetal heart rate pattern must be determined carefully every 15 minutes in order to diagnose fetal distress should this occur.

5. What preparations should be made for the infant at delivery?

The infant's mouth and pharynx must be well suctioned immediately after the head has been delivered. If the infant does not breathe well directly after delivery, intubation and further suctioning of the larger airways may be required before ventilation is started.

Monitoring and managing the first stage of labour

Take the chapter test before and after you read this chapter.

Objectives

When you have completed this unit you should be able to:

- Monitor and manage the first stage of labour.
- Evaluate accurately the progress of labour.
- Know the importance of the alert and action lines on the partogram.
- Recognise poor progress during the first stage of labour.
- Systematically evaluate a patient to determine the cause of the poor progress in labour.
- Manage a patient with poor progress in labour.
- Recognise patients at increased risk of prolapse of the umbilical cord.
- Manage a patient with cord prolapse.

The diagnosis of labour

8-1 When is a patient in labour?

A patient is in labour when she has *both* of the following:

1. Regular uterine contractions with at least 1 contraction every 10 minutes.
2. Cervical changes (i.e. cervical effacement and/or dilatation) *or* rupture of the membranes.

The two phases of the first stage of labour

The first stage of labour can be divided into two phases:

1. The latent phase.
2. The active phase.

> **The first stage of labour is divided into two phases: the latent phase and the active phase.**

8-2 What do you understand by the latent phase of the first stage of labour?

1. The latent phase starts with the onset of labour and ends when the patient's cervix is 3 cm dilated. With primigravidas the cervix should also be fully effaced to indicate that the latent phase has ended. However, in a multigravida the cervix need not be fully effaced.
2. During the latent phase, the cervix dilates slowly. Although no time limit need be set for cervical dilatation, this phase does not normally last longer than 8 hours. The time taken may vary widely.
3. During the latent phase there is a progressive increase in the duration and the frequency of uterine contractions.

8-3 What do you understand by the active phase of the first stage of labour?

1. This phase starts when the cervix is 3 cm dilated and ends when the cervix is fully dilated.
2. During the active phase, more rapid dilatation of the cervix occurs.
3. The cervix should dilate at a rate of at least 1 cm per hour.

NOTE
The average rate of dilatation of the cervix during the active phase is at least 1.5 cm per hour in multigravidas and 1.2 cm in primigravidas. Therefore, the lower limit of the normal rate of cervical dilatation is 1 cm per hour.

> The cervix should dilate at a rate of at least 1 cm per hour in the active phase of labour.

Monitoring of the first stage of labour

8-4 What do you understand by a complete physical examination during labour?

1. The routine observations (usually done hourly or half-hourly) of the condition of the mother, the condition of the fetus, and the contractions.
2. A careful abdominal examination.
3. A careful vaginal examination.

This examination is only complete when the findings have been charted on the partogram. If the findings are abnormal, a plan must be made regarding the further management of the patient.

8-5 When should you do a complete physical examination on a patient in labour?

1. On admission.
2. During the latent phase: Four hours after admission or when the patient starts to experience more painful, regular contractions.
3. During the active phase: 4-hourly, provided all observations indicate that progress is normal. If there is poor progress, the next complete examination will have to be done after 2 hours in most instances.

After the complete examination has been done and an assessment made about the progress of labour, a decision is taken on when the next complete examination should be done. The time of the next examination is marked on the partogram with an arrow. The next complete examination may, if the circumstances demand it, be done sooner (but not later) than the time indicated.

8-6 How should progress during the first stage of labour be monitored?

A *partogram* is used to monitor and record the progress of labour.

8-7 What is a partogram?

A partogram is a chart on which the progress of labour over time can be presented. You will notice that provision has been made on the chart to record all the important observations regarding the condition of the mother, the condition of the fetus, and the progress of labour.

An example of a partogram is shown in figure 8-1.

8-8 What is the first oblique line on the partogram called?

The *alert line*. It represents a rate of cervical dilatation of 1 cm per hour.

8-9 What is the importance of the alert line?

The alert line represents the minimum progress in cervical dilatation which is acceptable during the active phase of the first stage of labour.

8-10 What is the second oblique line on the partogram called?

This line is called the *action line*.

8-11 What is the importance of the action line?

1. Any patient whose graph of the cervical dilatation falls on or crosses the action line must have a complete examination by the doctor. Her further management must be under the doctor's supervision and direction. If a patient is not already in hospital, she will need to be transferred into a hospital where there are facilities for instrumental delivery and Caesarean section.
2. The progress of labour is very slow when the graph of cervical dilatation crosses or falls on this line. When this occurs, action must be taken in order to hasten the delivery of the infant.

If the cervical dilatation falls on, or crosses, the action line of the partogram, a doctor must be called to assess the patient.

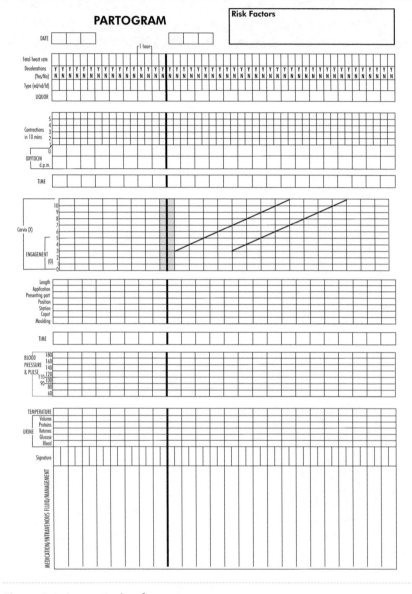

Figure 8-1: An example of a partogram

Management of a patient in the latent phase of the first stage of labour

The latent phase of labour should not last longer than 8 hours.

8-12 What is the initial management of a patient in the latent phase of labour?

When a patient is admitted in early labour, and on examination everything is found to be normal, only routine observations are done. The next complete examination is done 4 hours later, or sooner if the patient starts to experience more regular and painful contractions. The patient should eat and drink normally, and should be encouraged to walk around. She need not be admitted to the labour ward.

8-13 What should you do at the second complete examination?

At this time, the following must be assessed.

1. The contractions: If the contractions have stopped the patient is no longer in labour, and if the maternal and fetal conditions are normal, she may be discharged. However, if the contractions have remained regular, then you must assess the cervix.
2. The cervix:
   - If the effacement and dilatation of the cervix have remained unchanged, the patient is probably not in true labour. If she is experiencing painful contractions, she should be given an analgesic, e.g. pethidine 100 mg and promethazine (Phenergan) 25 mg or hydroxyzine (Aterax) 100 mg by intramuscular injection and, provided that all other observations are normal, the next complete physical examination is planned for 4 hours later.
   - If there has been progress in effacement and/or dilatation of the cervix, the patient is in labour and, provided that all other observations are normal, the next complete examination is planned for 4 hours later. If the cervix is 3 cm or more dilated, the patient has now progressed to the active phase of the first stage of labour.

8-14 What should you do if a patient has not progressed to the active phase of labour within 8 hours after admission?

1. The contractions may have stopped, in which case the patient is not in labour. If the membranes have not ruptured and if there is no indication to induce labour, the patient should be discharged.
2. The patient may still be having regular contractions. In this case, further management depends upon the state of the cervix:
   - If there has been no progress in effacement and/or dilatation of the cervix, the patient is probably not in labour. The responsible doctor should see and assess this patient, in order to decide whether labour should be induced.
   - If there has been progressive effacement and/or dilatation of the cervix, the patient is in labour. If the progress has been slow during the latent phase, it may be necessary to rupture the membranes or commence an oxytocin infusion if she is HIV positive as described in 8-35.

Management of a patient in the active phase of the first stage of labour

When a patient is admitted in the active phase of labour, she will probably be in normal labour. However, the possibility of cephalopelvic disproportion must be considered, especially if the patient is unbooked.

8-15 How do you manage a patient who is in normal labour?

When the condition of the mother and the condition of the fetus are normal, and there are no signs of cephalopelvic disproportion, the next complete examination must be done 4 hours later. The cervical dilatation, in centimetres, is recorded on the alert line of the partogram.

8-16 What represents normal progress during the active phase of the first stage of labour on the partogram?

1. The recording of cervical dilatation at the various vaginal examinations lie on or to the left of the alert line. In other words cervical dilatation is at least 1 cm per hour.
2. There is also progressive descent of the fetal head into the pelvis. This is detected by assessing the amount of the fetal head above the brim of the pelvis on abdominal examination. Descent of the head during the active phase of the first stage of labour may occur late, especially in multigravidas.

With normal progress during the active phase of the first stage of labour, the recording of the dilatation of the cervix will lie on or to the left of the alert line on the partogram. In addition, there will be progressively less of the fetal head palpable above the pelvic brim.

8-17 Why is it necessary to evaluate both cervical dilatation and the descent of the head in order to determine whether there has been progress in the active phase of the first stage of labour?

1. Cervical dilatation without associated descent of the head does not necessarily indicate progress in labour.
2. Cervical dilatation may occur when there are good contractions, in association with increasing caput succedaneum formation and moulding of the fetal skull, while the amount of fetal head palpable above the brim of the pelvis remains the same. In these circumstances no real progress has occurred, because the head is not descending into the pelvis.
3. The station of the presenting part of the head in relation to the spine, as felt on vaginal examination, can also improve *without further descent of the head and without real progress* having occurred. This is because of increasing caput succedaneum and moulding.

Descent of the head is assessed on abdominal and not on vaginal examination.

8-18 What circumstances will make it necessary to do vaginal examinations more frequently than 4-hourly in the active phase of the first stage of labour?

1. If cephalopelvic disproportion is suspected, the next vaginal examination must be done 2 hours later.
2. If a complete examination has revealed poor progress of labour, without the presence of cephalopelvic disproportion, the next complete examination should also be done 2 hours later, to assess the effectiveness of the measures taken to correct the poor progress.
3. If a patient's cervix is more than 6 cm dilated, the next complete examination would normally be done when the cervix is expected to be fully dilated. However, the examination may need to be done earlier if there are signs that the cervix is already fully dilated.

8-19 When should you rupture the patient's membranes?

1. It is possible to reduce the risk of transferring HIV from a mother to her infant by keeping the duration of ruptured membranes as short as possible. Do not rupture the membranes of patients whose HIV status is positive or unknown if they are still intact at the start of the active phase of labour. The following vaginal examination will not increase the risk of infection if the membranes are intact. The next complete examination should be done after 2 hours when the management should be as follows:
   - With normal progress do not rupture the membranes.
   - With poor progress the membranes should be ruptured and the next examination performed 4 hours later.

2. A patient who is HIV negative and in labour with a vertex presentation may have her membranes ruptured with safety if:
   - She is in the active phase of labour.
   - The fetal head is 3/5 or less palpable above the brim of the pelvis.

3. After rupturing the membranes, carefully feel around the fetal head to rule out the possibility of a cord prolapse.

If the fetal head is 4/5 or more above the pelvic brim, and the cervix is 6 cm or more dilated, it is safer to carefully rupture the membranes than to allow them to rupture spontaneously. This will reduce the risk of cord prolapse.

8-20 What should you do if a patient ruptures her membranes spontaneously during labour?

1. If the fetal head is 4/5 or more palpable above the pelvic inlet, or if there is a breech presentation, the patient is at high risk for a cord prolapse. A sterile vaginal examination must, therefore, be done to rule out this possibility.
2. If the fetal head is 3/5 or less palpable above the pelvic inlet, it is highly unlikely that a cord prolapse might happen. However, the fetal heart must be monitored to rule out the possibility of fetal distress due to cord compression.

8-21 What are the advantages of rupturing a patient's membranes?

1. Rupture of the membranes acts as a stimulus to labour, so that there is often better progress.
2. Meconium staining of the liquor will be detected.
3. If the cord prolapses when the membranes are ruptured, this can be detected immediately, and the appropriate management can therefore be started without delay.

It is important to make sure that the patient is in the active phase of the first stage of labour before rupturing the membranes.

Poor progress in the active phase of the first stage of labour

8-22 How would you recognise poor progress in the active phase of labour?

Poor progress is present when the graph showing cervical dilatation crosses the alert line. In other words, cervical dilatation in the active phase of the first stage of labour is less than 1 cm per hour.

8-23 What should you do if the graph showing cervical dilatation crosses the alert line?

A systematic assessment of the patient must be made in order to determine the cause of the poor progress in labour.

8-24 How should you systematically examine a patient with poor progress in the active phase of the first stage of labour?

Step 1: Two questions must be asked:

1. Is the patient in the active phase of the first stage of labour?
2. Are the membranes ruptured?

If the answer to both questions is 'yes', proceed to step 2.

Step 2: The cause of the poor progress of labour must be determined by examining the patient using the 'Rule of the 4 Ps'. The 4 Ps are:

1. The patient.
2. The powers.
3. The passenger.
4. The passage.

> The cause of poor progress of the active phase of the first stage of labour is determined by assessing the 4 Ps.

8-25 How may problems with the patient cause poor progress of labour and how should these problems be managed?

Any of the following factors may interfere with the normal progress of labour.

1. *The patient needs pain relief.* Patients who experience very painful contractions, especially if associated with excessive anxiety, may have poor progress of labour as a result. Pain relief, emotional support and reassurance can be of great value in speeding up the progress of labour.

2. *The patient has a full bladder.* A full bladder not only causes mechanical obstruction, but also depresses uterine muscle activity. A patient must be encouraged to pass urine frequently but may need catheterisation, and sometimes an indwelling catheter, until after delivery.

3. *The patient is dehydrated.* Dehydration is recognised by the fact that the patient is thirsty, has a dry mouth, passes small amounts of concentrated urine and may have ketonuria. Dehydration must be corrected as it may be the cause of the poor progress. With good care during labour the patient will not become dehydrated, because she can eat and drink during the latent phase of labour and take oral fluids during the active phase of labour. If there is poor progress during the active phase of labour, an intravenous infusion must be started.

8-26 How may problems with the powers cause poor progress of labour?

The powers (i.e. the uterine contractions) may either be inadequate or ineffective. Any patient in whom labour progresses normally has both adequate and effective contractions, irrespective of the duration and frequency of contractions.

1. *Inadequate uterine contractions.* Inadequate uterine contractions can be the cause of poor progress of labour. Such contractions:
   ○ Last less than 40 seconds, and/or
   ○ There are fewer than 2 contractions per 10 minutes.

2. *Ineffective uterine contractions.* The uterine contractions may be adequate but not effective, as poor progress can occur even in the presence of apparently good, painful contractions (i.e. 2 or more in 10 minutes with each contraction lasting 40 seconds or longer), without disproportion being present (i.e. no moulding of the fetal skull). The problem of ineffective contractions occurs only in primigravidas. Any patient whose labour progresses normally must have effective uterine contractions.

NOTE
Dysfunctional uterine contractions are diagnosed when the uterine contractions appear to be ineffective.

8-27 How may problems with the passenger cause poor progress of labour and how should these problems be managed?

The cause of poor progress of labour may be due to a problem with the passenger (i.e. the fetus). These problems can be identified by performing an abdominal examination followed by a vaginal examination.

On abdominal examination the following problems causing poor progress may be identified.

1. *The lie of the fetus is abnormal.* If the lie of the fetus is transverse the patient will need a Caesarean section.
2. *The presenting part of the fetus is abnormal.* With a breech presentation, the patient must be assessed by a doctor to decide whether a vaginal delivery will be possible or whether a Caesarean section is required. If the presentation is cephalic, the part of the head which is presenting must be determined on vaginal examination.

   NOTE
   Fetuses who present by the breech and who comply with the criteria for vaginal delivery, are only delivered vaginally if there is normal progress during the first stage of labour.

3. *The fetus is large.* A large fetus (i.e. estimated as 4 kg or more), with signs of cephalopelvic disproportion (i.e. 2+ or 3+ moulding) must be delivered by Caesarean section.
4. *There are 2 or more fetuses.* Poor progress may also occur in a patient with a multiple pregnancy, usually due to inadequate uterine contractions.
5. *The fetal head has not engaged.* The number of fifths of the head palpable above the pelvis must always be assessed:
   ○ Engagement has occurred only when 2/5 or less of the head is palpable above the brim of the pelvis. In this case the problem of cephalopelvic disproportion at the pelvic inlet is excluded.
   ○ With 3/5 or more of the head above the pelvic brim, plus 2+ or 3+ moulding, a Caesarean section is indicated for cephalopelvic disproportion at the pelvic inlet.

An abdominal examination, to assess the lie and the presenting part of the fetus, as well as the amount of fetal head palpable above the pelvic brim, must always be done before performing a vaginal examination.

On vaginal examination the following problems causing poor progress may be identified.

1. *The presenting part is abnormal.* Vertex (i.e. occipital) presentation of the fetal head is the most favourable presentation for the normal progress of labour. With any other presentation of the fetal head in early labour (e.g. brow), there is no urgency to interfere, as the presentation may become more favourable when the patient is in established labour. However, in established labour, if moulding is present in any presentation other than a vertex, a Caesarean section will have to be done.

2. *The position of the fetal head in relation to the pelvis is abnormal.* An occipito-anterior (right or left) is the most favourable position for normal progress of labour. Positions other than this (i.e. left or right occipito-posterior) will progress more slowly. Labour can be allowed to continue provided there is progress, and no progressive evidence of disproportion. The patient will also need adequate pain relief and an intravenous infusion to prevent dehydration.

3. *Cephalopelvic disproportion is present.*

   ○ The head is examined for the amount of caput succedaneum present. Caput is not an accurate indicator of disproportion as it can also be present in the absence of disproportion, for example, in a patient who bears down before the cervix is fully dilated.

   ○ The sutures are examined for moulding, which is the best indication of the presence of disproportion. 3+ of moulding is a definite sign of disproportion. In a vertex presentation, the sagittal and lambdoid (occipito-parietal) sutures are examined. The worst degree of moulding noted in any of the sutures is that which is recorded on the partogram as the amount of moulding present.

   ○ Improvement in the station of the presenting part (i.e. the level of the presenting part relative to the ischial spines) is not a reliable method of assessing progress in labour, compared to descent and engagement of the fetal head as determined on abdominal examination.

> Improvement in the station of the presenting part of the fetal head, in relation to the ischial spines, is not a reliable method of assessing progress in the first stage of labour.

8-28 How may problems with the passage cause poor progress in labour and how should these problems be managed?

The following problems with the passage may cause poor progress in labour:

1. *The membranes are still intact.* Should the membranes still be intact, they must be ruptured and the patient reassessed after 4 hours before poor progress can be diagnosed.
2. *The pelvis is small.* A pelvic assessment which shows a small pelvis, together with 2+ or 3+ moulding of the fetal skull means that there is cephalopelvic disproportion, and is an indication for Caesarean section.

8-29 What are the two important causes of poor progress of labour?

1. *Cephalopelvic disproportion.* This is a dangerous condition if it is not recognised early and not correctly managed.
2. *Inadequate uterine action.* This is a common cause of poor progress in primigravidas. It can be easily corrected with an oxytocin infusion.

8-30 What must be done after the patient has been systematically evaluated to determine the cause of the poor progress of labour?

1. The nurse attending to the patient must inform the doctor about the clinical findings. Together they must decide on the cause of the slow progress and what action must be taken to correct this problem.
2. A decision must also be made as to when the next complete examination of the patient will be done. Usually this will be in 2 hours, but sometimes in 4 hours. This consultation may be done by telephone and it is not necessary for the doctor to see the patient at this stage.
3. If labour progresses satisfactorily following the action taken, labour is allowed to continue. However, if poor progress continues, or if the

action line has been reached or crossed, the patient must be examined by the responsible doctor who must then decide on further management.

The following are examples of causes of poor progress in labour together with their management:

Cause	Action
Cephalopelvic disproportion	Caesarean section
An anxious patient unable to cope with painful contractions	Reassurance and analgesia
Inadequate uterine contractions	An oxytocin infusion
Occipito-posterior position	Analgesia and an intravenous infusion
Ineffective uterine contractions	Analgesia followed by an oxytocin infusion

Cephalopelvic disproportion

8-31 How will you know when poor progress is due to cephalopelvic disproportion?

This can be recognised by the following findings:

1. On abdominal examination, the fetal head is not engaged in the pelvis. Remember, this is diagnosed by finding 3/5 or more of the head palpable above the brim of the pelvis.
2. On vaginal examination, there is severe moulding (i.e. 3+) of the fetal skull. Severe moulding must always be regarded as serious, as it confirms that cephalopelvic disproportion is present.

Cephalopelvic disproportion may already be present when the patient is admitted.

A high fetal head (3/5 or more above the brim) on abdominal examination, with 3+ moulding on vaginal examination, indicates cephalopelvic disproportion.

8-32 Does a patient's cervix always dilate at a rate slower than 1 cm per hour if cephalopelvic disproportion is present?

When there is cephalopelvic disproportion, the cervix usually dilates at a rate slower than 1 cm per hour, but the cervix may dilate normally, even though the fetal head remains high due to cephalopelvic disproportion. This is a dangerous situation as it may be incorrectly concluded that labour is progressing normally.

8-33 What features would make you diagnose cephalopelvic disproportion when the fetal head is not descending into the pelvis?

Often, especially in multiparous patients, the head does not descend into the pelvis until late in the active phase of the first stage of labour. However, when the head does not descend into the pelvis, you should look for possible causes:

1. A malpresentation, e.g. a face or a brow presentation.
2. Moulding (i.e. 2+ or 3+).

If either of these are present, there is cephalopelvic disproportion, and a Caesarean section should be done.

On the other hand, labour can be allowed to continue if:

1. There is no malpresentation.
2. There is no more than 1+ moulding.
3. The maternal and fetal conditions are good.

The next complete physical examination must be repeated within 2 hours.

8-34 What should you do if you decide that the poor progress is due to cephalopelvic disproportion?

1. Once the diagnosis of cephalopelvic disproportion has been made, the infant must be delivered as soon as possible. This means that a Caesarean section will have to be done.
2. While the preparations for Caesarean section are being made, it is of value to both the mother and fetus to suppress uterine contractions. This is done by giving 3 nifedipine (Adalat) 10 mg capsules by mouth (a total

of 30 mg) or give 250 µg (0.5 ml) salbutamol (Ventolin) slowly intravenously, the 0.5 ml salbutamol is diluted with 9.5 ml sterile water and given slowly intravenously over 5 minutes, provided that there are no contraindications.

Inadequate uterine action

8-35 What should you do if you decide that the poor progress is due to inadequate or ineffective uterine contractions?

1. Provided there are no contraindications, the patient must be given an oxytocin infusion in order to strengthen the contractions.
2. The patient's progress must be reassessed after 2 hours.
3. If cervical dilatation has proceeded at the rate of 1 cm per hour or more, progress has been satisfactory and labour is allowed to continue.
4. If cervical dilatation has been slower than 1 cm per hour once the patient has adequate uterine contractions, the patient must be reassessed by the responsible doctor. Cephalopelvic disproportion may be present.
5. If at this stage the patient is still in a peripheral clinic, there should be enough time to refer her to hospital before the action line is crossed.
6. Patients who complain of painful contractions need analgesia before oxytocin is started.

8-36 What are the contraindications to the use of oxytocin in order to strengthen contractions in the first stage of labour?

1. Evidence of cephalopelvic disproportion. Oxytocin must, therefore, *not* be given if there is already moulding (i.e. 2+ or 3+) present.
2. Any patient with a scar of the uterus, e.g. from a previous Caesarean section.
3. Any patient with a fetus in whom the presenting part is not a vertex.
4. Multiparas with poor progress during the active phase of labour of the first stage of labour.
5. Grande multiparity during the latent or active phase of the first stage of labour.

6. When there is fetal distress.
7. Patients with poor kidney function or heart valve disease.

8-37 How must oxytocin be administered when it is used during the first stage of labour?

The following is a good method:

1. Begin with 1 unit of oxytocin in 1 litre of Plasmalyte B, Ringer's lactate or rehydration fluid.
2. Use a giving set which delivers 20 drops per ml.
3. Start with 15 drops per minute and increase the rate at intervals of 30 minutes to 30 drops, and then to 60 drops per minute, until the patient gets at least 3 contractions lasting at least 40 seconds every 10 minutes.
4. If there are still inadequate contractions with 1 unit of oxytocin per litre at 60 drops per minute, a new litre of intravenous fluid containing 8 units per litre is started at a rate of 15 drops per minute. The rate is increased in the same way as above until 30 drops per minute are being given. This is the maximum amount of oxytocin which should be used during the first stage of labour.

8-38 What are the effects of a long labour?

Both the mother and fetus may be affected.

1. The mother. A patient in whom the progress of labour is slow is more likely to become anxious and to be dehydrated. If the poor progress is due to cephalopelvic disproportion (i.e. obstructed labour), and labour is allowed to continue, then there is the danger of the mother developing any or all of the following:
    ◦ A ruptured uterus.

- A vesicovaginal fistula.
- A rectovaginal fistula.

2. The fetus. The stress of a long labour results in progressive fetal hypoxia, which causes fetal distress and eventually in intra-uterine death.

The referral of patients with poor progress during the active phase of the first stage of labour

The guidelines for referral will vary from region to region, depending on the distances between clinics and hospitals, and the availability of transport. In general, arrangements must be made so that the patient will be under the care of the responsible doctor by the time the graph depicting cervical dilatation crosses the action line.

8-39 What arrangements should you make to ensure the patient's safety during transfer to hospital, if there is poor progress of labour?

1. An intravenous infusion must be started.
2. The patient must lie on her side while being transferred to hospital.
3. A nurse should accompany the patient, unless there is a trained ambulance crew.
4. If cephalopelvic disproportion is the cause of the poor progress of labour, the contractions must be stopped. To stop contractions, 3 nifedipine (Adalat) 10 mg capsules (total of 30 mg) can be taken orally or 250 µg (0.5 ml) salbutamol (Ventolin) slowly intravenously, the 0.5 ml salbutamol is diluted with 9.5 ml sterile water and given slowly intravenously over 5 minutes. If indicated, the same dose of salbutamol may be repeated after 30 minutes. Both drugs should only be used if there are no contraindications.

Prolapse of the umbilical cord

8-40 Why is prolapse of the umbilical cord a serious complication?

Because the flow of blood between the fetus and placenta is severely reduced and may stop completely, causing fetal distress and possibly fetal death.

8-41 What is the difference between a cord presentation and a cord prolapse?

1. With a cord presentation, the umbilical cord lies in front of the presenting part with the *membranes still intact.*
2. With a cord prolapse, the cord lies in front of the presenting part and the *membranes have ruptured.* The loose cord may lie between the presenting part of the fetus and the cervix, in the vagina or outside the vagina.

8-42 How should a cord presentation be managed?

If the cord is felt between the membranes and the presenting part of the fetus, if the fetus is alive and is viable and if the patient is in labour, a Caesarean section must be done. This will prevent a cord prolapse when the membranes rupture.

8-43 Which patients are at risk of a prolapsed cord?

1. Patients in labour with an abnormal lie (e.g. transverse lie) or an abnormal presentation (e.g. breech presentation).
2. Patients who rupture their membranes when the fetal head is still not engaged (i.e. 4/5 or more above the pelvic brim, e.g. in a grande multipara).
3. Patients with polyhydramnios where the increased volume of liquor may wash the cord out of the uterus.
4. Patients in preterm labour where the presenting part is small relative to the pelvis when the membranes rupture.
5. Patients with a multiple pregnancy, where preterm labour, abnormal lie and polyhydramnios are common.

8-44 What should be done when a patient, who is at high risk of prolapse of the cord, ruptures her membranes?

A sterile vaginal examination must immediately be done to determine whether the cord has prolapsed.

8-45 What is the management of a prolapsed cord?

A vaginal examination must be done immediately.

1. If the cervix is 9 cm or more dilated and the fetal head is on the perineum, the patient must bear down and the infant must be delivered as soon as possible.
2. Otherwise the patient must be managed as follows:
   - Replace the cord carefully into the vagina.
   - Give the patient mask oxygen and give 250 µg (0.5 ml) salbutamol (Ventolin) slowly intravenously, the 0.5 ml salbutamol is diluted with 9.5 ml sterile water and given slowly intravenously over 5 minutes to stop labour.
   - Put a Foley catheter into the patient's bladder and fill the bladder with 500 ml saline.
   - If the full bladder does not lift the presenting part off the prolapsed cord, the presenting part must be pushed up by an assistant's hand in the vagina, and by turning the patient into the knee-chest position.

8-46 Why should the cord carefully be replaced in the vagina?

The cord must not be allowed to become cold or dry as this will produce vasospasm and, thereby, further reduce the blood flow through the cord.

8-47 Why are oxygen and salbutamol given to a patient with a prolapsed cord?

1. Giving oxygen to the patient may improve the oxygen supply to the fetus.
2. Stopping uterine contractions will reduce the pressure of the presenting part on the prolapsed cord.

8-48 Should a Caesarean section be done on all women with a prolapsed cord if the infant cannot be rapidly delivered vaginally?

No. A Caesarean section is only done if the infant is potentially viable (28 weeks or more) and the cord is still pulsating. Otherwise the infant should be delivered vaginally as the chances of survival are then extremely small.

HIV positive women

On admission to the labour ward the HIV status of all pregnant women must be established, documented and the correct antiretroviral (ARV) medication prescribed.

8-49 How should antiretroviral medication be administered to HIV positive women during labour?

Women who have been on ARV prophylaxis or treatment during pregnancy should continue taking their daily dose of FDC throughout labour. They do not need any additional ARV drugs in labour.

However HIV positive women who have not taken ARV prophylaxis or treatment during pregnancy or who only started FDC in the last weeks of pregnancy are at high risk of transmitting HIV to their infant. Therefore they should receive 300mg of AZT 3 hourly by mouth and a single dose of 200 mg nevirapine (NVP) as well as a single dose of TDF/FTC (Truvada). The Truvada is given to prevent resistance against nevirapine developing.

Case study 1

A primigravida patient at term, who is HIV negative, is admitted to the labour ward. She has 1 contraction, lasting 30 seconds, every 10 minutes. The cervix is 1 cm dilated and 1.5 cm long. The maternal and fetal observations are normal. After 4 hours she is having 2 contractions, each lasting 40 seconds, every 10 minutes. On vaginal examination the cervix is now 2 cm dilated and 0.5 cm long with bulging membranes. The diagnosis of poor progress of labour due to poor uterine contractions is made and an oxytocin infusion is started to improve contractions.

1. Do you agree with the diagnosis of poor progress of labour?

The diagnosis is incorrect as the patient is still in the latent phase of the first stage of labour. Poor progress of labour can only be diagnosed in the active phase of labour.

2. Why can it be said with certainty that the patient is in the latent phase of labour?

- The cervix is still less than 3 cm dilated.
- The cervix is dilating slowly.
- The cervix is effacing.
- The frequency of the uterine contractions is increasing.

3. What is your assessment of the patient's management?

Apart from the wrong diagnosis, oxytocin should not be given before the membranes have been ruptured.

4. Should the patient's membranes have been artificially ruptured when the second vaginal examination was done?

No. If the maternal and fetal condition are good, you should wait until the cervix is 3 cm or more dilated. The membranes may also be ruptured if the patient has been in the latent phase of labour for 8 hours without any progress.

Case study 2

A patient at term is admitted in labour with a vertex presentation. The cervix is already 4 cm dilated. The cervical dilatation is recorded on the alert line. At the next vaginal examination the cervix has dilated to 8 cm. Caput can be palpated over the fetal skull. It is decided that the progress is favourable and that the next vaginal examination should be done after a further 4 hours.

1. On admission, should the woman's cervical dilatation have been entered on the alert line?

Yes. The patient is in the active phase of the first stage of labour as her cervix is 4 cm dilated. Therefore, the cervical dilatation must be plotted on the alert line. The future observations should fall on or to the left of the alert line.

2. Do the findings of the second examination indicate normal progress of labour?

Not necessarily, as no information is given about the amount of fetal head palpable above the pelvic brim. Cervical dilatation without descent of the head does not always indicate normal progress of labour.

3. Is normal cervical dilatation with improvement in the station of the presenting part possible if cephalopelvic disproportion is present?

Yes. The uterine contractions cause an increasing amount of caput and moulding, which is incorrectly interpreted as normal progress of labour. In this case, caput was noted during the second examination. However, further information about any moulding and the amount of fetal head palpable above the pelvic brim are essential before it can be decided whether normal progress is present or not.

4. Was the correct decision made at the time of the second examination to repeat the vaginal examination after 4 hours?

No. If the cervix is 8 cm dilated, the next examination must be done 2 hours later, or even sooner if there are indications that the woman's cervix is fully dilated. If it is uncertain whether the progress of labour is normal then the examination should also be repeated in 2 hours.

Case study 3

A primigravida patient at term is admitted in labour. At the first examination the fetal head is 2/5 above the pelvic brim and the cervix is 6 cm dilated. 3 contractions in 10 minutes, each lasting 45 seconds, are palpated. At the next examination 4 hours later, the head is still 2/5 above the brim and the cervix is still 6 cm dilated. No moulding can be felt. The patient is still having 3 contractions in 10 minutes, each lasting 45 seconds and complains that the contractions are painful. Because there has been no progress in spite of painful contractions of adequate frequency and duration, it is decided that cephalopelvic disproportion is present and that, therefore, a Caesarean section must be done.

1. Do you agree that the poor progress of labour is due to cephalopelvic disproportion?

No. To diagnose poor progress due to cephalopelvic disproportion, severe moulding (3+) must be present.

2. What is most probably the reason for the poor progress of labour?

The patient is a primigravida with strong, painful contractions and no signs of cephalopelvic disproportion. A diagnosis of ineffective uterine contractions (dysfunctional uterine contractions) can, therefore, be made with confidence.

3. What should be the management of the patient's poor progress of labour?

Firstly, the patient should be reassured and given analgesia with pethidine and promethazine (Phenergan) or hydroxyzine (Aterax). Then an oxytocin infusion should be started to make the contractions more effective.

4. Why is reassuring the patient so important?

Anxious patients often progress slowly in labour and have painful contractions. Emotional support during labour is a very important part of patient care.

5. When must the next vaginal examination be done?

The next vaginal examination should be done 2 hours later to determine whether the treatment has been effective. During the examination it is very important to exclude cephalopelvic disproportion.

Case study 4

A patient who is in labour at term has progressed slowly and the alert line has been crossed. During a systematic evaluation of the patient by the midwife for poor progress of labour, a diagnosis of an occipito-posterior position is made. As the patient is making some progress, she decides to allow labour to continue. After 4 hours, the cervical dilatation falls on the action line. Although there is still slow progress, she again decides to allow labour to continue and to repeat the vaginal examination in a further 2 hours.

1. Was the patient managed correctly when she crossed the alert line?

Yes. She was systematically examined and a diagnosis of slow progress of labour due to an occipito-posterior position was made.

2. What should be done if a long first stage of labour is expected due to an occipito-posterior position?

An intravenous infusion must be started to ensure that the patient does not become dehydrated. In addition, adequate analgesia must be given.

3. Was the patient correctly managed when she reached the action line?

No. A doctor should have evaluated the patient. Further management should have been under his/her direction.

4. Under what conditions should the doctor allow labour to progress further?

If there is steady progress of labour, the maternal and fetal conditions are good, and there is less than 3+ moulding.

8A

Skills: Examination of the abdomen in labour

Objectives

When you have completed this skills chapter you should be able to:

- Assess the size of the fetus.
- Determine the fetal lie and presentation.
- Determine the descent of the head.
- Grade the uterine contractions.

Abdominal palpation

A. When should you examine the abdomen of a patient who is in labour?

The abdominal examination forms an important part of every complete physical examination in labour. The examination is done:

1. On admission.
2. Before *every* vaginal examination.
3. At any other time when it is considered necessary.

B. What should be assessed on examination of the abdomen of a patient who is in labour?

1. The shape of the abdomen.
2. The height of the fundus.
3. The size of the fetus.
4. The lie of the fetus.
5. The presentation of the fetus.

6. The fetal heart rate pattern.
7. The descent and engagement of the head.
8. The presence or absence of hardness and tenderness of the uterus.
9. The contractions.

C. Shape of the abdomen

It is helpful to look at the shape and contour of the abdomen.

1. The shape of the uterus will be oval with a singleton pregnancy and a longitudinal lie.
2. The shape of the uterus will be round with a multiple pregnancy or polyhydramnios.
3. A 'flattened' lower abdomen suggests a vertex presentation with an occipito-posterior position (ROP or LOP).
4. A suprapubic bulge suggests a full bladder.

D. Height of the fundus

It is important to ask yourself whether the height of the fundus is in keeping with the patient's dates and the findings at previous antenatal attendances.

E. Size of the fetus

It is important on palpation to assess the size of the fetus. This is best done by feeling the size of the fetal head. Is the size of the fetus in keeping with the patient's dates and the size of the uterus? A fetus which feels smaller than expected is likely to be associated with:

1. Incorrect dates.
2. Intra-uterine growth restriction.
3. Multiple pregnancy.

F. Lie and presentation of the fetus

The lie and presentation of the fetus is decided on abdominal palpation by using the four steps described for antenatal care.

It is important to know whether the lie is longitudinal (cephalic or breech presentation), oblique, or transverse. With an abnormal lie, there is an increased risk of umbilical cord prolapse. An abnormal lie may suggest that there is a multiple pregnancy or a placenta praevia.

It is also important to know the presentation of the fetus. If a breech presentation is present, it must be decided whether a vaginal delivery is possible. With breech presentation, there is an increased risk of cord prolapse or a placenta praevia.

G. Cephalic presentation of the fetus

If the presentation is cephalic, it is sometimes possible when palpating the abdomen to determine the presenting part of the fetal head (vertex, face or brow). Figure 8A-1 indicates some features that can assist you in determining the presentation.

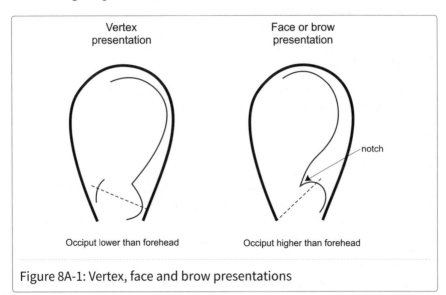

Figure 8A-1: Vertex, face and brow presentations

H. Descent and engagement of the head

This assessment is an essential part of *every* examination of a patient in labour. The descent and engagement of the head is an important part of assessing the progress of labour and must be assessed before each vaginal examination.

The amount of descent and engagement of the head is assessed by feeling how many fifths of the head are palpable *above* the brim of the pelvis:

1. 5/5 of the head palpable means that the whole head is above the inlet of the pelvis.
2. 4/5 of the head palpable means that a small part of the head is below the brim of the pelvis and can be lifted out of the pelvis with a deep pelvic grip.
3. 3/5 of the head palpable means that the head cannot be lifted out of the pelvis. On doing a deep pelvic grip, your fingers will move outwards from the neck of the fetus, then inwards before reaching the pelvic brim.
4. 2/5 of the head palpable means that most of the head is below the pelvic brim, and on doing a deep pelvic grip, your fingers only splay outwards from the fetal neck to the pelvic brim.
5. 1/5 of the head palpable means that only the tip of the fetal head can be felt above the pelvic brim.

It is very important to be able to distinguish between 3/5 and 2/5 head palpable above the pelvic brim. If only 2/5 of the head is palpable, then engagement has taken place and the possibility of disproportion at the pelvic inlet can be ruled out.

Descent and engagement of the head are assessed on abdominal and not on vaginal examination.

I. Hardness and tenderness of the uterus

A uterus may be regarded as abnormally hard:

1. When it is difficult to palpate fetal parts.
2. When the uterus feels harder than usual.

This may occur:

1. In some primigravidas.
2. During a contraction.
3. When there has been an abruptio placentae.
4. When the uterus has ruptured.
5. When there is polyhydramnios.

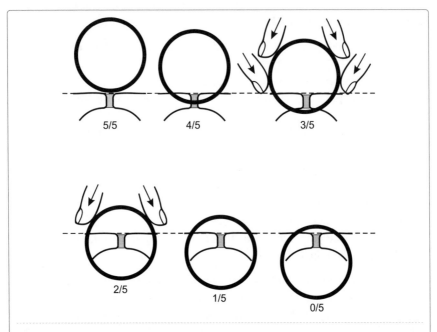

Figure 8A-2: An accurate method of determining the amount of head palpable above the brim of the pelvis

When there is both hardness and tenderness of the uterus, without period of relaxation during which the uterus is not tender, the commonest causes are:

1. An abruptio placentae.
2. A ruptured uterus.

Therefore, there is likely to be a serious problem if the uterus is harder than normal *and* there is also tenderness without periods of relaxation. Hardness or tenderness of the uterus must be recorded on the partogram and reported immediately to the responsible doctor.

Assessing contractions

J. Contractions

Contractions can be felt by placing a hand on the abdomen and feeling when the uterus becomes hard, and when it relaxes. It is therefore possible to assess the length of a contraction by taking the time at the beginning and end of the contraction. The strength of contractions is assessed by measuring their duration, and also the frequency with which they occur in a period of 10 minutes.

K. Grading the duration of contractions

1. Contractions lasting less than 20 seconds ('weak contractions').
2. Contractions lasting 20–40 seconds ('moderate contractions')
3. Contractions lasting more than 40 seconds ('strong contractions').

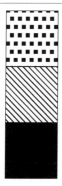

A contraction lasting less than 20 seconds

A contraction lasting 20 - 40 seconds

A contraction lasting more than 40 seconds

Figure 8A-3: Method of grading the duration of uterine contractions for recording on the partogram

L. Grading the frequency and duration of contractions

The frequency of contractions is assessed by counting the number of contractions that occur in a period of 10 minutes

Assessing the fetal heart rate

M. Fetal heart rate pattern

The fetal heart rate must be detected and the fetal heart rate pattern assessed and recorded every time the abdomen is examined in labour.

Skills: Vaginal examination in labour

Objectives

When you have completed this skills chapter you should be able to:

- Perform a complete vaginal examination during labour.
- Assess the state of the cervix.
- Assess the presenting part.
- Assess the size of the pelvis.

Preparation for a vaginal examination in labour

A. Equipment that should be available for a sterile vaginal examination

A vaginal examination in labour is a sterile procedure if the membranes have ruptured or are going to be ruptured during the examination. Therefore, a sterile tray is needed. The basic necessities are:

1. Swabs.
2. Tap water for swabbing.
3. Sterile gloves.
4. A suitable instrument for rupturing the membranes.
5. An antiseptic vaginal cream or sterile lubricant.

An ordinary surgical glove can be used and the patient does not need to be swabbed if the membranes have not ruptured yet and are not going to be ruptured during the examination.

B. Preparation of the patient for a sterile vaginal examination

1. Explain to the patient what examination is to be done, and why it is going to be done.
2. The woman needs to know that it will be an uncomfortable examination, and sometimes even a little painful.
3. The patient should lie on her back, with her legs flexed and knees apart. Do not expose the patient until you are ready to examine her. It is sometimes necessary to examine the patient in the lithotomy position.
4. The patient's vulva and perineum are swabbed with tap water. This is done by first swabbing the labia majora and groin on both sides and then swabbing the introitus while keeping the labia majora apart with your thumb and forefinger.

C. Preparation needed by the examiner

1. The person to do the vaginal examination must have either scrubbed or thoroughly washed his/her hands.
2. Sterile gloves must be worn.
3. The examiner must *think* about the findings, and their significance for the patient and the management of her labour.

Procedure of examination

A vaginal examination in labour is a systematic examination, and the following should be assessed:

1. Vulva and vagina.
2. Cervix.
3. Membranes.
4. Liquor.
5. Presenting part.
6. Pelvis.

Always examine the abdomen before performing a vaginal examination in labour.

> An abdominal examination should always be done before a vaginal examination.

The vulva and vagina

D. Important aspects of the examination of the vulva and vagina

This examination is particularly important when the patient is first admitted:

1. When you examine the vulva you should look for ulceration, condylomata, varices and any perineal scarring or rigidity.
2. When you examine the vagina, the presence or absence of the following features should be noted:
   ◦ A vaginal discharge.
   ◦ A full rectum.
   ◦ A vaginal stricture or septum.
   ◦ Presentation or prolapse of the umbilical cord.
3. A speculum examination, *not* a digital examination, must be done if it is thought that the patient has preterm or prelabour rupture of the membranes.

The cervix

When you examine the cervix you should observe:

1. Length.
2. Dilatation.

E. Measuring cervical length

The cervix becomes progressively shorter in early labour. The length of the cervix is measured by assessing the length of the endocervical canal. This is the distance between the internal os and the external os on digital examination. The endocervical canal of an uneffaced cervix is approximately

3 cm long, but when the cervix is fully effaced there will be no endocervical canal, only a ring of thin cervix. The length of the cervix is measured in centimetres. In the past the term 'cervical effacement' was used and this was measured as a percentage.

F. Dilatation

Dilatation must be assessed in centimetres, and is best measured by comparing the degree of separation of the fingers on vaginal examination, with the set of circles in the labour ward. In assessing the dilatation of the cervix, it is easy to make two mistakes:

1. If the cervix is very thin, it may be difficult to feel, and the patient may be said to be fully dilated, when in fact she is not.
2. When feeling the rim of the cervix, it is easy to stretch it, or pass the fingers through the cervix and feel the rim with the side of the fingers. Both of these methods cause the recording of dilatation to be more than it really is. The correct method is to place the tips of the fingers on the edges of the cervix.

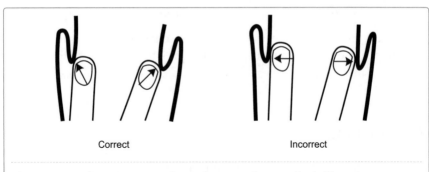

Correct   Incorrect

Figure 8B-1: The correct method of measuring cervical dilatation

The membranes and liquor

G. Assessment of the membranes

Rupture of the membranes may be obvious if there is liquor draining. However, one should always feel for the presence of membranes overlying the presenting part. If the presenting part is high, it is usually quite easy to feel intact membranes. It may be difficult to feel them if the presenting part is well applied to the cervix. In this case, one should wait for a contraction, when some liquor often comes in front of the presenting part, allowing the membranes to be felt. Sometimes the umbilical cord can be felt in front of the presenting part (a cord presentation).

If the membranes are intact, the following two questions should be asked:

1. Should the membranes be ruptured?
   - In most instances, if the patient is in the active phase of labour, the membranes should be ruptured.
   - When the presenting part is high, there is always the danger that the umbilical cord may prolapse. However, it is better for the cord to prolapse while the hand of the examiner is in the vagina, when it can be detected immediately, than to have the cord prolapse with spontaneous rupture of the membranes while the patient is unattended.
   - HIV-positive patients should not have their membranes ruptured unless there is poor progress of labour.
2. What is the condition of the liquor when the membranes rupture?

   The presence of meconium may change the management of the patient as it indicates that fetal distress has been and may still be present.

The presenting part

An abdominal examination must have been done before the vaginal examination to determine the lie of the fetus and the presenting part. If the presenting part is the fetal head, the number of fifths palpable above the pelvic brim must first be determined.

When palpating the presenting part on vaginal examination, there are four important questions that you must ask yourself:

1. What is the presenting part, e.g. head, breech or shoulder?
2. If the head is presenting, what is the presentation, e.g. vertex, brow or face presentation?

3. What is the position of the presenting part in relation to the mother's pelvis?
4. If the presentation is occiput, vault or brow, is moulding present?

H. Assessing the presenting part

The presenting part is usually the head but may be the breech, the arm, or the shoulder.

1. *Features of an occiput presentation.* The posterior fontanelle is normally felt. It is a small triangular space. In contrast, the anterior fontanelle is diamond shaped. If the head is well flexed, the anterior fontanelle will not be felt. If the anterior fontanelle can be easily felt, the head is deflexed and the presenting part the vault.
2. *Features of a face presentation.* On abdominal examination the presenting part is the head. However, on vaginal examination:
   ○ Instead of a firm skull, something soft is felt.
   ○ The gum margins distinguish the mouth from the anus.
   ○ The cheek bones and the mouth form a triangle.
   ○ The orbital ridges above the eyes can be felt.
   ○ The ears may be felt.
3. *Features of a brow presentation.* The presenting part is high. The anterior fontanelle is felt on one side of the pelvis, the root of the nose on the other side, and the orbital ridges may be felt laterally.
4. *Features of a breech presentation.* On abdominal examination the presenting part is the breech (soft and triangular). On vaginal examination:
   ○ Instead of a firm skull, something soft is felt.
   ○ The anus does not have gum margins.
   ○ The anus and the ischial tuberosities form a straight line.
5. *Features of a shoulder presentation.* On abdominal examination the lie will be transverse or oblique. Features of a shoulder presentation on vaginal examination will be quite easy if the arm has prolapsed. The shoulder is not always that easy to identify, unless the arm can be felt. The presenting part is usually high.

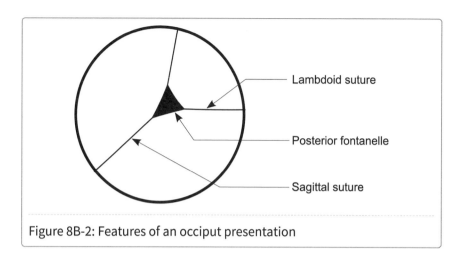

Figure 8B-2: Features of an occiput presentation

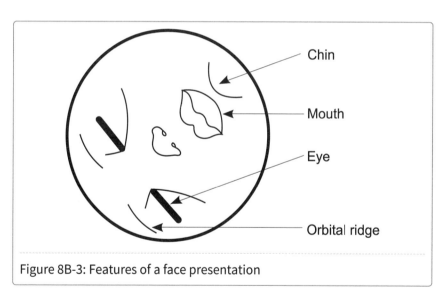

Figure 8B-3: Features of a face presentation

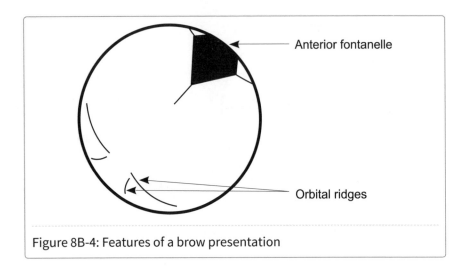

Figure 8B-4: Features of a brow presentation

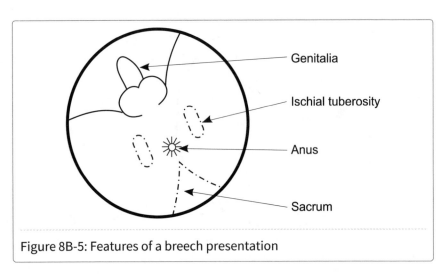

Figure 8B-5: Features of a breech presentation

I. Determining the position of the presenting part

Position means the relationship of a fixed point on the presenting part (i.e. the point of reference or the denominator) to the mother's pelvis. The position is determined on vaginal examination.

1. In a vertex presentation the point of reference is the posterior fontanelle (i.e. the occiput).
2. In a face presentation the point of reference is the chin (i.e. the mentum).
3. In a breech presentation the point of reference is the sacrum of the fetus.

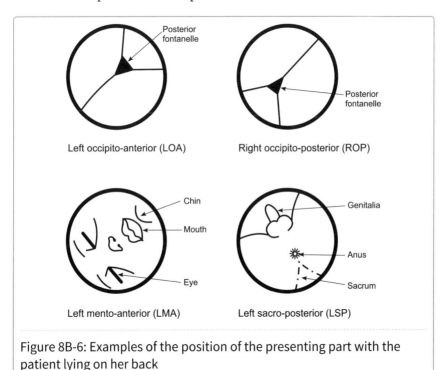

Figure 8B-6: Examples of the position of the presenting part with the patient lying on her back

J. Determining the descent and engagement of the head

The descent and engagement of the head is assessed on abdominal and not on vaginal examination.

Moulding

Moulding is the overlapping of the fetal skull bones at a suture which may occur during labour due to the head being compressed as it passes through the pelvis of the mother.

K. The diagnosis of moulding

In a cephalic (head) presentation, moulding is diagnosed by feeling the overlap of the sutures of the skull on vaginal examination, and assessing whether or not the overlap can be reduced (corrected) by pressing gently with the examining finger.

The presence of caput succedaneum can also be felt as a soft, boggy swelling, which may make it difficult to identify the presenting part of the fetal head clearly. With severe caput the sutures may be impossible to feel.

L. Grading the degree of moulding

The occipito-parietal and the sagittal sutures are palpated and the relationship or closeness of the two adjacent bones assessed. The amount of moulding recorded on the partogram should be the most severe degree found in any of the sutures palpated.

The degree of moulding is assessed according to the following scale:

0 = Normal separation of the bones with open sutures.

1+ = Bones touching each other.

2+ = Bones overlapping, but can be separated with gentle digital pressure.

3+ = Bones overlapping, but cannot be separated with gentle digital pressure. (3+ is regarded as severe moulding.)

M. Assessing the pelvis

When assessing the pelvis, the size and shape of the pelvic inlet, the mid-pelvis, and the pelvic outlet must be determined.

1. To assess the size of the pelvic inlet, the sacral promontory and the retropubic area are palpated.

2. To assess the size of the mid-pelvis, the curve of the sacrum, the sacrospinous ligaments and the ischial spines are palpated.
3. To assess the size of the pelvic outlet, the subpubic angle, intertuberous diameter and mobility of the coccyx are determined.

It is important to use a step-by-step method to assess the pelvis.

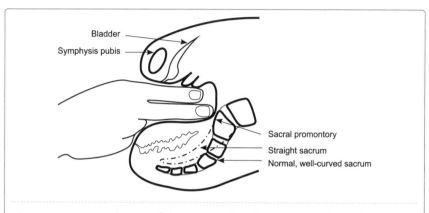

Figure 8B-7: Lateral view of the pelvis, showing the examining fingers just reaching the sacral promontory

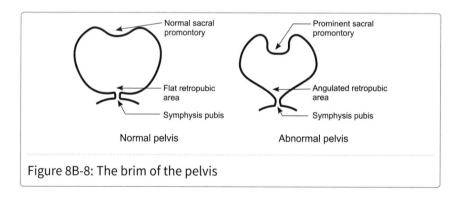

Figure 8B-8: The brim of the pelvis

Step 1. The sacrum

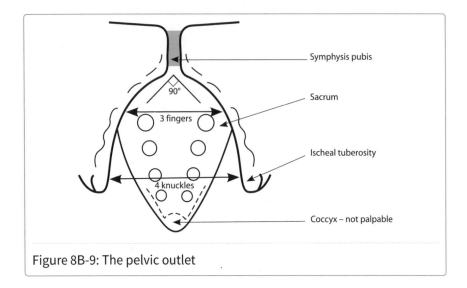

Figure 8B-9: The pelvic outlet

Start with the sacral promontory and follow the curve of the sacrum down the midline.

1. An adequate pelvis: The promontory cannot be easily palpated, the sacrum is well curved and the coccyx cannot be felt.
2. A small pelvis: The promontory is easily palpated and prominent, the sacrum is straight, and the coccyx is prominent and/or fixed.

Step 2. The ischial spines and sacrospinous ligaments

Lateral to the midsacrum, the sacrospinous ligaments can be felt. If these ligaments are followed laterally, the ischial spines can be palpated.

1. An adequate pelvis: 2 fingers can be placed on the sacrospinous ligaments (i.e. they are 3 cm or longer) and the spines are small and round.
2. A small pelvis: The ligaments allow less than 2 fingers and the spines are prominent and sharp.

Step 3. Retropubic area

Put 2 examining fingers, with the palm of the hand facing upwards, behind the symphysis pubis and then move them laterally to both sides:

1. An adequate pelvis: The retropubic area is flat.
2. A small pelvis: The retropubic area is angulated.

Step 4. The subpubic angle and intertuberous diameter

To measure the subpubic angle, the examining fingers are turned so that the palm of the hand faces upward, a third finger is held at the entrance of the vagina (introitus) and the angle under the pubis felt. The intertuberous diameter is measured with the knuckles of a closed fist placed between the ischial tuberosities.

1. An adequate pelvis: The subpubic angle allows 3 fingers (i.e. an angle of about 90°) and the intertuberous diameter allows four knuckles.
2. A small pelvis: The subpubic angle allows only 2 fingers (i.e. an angle of about 60°) and the intertuberous diameter allows only three knuckles.

8C

Skills: Recording observations on the partogram

Objectives

When you have completed this skills chapter you should be able to:

- Record and assess the condition of the mother.
- Record and assess the condition of the fetus.
- Record and assess the progress of labour.

The partogram

The condition of the mother, the condition of the fetus, and the progress of labour are recorded on the partogram.

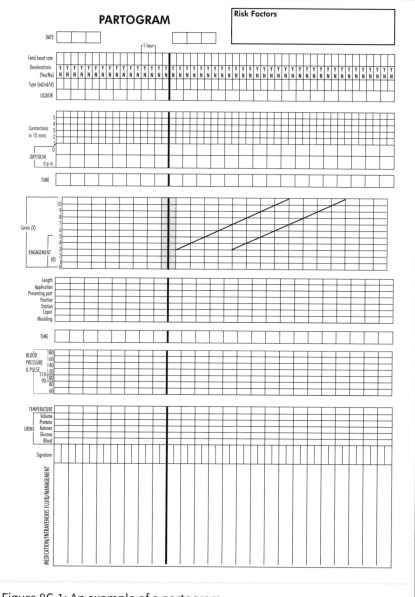

Figure 8C-1: An example of a partogram

Recording the condition of the mother

A. Recording the blood pressure, pulse and temperature

The maternal blood pressure, pulse and temperature should be recorded on the partogram.

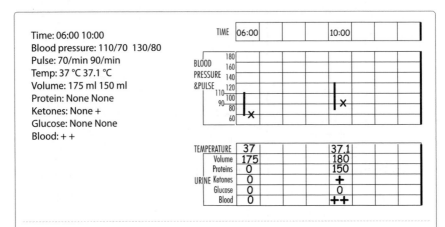

Figure 8C-2: Recording blood pressure, pulse, temperature and urine results on the partogram

B. Recording the urinary data

1. Volume is recorded in ml.
2. Protein is recorded as 0 to 4+.
3. Ketones are recorded as 0 to 4+.

Recording the condition of the fetus

C. Recording the fetal heart rate pattern

The following two observations must be recorded on the partogram:

1. The baseline heart rate.
2. The presence or absence of decelerations. If decelerations are present, you must record whether they are early or late decelerations (see figure 8C-3).

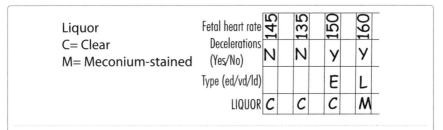

Liquor	Fetal heart rate	145	135	150	160
C= Clear	Decelerations				
M= Meconium-stained	(Yes/No)	N	N	Y	Y
	Type (ed/vd/ld)			E	L
	LIQUOR	C	C	C	M

Figure 8C-3: Recording the fetal heart rate pattern and the liquor findings on the partogram

D. Recording the liquor findings

Three symbols are used:

I = *Intact* membranes.

C = *Clear* liquor draining.

M = *Meconium-stained* liquor draining (see figure 8C-3).

E. How often should you record the liquor findings?

The recordings should be made:

1. At each vaginal examination.
2. Whenever a change in the liquor is noted, e.g. when the membranes rupture or if the patient starts to drain meconium-stained liquor after having had clear liquor before.

Recording the progress of labour

F. Recording the cervical dilatation

Cervical dilatation is measured in cm and then recorded by marking an 'X' on the partogram.

G. Recording the length of the cervix (effacement)

The length of the cervix is recorded by drawing a thick, vertical line on the same part of the chart that is used for the cervical dilatation. The length of the line drawn indicates the length of the endocervical canal in cm. It is drawn on the chart whenever the cervical dilatation is recorded. Alternatively, the length of the endocervical canal, measured in cm or mm, can be noted in the space provided.

H. Recording the amount of the head palpable above the brim of the pelvis (descent and engagement)

The findings are recorded by marking an 'O' on the partogram (see figure 8C-4).

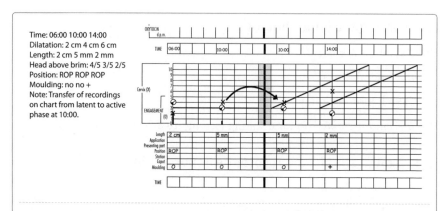

Figure 8C-4: Recording the cervical dilatation, cervical length, the amount of fetal head above the brim, position of the head, and moulding on the partogram

I. Recording the position of the fetal head

The position of the fetal head is recorded by marking the 'O' with fontanelles and the sagittal suture. Alternatively, the position can be noted (e.g. ROA) in the space provided (see figure 8C-4). This is recorded at every vaginal examination.

J. Recording moulding of the fetal head

The degree of moulding (i.e. 0 to 3+) is also recorded on the partogram.

K. Recording the duration of contractions

The duration of contractions is also recorded on the partogram. The block is stippled if the contractions last less than 20 seconds (i.e. weak contractions), the block is striped if the contractions last between 20 and 40 seconds (i.e. moderate contractions) and the block is coloured in completely if the contractions last more than 40 seconds each (i.e. strong contractions).

L. Recording the frequency of contractions

The number of contractions occurring within 10 minutes is recorded by marking off 1 block for each contraction, e.g. 2 blocks marked off equals 2 contractions in 10 minutes, 4 blocks marked off equals 4 contractions in 10 minutes, and 5 blocks if 5 or more contractions in 10 minutes (see figure 8C-5).

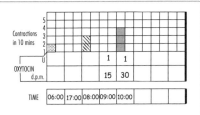

06:00: One weak contraction in ten minutes
08:00: Two moderate contractions in ten minutes
10:00: Three strong contractions in ten minutes
An infusion of one unit of oxytocin in one litre at 15 drops per minute is being administered from 9:00 and at 30 drops per minute from 10:00.

Figure 8C-5: Recording the duration and frequency of contractions on the partogram

M. Recording drugs and intravenous fluid given during labour

In the space provided on the partogram you should record:

1. The name of the drug.
2. The dose of the drug given.
3. The time the drug was given.
4. The type of intravenous fluid.
5. The time the intravenous fluid was started.
6. The rate of administration.
7. The amount of intravenous fluid given (after completion).

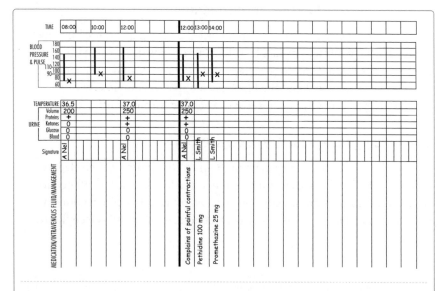

Figure 8C-6: Documenting medication, assessment, management and time on the partogram

N. Assessment and management

After each examination an assessment must be made and recorded on the partogram. All management in labour must also be recorded on the partogram.

O. Recording the time on the partogram

The time, to the nearest half hour, should also be entered on the partogram whenever an observation is recorded, medication is given, an assessment is made or management is altered.

Exercises on the correct use of the partogram

Only the information given in the cases will be shown on the partogram. In practice, all the appropriate spaces on the partogram must be filled in.

Case study 1

A primigravida at term is admitted to a primary-care perinatal clinic at 06:00 with a history of painful contractions for several hours. She received antenatal care and is known to be HIV negative. The maternal and fetal conditions are satisfactory. On abdominal examination a single fetus with a longitudinal lie is found. The presenting part is the fetal head, and 4/5 is palpable above the brim of the pelvis. 2 contractions in 10 minutes, each lasting 15 seconds are noted. On vaginal examination the cervix is 1 cm long and 2 cm dilated. The fetal head is in the right occipito-lateral position.

1. Is the patient in active labour?

No. The cervix is less than 3 cm dilated. The patient is, therefore, still in the latent phase of labour.

2. How should you enter your findings on the partogram?

As the patient is still in the latent phase of labour, the descent and amount of fetal head palpable above the brim, the presenting part and the position of the head, and the length and dilatation of the cervix, must be recorded on the vertical line forming the left-hand margin of the latent phase part of the partogram. The correct way of entering the above data on the partogram is shown in figure 8C-7.

3. How should you manage this patient further?

The patient must have the routine observations (such as pulse rate, blood pressure and fetal heart) performed at the usual intervals. She must be offered analgesia and sedation. Adequate analgesia, e.g. pethidine 100 mg and promethazine 25 mg or hydroxyzine 100 mg, should be given by intramuscular injection as soon as the patient asks for pain relief. A second complete examination should be done at 10:00, i.e. 4 hours after the first complete examination. The patient must be encouraged to walk about as this will help the progress towards the active phase of the first stage of labour.

At the second complete examination the maternal and fetal conditions are satisfactory. On abdominal examination 2/5 of the fetal head is palpable above the brim of the pelvis. 3 contractions in 10 minutes, lasting between 30 seconds each, are noted. On vaginal examination the cervix is 2 mm long and 5 cm dilated. The head is in the right occipito-anterior position. The membranes are artificially ruptured and the liquor is found to be clear.

4. Is the patient still in the latent phase of labour?

No. The cervix is more than 3 cm dilated. The patient is, therefore, in the active phase of labour.

5. Where should you enter the findings obtained at 10:00?

The findings must be entered on the latent phase part of the partogram, 4 hours to the right of the findings at 06:00. However, as the patient is now in active labour, the data must then be transferred to the active phase part of the partogram. This must be indicated with an arrow.

6. How should you transfer the findings at 10:00 from the latent to the active phase part of the partogram?

The X (cervical dilatation) must be moved horizontally to the right until it lies on the alert line. This will again be at 5 cm dilatation. The O (number of fifths of the head above the pelvic brim) is similarly transferred to lie on the same vertical line opposite the 2 lines on the vertical axis. The new position of the head (ROA) must be indicated on the O. The length of the cervix is recorded by a 5 mm thick black column on the base line vertically below the X and O. The fact that the membranes have been ruptured is entered in the block provided for medication/ I.V. fluids/management. A 'C' in the block provided for liquor indicates that the liquor is clear. The correct method of transferring the above findings from the latent to the active part of the partogram is shown in figure 8C-7. (The length of the cervix and the position of the fetal head may also be entered in the appropriate blocks provided elsewhere on the partogram).

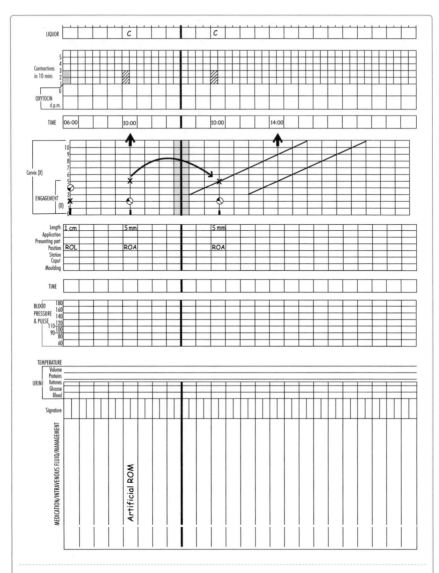

Figure 8C-7: Information from case study 1 correctly entered onto the partogram

Case study 2

A multigravida is admitted to the labour ward at 08:00 in labour at term. She received antenatal care and is known to be HIV negative. The maternal and fetal conditions are satisfactory. On abdominal examination the head is 5/5 palpable above the brim of the pelvis. 3 contractions in 10 minutes, each lasting 25 seconds are noted. On vaginal examination the cervix is 1 cm long (and thus not fully effaced) and 4 cm dilated. The presenting part is in the left occipito-posterior position. The patient complains that her contractions are painful.

1. Is the patient in the active phase of labour?

Yes, as the cervix is more than 3 cm dilated.

2. How should you record your findings?

As the patient is in the active phase of labour, the findings must be entered on the active phase part of the partogram. The X (cervical dilatation) is recorded on the alert line, opposite the 4 on the vertical axis indicating 4 cm dilatation. The O (number of fifths palpable above the pelvic brim) is recorded above the X opposite the 5 on the vertical line. The length of the cervix is recorded by a 1 cm column on the base line, vertically below the X and O. The correct way of recording the above findings is in figure 8C-8.

3. How should you manage the patient further?

The routine observations (e.g. pulse rate, blood pressure, fetal heart, and urine output) must be performed at the usual intervals. The patient must be offered analgesia. Pethidine 100 mg and promethazine 25 mg or hydroxyzine 100 mg should be given by intramuscular injection as soon as the patient requests pain relief. A second complete examination should be done at 12:00, i.e. 4 hours after the first complete examination.

At the second complete examination the maternal and fetal conditions are satisfactory. On abdominal examination the head is 3/5 palpable above the brim of the pelvis. 3 contractions in 10 minutes, each lasting 25 seconds, are noted. On vaginal examination the cervix is 5 mm long and 5 cm dilated with bulging membranes.

The presenting part is in the left occipito-transverse position. Poor progress is diagnosed and a systemic assessment of the patient is made in order to determine the cause. Intact membranes and inadequate uterine contractions are diagnosed as the causes of the poor progress.

4. How should you record these findings on the partogram?

The X must be recorded on the horizontal line corresponding to 5 cm cervical dilatation, 4 hours to the right of the record at 08:00. The position of the fetal head and length of the cervix are recorded on the same vertical line as the X. The correct way of recording these observations is shown in figure 8C-8.

5. Is the progress of labour satisfactory?

No. This is immediately apparent by observing that the second X has crossed the alert line. For labour to have progressed satisfactorily, the cervix should have been at least 8 cm dilated (4 cm initially plus 1 cm per hour over the past 4 hours).

6. How should you manage this patient further?

The membranes must be ruptured. Rupture of the membranes will result in stronger uterine contractions. Because there has been inadequate progress of labour, a third complete examination should be performed at 14:00, i.e. 2 hours after the second complete examination.

At the third complete examination the maternal and fetal conditions are satisfactory. On abdominal examination the head is 1/5 palpable above the pelvic brim. 4 contractions in 10 minutes, each lasting 50 seconds are observed. On vaginal examination the cervix is 1 mm long and 9 cm dilated. The presenting part is in the left occipito-anterior position. The findings are recorded as shown in figure 8C-8.

7. What is your assessment of the progress of labour at 14:00?

Labour is progressing satisfactorily. This is shown by the third X having moved closer to the alert line. The head, which has rotated from the left occipito-posterior to the left occipito-anterior position, is also engaged. A spontaneous vertex delivery may be expected within an hour.

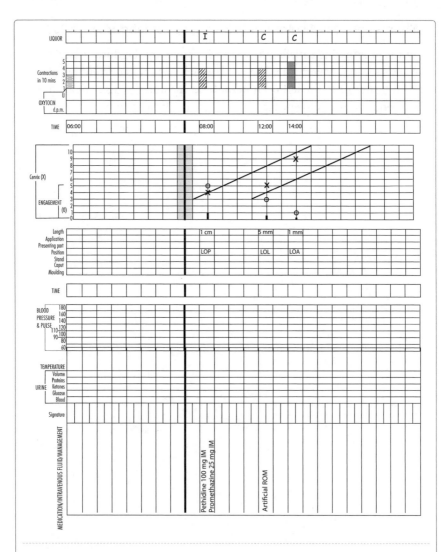

Figure 8C-8: Information from case study 2 correctly entered onto the partogram

Case study 3

A gravida 2 para 1 is admitted to the labour ward at 09:00 in labour at term. She has already had painful contractions for the past 2 hours. Two years before she had a difficult forceps delivery for a prolonged second stage of labour. The infant's birth weight was 3000 g. The maternal and fetal conditions are satisfactory. On abdominal examination the head is 4/5 palpable above the brim of the pelvis. The cervix is 2 mm long and 5 cm dilated. There is 1+ of moulding present and the presenting part is in the right occipito-posterior position. The patient is HIV negative and an artificial rupture of the membranes is performed and a small amount of meconium-stained liquor is drained. The patient is given pethidine 100 mg and promethazine 25 mg or hydroxyzine 100 mg. A second complete examination is scheduled for 13:00.

1. How should you record the above findings?

As the patient is in the active phase of labour, the findings must be entered on the active phase part of the partogram. The X (cervical dilatation) is recorded on the alert line opposite the 5 on the vertical line. The other findings are entered in their appropriate places as shown in figure 8C-9.

2. Is the decision to schedule the next complete examination at 13:00 correct?

Yes. There are no signs of cephalopelvic disproportion (e.g. 3+ moulding) on admission, and the maternal and fetal conditions are satisfactory.

3. What observations must be done carefully during the next 4 hours?

Meconium in the liquor indicates that the fetus is at an increased risk for fetal distress. Therefore, the fetal heart rate pattern must be observed carefully for signs of fetal distress (e.g. late decelerations).

4. What is likely to happen to this patient's progress of labour?

The most likely outcome is the development of cephalopelvic disproportion. On abdominal examination the head will remain 3/5 or more palpable above the pelvic brim (i.e. unengaged) and on vaginal examination there will be 3+ moulding. An urgent Caesarean section should then be performed.

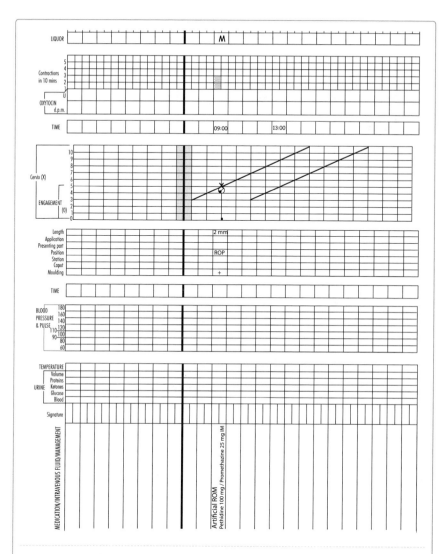

Figure 8C-9: Information from case study 3 correctly entered onto the partogram

9

The second stage of labour

Take the chapter test before and after you read this chapter.

Objectives

When you have completed this unit you should be able to:

- Identify the onset of the second stage of labour.
- Decide when the patient should start to bear down.
- Communicate effectively with the patient during labour.
- Use the maternal effort to the best advantage when the patient bears down.
- Make careful observations during the second stage of labour.
- Accurately evaluate progress in the second stage of labour.
- Manage a patient with a prolonged second stage of labour.
- Diagnose and manage impacted shoulders.

The normal second stage of labour

9-1 What clinical signs indicate the start and end of the second stage of labour?

The second stage of labour starts when the patient's cervix is fully dilated and ends when the infant is completely delivered.

9-2 What symptoms and signs indicate that the second stage of labour has begun?

One or more of the following may occur:

1. Uterine contractions increase in both frequency and duration, i.e. they are more frequent and last longer.
2. The patient becomes restless.
3. Nausea and vomiting often occur.
4. The patient has an uncontrollable urge to bear down (push).
5. The perineum bulges during a contraction as it is stretched by the fetal head.

If the symptoms and signs suggest that the second stage of labour has begun, an abdominal examination to assess the amount of head palpable above the pelvic brim, followed by a vaginal examination, must be done.

9-3 Is there a difference between primigravidas and multigravidas at the start of the second stage of labour?

Yes. In primigravidas the head is usually engaged when the cervix reaches full dilatation. In contrast, multigravidas often reach full cervical dilatation when the fetal head is still 3/5 or more palpable above the pelvic brim (i.e. the head is still not engaged).

A patient should only start bearing down when the fetal head distends the perineum and she has a strong urge to bear down.

9-4 What is the definition of engagement of the fetal head?

The fetal head is engaged when the largest transverse diameter of the head (the biparietal diameter) has passed through the pelvic inlet. When the fetal head is engaged, 2/5 or less of the head is palpable above the pelvic brim.

The fetal head is engaged when only 2/5 or less of the head is palpable above the brim of the pelvis.

Engagement usually starts before the onset of labour. Initially 5/5 of the head is palpable above the pelvic brim, but when engagement has been completed, the head is no longer palpable on abdominal examination. Engagement of the head *cannot* be determined on vaginal examination.

Managing the second stage of labour

9-5 Should the patient start bearing down as soon as the cervix is fully dilated?

No. The patient should wait until the fetal head starts to distend the perineum, when she will experience a strong urge to bear down. The fetal head will be engaged with 1/5 of the fetal head palpable above the brim of the pelvis.

9-6 In a patient with a fully dilated cervix, but an unengaged fetal head, when is it safe to wait for engagement before allowing the patient to bear down?

1. If there are no signs of fetal distress.
2. If there are no signs of cephalopelvic disproportion.

> Waiting for engagement of the head in a patient with a fully dilated cervix should only be allowed if there are no signs of fetal distress or cephalopelvic disproportion.

9-7 How long should you wait before asking the patient to bear down if the cervix is fully dilated but the head is not yet engaged?

1. The patient should be assessed after an hour if there are no signs of fetal distress and the maternal observations are normal.
2. Usually engagement of the head will occur during this time and the patient will feel a strong urge to bear down within an hour.

3. If the head has still not engaged after an hour, you can wait a further hour provided that all other observations are normal and there are no signs of cephalopelvic disproportion.
4. If the head has not engaged after waiting 2 hours, a doctor must carefully examine the patient for cephalopelvic disproportion which may be present as a result of a big fetus or an abnormal presentation of the fetal head. A Caesarean section is most likely indicated.

9-8 In what position should the patient be delivered?

1. The patient is usually delivered on her back (i.e. the dorsal position) because it is easier for the person managing the delivery. However, this position has the disadvantage that it may cause postural hypotension which may result in fetal distress. This problem can be avoided if a firm pillow is placed under one of the patient's hips so that she is turned 15° onto her side and does not lie flat on her back.
2. The lateral position (i.e. on her side) prevents the problem of postural hypotension. In addition, the person conducting the delivery has a good view of the vulva and perineum, the pelvic muscles are relaxed, and the delivery can be better controlled. The lateral position is particularly useful when the patient will not give her full co-operation.
3. The upright position (i.e. vertical or squatting position) is becoming more frequently used. The patient sits on her heels and supports herself on outstretched arms. This position has the following advantages:
   ○ The maternal effort becomes more effective.
   ○ The duration of the second stage is shortened.
   ○ Fewer patients need an assisted delivery.
4. The semi-Fowler's position, where the patient's back is lifted to 45° from the horizontal, may be used instead of the upright position. This partial-sitting position is comfortable both for the patient and the person conducting the delivery.

The position used during the second stage of labour depends on the patient's choice and the circumstances under which the delivery is conducted. The position chosen should allow for the best maternal effort at bearing down.

9-9 How would you get the best maternal co-operation during the second stage of labour?

1. Good communication between the patient and the midwife or doctor is very important. A relationship of trust developed during the first stage of labour will encourage good communication and co-operation during the second stage.
2. The patient must know what is expected of her during the second stage. The person conducting the delivery should encourage and support the patient and inform her about the progress. Good co-operation and attempts at bearing down should be praised.

9-10 How should you ensure that a patient bears down as effectively as possible?

1. While the patient is passive in the first stage, she must actively use her strength during the second stage of labour to assist the uterine contractions. The more effectively she uses her strength, the shorter the second stage will be.
2. The midwife or doctor must make sure that the patient knows when and how to bear down.
3. It is important that she rests between contractions and bears down during contractions.
4. At the height of the contraction, the patient is asked to take a deep breath, to put her chin on her chest, and to bear down as if she were going to empty her rectum. This action is most effective and easiest if the patient holds onto her legs or some other firm object.
5. Each bearing down effort should last as long as possible. This is better than a number of short efforts.
6. When the patient needs to breathe while pushing, she must quickly breathe out, take a deep breath and bear down again.
7. With multigravidas, it is sometimes necessary for the patient to breathe rather than push during a contraction to prevent the fetal head from delivering too quickly.

> Good communication between the patient and the person conducting the delivery is very important during labour.

9-11 What observations must be made during the second stage of labour?

If the head is still not engaged and it is decided to wait for engagement, the same observations usually made during the first stage of labour should be continued.

If the head is engaged and the patient is asked to bear down, the following observations must be done:

1. Listen to the fetal heart between contractions to determine the baseline fetal heart rate.
2. Listen to the fetal heart immediately after *each* contraction. If the fetal heart rate remains the same as that of the baseline rate, you are reassured that the fetus is in good condition. However, if the fetal heart is slower at the end of the contraction, and the slow heart rate takes more than 30 seconds to return to the baseline rate (i.e. a late deceleration), the fetus must be delivered as rapidly as possible because fetal distress has developed.
3. Observe the frequency and duration of the uterine contractions.
4. Look for any vaginal bleeding.
5. Record the progress of labour.

9-12 How is progress monitored in the second stage of labour?

With every uterine contraction and attempt at bearing down there should be some progress in the descent of the fetal head onto the perineum.

9-13 What should be done if there is no progress in the descent of the head onto the perineum?

1. If the patient has at least 2 contractions in 10 minutes, each lasting 40 seconds or more and there is no progress in the descent of the head after four attempts at bearing down, a doctor must assess the patient for a possible assisted delivery.

2. If a primigravida has inadequate uterine contractions and there are no signs of cephalopelvic disproportion (i.e. 2+ moulding or less), an oxytocin infusion should be started. When strong contractions are obtained, the patient must start bearing down.
3. If there is no progress in the descent of the head, and signs of cephalopelvic disproportion are present (i.e. 3+ moulding), the patient should not bear down. Instead she should concentrate on her breathing during contractions. The doctor must urgently assess the patient as an emergency Caesarean section is indicated. While preparing the patient, intra-uterine resuscitation must be done.

> With strong contractions and good bearing down there should be progress in the descent of the presenting part onto the perineum.

9-14 How should you manage fetal distress in the second stage of labour?

1. An episiotomy should be done, if the fetal head distends the perineum when the patient bears down, so that the fetus can be delivered with the next contraction.
2. If the perineum does not bulge with contractions and it appears as if the fetus will not be delivered after the next two efforts at bearing down, then the doctor must be called to assess the patient and possibly perform an assisted delivery. If the prerequisites for an assisted delivery cannot be met an emergency Caesarean section must be done. While preparing the patient, intra-uterine resuscitation must be done.

9-15 How should a normal vaginal delivery be managed?

The midwife or doctor managing the second stage of labour must always be prepared for possible complications. Equipment which may be required must be at hand and in good working order. Drugs which may be needed must be easily available.

1. *Emptying the bladder.* Any factor, such as a full bladder, that prevents descent of the fetal head or decreases the strength of uterine

contractions should be corrected. Therefore, it is very important for the patient to empty her bladder before starting to bear down.

2. *Supporting the perineum*: A swab should be placed over the patient's anus to prevent the vulva, and later the fetal head, being soiled with stool (i.e. faeces). It is important to support the perineum in order to:
   ○ Increase flexion of the fetal head so that the smallest possible diameter passes through the vagina. This can be done by pressing immediately above the anus.
   ○ Relieve the pressure on the perineum. Remember that the perineum must be in view all the time.

3. *Crowning of the head*: When the head is crowning, the vaginal outlet is stretched and an episiotomy may be indicated. The midwife or doctor should place one hand on the vertex to prevent sudden delivery of the head. The other hand, supporting the perineum, is now moved upwards to help extend the head. It is important that the fetal head is only controlled and not held back.

4. *Feeling for a cord*: Check that the umbilical cord is not wrapped tightly around the infant's neck. A loose cord can be slipped over the head, but a tight cord should be clamped and cut.

5. *Delivering of the shoulders and body*: With gentle continuous posterior traction on the head and lateral flexion, the anterior shoulder is delivered from under the symphysis pubis. The posterior shoulder is then lifted over the perineum. The rest of the infant's body is now delivered, following the curve of the birth canal and not by simply pulling it straight out of the vagina.

Episiotomy

9-16 What is the place of an episiotomy in modern midwifery?

An episiotomy is not done routinely but only if there is a good indication, such as:

1. When the infant needs to be delivered without delay.
   ○ Fetal distress during the second stage of labour.
   ○ Maternal exhaustion.

- A prolonged second stage of labour when the fetal head bulges the perineum and it is obvious that an episiotomy will hasten the delivery.
- When a quick and easy second stage is needed, e.g. in a patient with heart valve disease.

2. With the delivery of a preterm infant when an easy delivery is wanted.
3. When there is a high risk of a third-degree tear.
   - A thick, tight perineum.
   - A previous third-degree tear.
   - A repaired rectocoele.
4. When a breech or forceps delivery is done.

9-17 Does a second-degree tear heal faster and with fewer complications than an episiotomy?

Yes. A second-degree tear is easier to repair and heals quicker with less pain and discomfort than an episiotomy. Therefore, a second-degree tear is preferable to an episiotomy. A episiotomy should not be done routinely in primigravidas.

> An episiotomy should only be done if there is a definite indication.

9-18 Which type of episiotomy should be done?

Usually a mediolateral episiotomy is done. However, if the midwife or doctor has experience with the technique, a median episiotomy can be done.

Prolonged second stage of labour

9-19 What is the definition of a prolonged second stage of labour?

When diagnosing a prolonged second stage the time is usually measured from the start of bearing down. If a primigravida bears down for more than

45 minutes, or a multigravida for more than 30 minutes, without the infant being delivered, a prolonged second stage of labour is diagnosed.

> The second stage of labour is prolonged if it lasts longer than 45 minutes in a primigravida or 30 minutes in a multigravida.

9-20 What factors during the antenatal period, or first stage of labour, would indicate that the patient is at an increased risk of a prolonged second stage of labour?

1. Factors during the antenatal period which suggest that the patient will deliver a large infant:
   o A patient with a symphysis-fundus height measurement above the 90th centile, when multiple pregnancy and polyhydramnios have been excluded, i.e. there appears to be a large fetus.
   o A patient with impaired glucose tolerance or diabetes mellitus.
   o A patient who weighs more than 85 kg.
   o A patient with a previous infant weighing 4 kg or more at birth.

2. Factors during the first stage of labour:
   o An estimated fetal weight, assessed on abdominal examination, of 4 kg or more.
   o A patient with poor progress in the first stage of labour before eventually reaching full cervical dilatation.
   o A patient who progressed normally during the active phase of the first stage of labour, but whose progress was slower from 7 or 8 cm until full dilatation.

> Slow progress in the first stage of labour may be followed by a prolonged second stage of labour.

9-21 How should you manage a patient with a prolonged second stage of labour?

1. If a doctor is available, the doctor should assess the patient. Usually an assisted delivery is done once cephalopelvic disproportion has been excluded and 1/5 or no fetal head remains above the pelvic brim. A

Caesarean section should be done if cephalopelvic disproportion is present.

2. If a doctor is not available, the patient should be referred to a level 1 or 2 hospital with facilities to perform a Caesarean section.

> A prolonged second stage of labour is a dangerous complication which requires immediate and appropriate management.

9-22 How should a patient with a prolonged second stage of labour be managed during transfer to a hospital for Caesarean section?

1. The patient should lie on her side and not bear down with contractions. Instead, she should concentrate on her breathing.
2. An intravenous infusion should be started and 250 µg (0.5 ml) salbutamol (Ventolin) given slowly intravenously or 3 nifedipine (Adalat) 10 mg capsules (30 mg in total) orally, provided there are no contraindications.
3. If there are any signs of fetal distress the patient should be given oxygen by face mask.

Management of impacted shoulders

9-23 Which patients are at high risk of developing impacted shoulders?

The same patients who are at high risk of a prolonged second stage of labour are also at risk of developing impacted shoulders (shoulder dystocia), i.e. women who probably have a large infant.

9-24 What signs during the second stage of labour indicate that the shoulders are impacted?

1. Normally the infant's head is delivered by extension. However, with impacted shoulders the head is held back, does not fall forward on the perineum and does not undergo the normal rotation.
2. The size of the infant's head and cheeks at delivery indicate that the infant is big and fat. Usually the patient is also obese.
3. Attempts at external rotation, lateral flexion and traction fail to deliver the shoulders.

The earlier these signs of impacted shoulders are recognised, the better is the chance that this complication will be successfully managed.

9-25 How should a patient with impacted shoulders be managed?

The following management should be carefully followed in a step-by-step manner:

1. The patient must be told that a serious complication has developed and that she must give the midwife or doctor her full co-operation.
2. The patient should be moved so that her buttocks are over the edge of the bed to allow good downward traction on the fetal head. This can be done rapidly by removing the end of the bed or by turning the patient across the bed.
3. The patient's hips and knees must be fully flexed so that her knees almost touch her shoulders. The midwife or doctor must hold the infant's head between both hands and firmly pull the head down (posteriorly) while an assistant must at the same time press firmly just above the patient's symphysis pubis. The amount of downward traction applied should be gradually increased until a reasonable amount of traction is used. This reduces the risk of a brachial plexus injury. The suprapubic pressure must be firm enough to allow the assistant's hand to pass behind the symphysis pubis. This procedure helps to get the infant's anterior shoulder to pass under the symphysis pubis. The patient must bear down as strongly as possible during these attempts to deliver the shoulders.

4. If the infant is not delivered after two attempts, you should deliver the posterior shoulder:

   ○ The midwife or doctor should place a right hand (if right-handed) or a left hand (if left-handed) posterior to the fetus in the vagina to reach the infant's shoulder. The cavity of the sacrum is the only area which provides space for manipulation.

   ○ The posterior arm of the infant should be followed until the elbow is reached. The arm must be flexed at the elbow and then pulled anteriorly over the chest and out of the vagina. Delivery of the posterior arm also delivers the posterior shoulder.

   ○ The anterior shoulder can now be freed by pulling the infant's head down (posteriorly).

   ○ If the anterior shoulder cannot be released, the infant must be rotated through 180°. During the rotation the infant's head and freed arm should be firmly held. The freed arm will indicate the direction of the rotation, i.e. turn the infant so that the shoulder follows the freed arm. Once the anterior shoulder has been rotated into the hollow of the sacrum, the trapped shoulder can be released by inserting a hand posteriorly, flexing the arm at the elbow, and pulling the arm out of the vagina.

The rules of delivering impacted shoulders must be followed carefully without panicking. If the infant is delivered within 5 minutes of detecting the complication, no brain damage should occur. While the above management helps to reduce the risk of birth injury, fracture of the clavicle or humerus may occur with delivery of the posterior shoulder. This is preferable to an Erb's (brachial) palsy. Time should not be wasted trying other methods which are not effective.

Impaction of the shoulders is a serious complication and requires fast and effective management according to a clear plan.

Managing the newborn infant

9-26 When should you first suction the infant's airways at delivery?

1. An infant with meconium-stained liquor: Once the infant's head has been delivered, do not carry on with the delivery until the infant's mouth and throat have been well suctioned. If necessary hold the shoulders back until the airways have been cleared. Always suction the mouth first before clearing the nose.
2. An infant with clear liquor: Suctioning the infant's airways is not necessary before delivering the shoulders. After delivery suctioning is only needed if the infant does not breathe well.

9-27 What is the immediate management of the infant after a vaginal delivery?

Dry the infant very well and assess whether the infant cries or breathes well. If the infant breathes well, leave the infant on the mother's abdomen and only clamp and cut the umbilical cord after 2 to 3 minutes. If the infant does not breathe well, clamp and cut the cord immediately and move the infant to a convenient place for resuscitation.

Case study 1

A multiparous patient presents in labour at 18:00. The fetal head is palpable 3/5 above the pelvic brim and the cervix is found to be 7 cm dilated. The vaginal examination is repeated at 21:00 when the alert line indicates that the cervix should be fully dilated. The examination confirms that the cervix is fully dilated. However, the fetal head is still not engaged. Preparations are made for the patient to start bearing down.

1. Do you agree that the patient should start bearing down now that she has reached full dilatation of the cervix?

No. She should not start bearing down until the fetal head is fully engaged and has reached the perineum.

2. What symptoms and signs would indicate to you that the patient should start bearing down?

The patient will have an uncontrollable urge to bear down. In addition the fetal head will be engaged on abdominal examination and the fetal head will distend the perineum when the patient bears down.

3. If the abdominal examination shows that the fetal head is not engaged, what conditions must be met when deciding to wait before allowing the patient to bear down?

Fetal distress must be excluded by making sure that there are no late fetal heart rate decelerations. Cephalopelvic disproportion must also be excluded by finding 2+ moulding or less on vaginal examination.

4. How long is it safe to wait for the fetal head to engage?

The patient should be examined again after an hour. If the head is still not engaged, you can wait for a further hour provided that there are still no signs of either cephalopelvic disproportion or fetal distress. Thereafter, a doctor must be called to evaluate the patient. If the prerequisites for an assisted delivery cannot be met, an emergency Caesarean section must be done.

5. Would you manage a primigravida patient in the same way as a multigravida if she reached full cervical dilatation without engagement of the fetal head?

Usually primigravidas only reach full cervical dilatation after the fetal head has engaged. Therefore, there is a greater chance of cephalopelvic disproportion in a primigravida than in a multigravida who may reach full cervical dilatation with an unengaged fetal head.

Case study 2

A patient who progressed normally during the first stage of labour until a cervical dilatation of 7 cm reaches full dilatation of the cervix after a further 5 hours. At the last examination 3/5 of the fetal head is still palpable above the pelvic brim while 3+ moulding is found on vaginal examination. The patient is prepared for the second stage of labour and is asked to bear down with contractions.

1. What complications would you expect when you consider the patient's progress during the first stage of labour?

A prolonged second stage of labour as the patient's progress in labour was slower than expected between 7 cm and full dilatation.

2. What would be the most likely cause of a prolonged second stage in this patient?

Cephalopelvic disproportion as indicated by an unengaged fetal head and 3+ moulding.

3. Do you agree with the decision to allow the patient to bear down because she is fully dilated?

No. As the patient has cephalopelvic disproportion, a Caesarean section must be performed.

4. How should this patient be managed further if she is at a clinic?

She must be referred to a hospital with facilities to perform a Caesarean section.

5. What arrangements must be made to make the transfer of this patient as safe as possible?

The patient must lie on her side and an intravenous infusion must be started. If there are no contraindications, the contractions must be stopped with intravenous salbutamol (Ventolin) or oral nifedipine (Adalat). If there is any concern about the condition of the fetus, the patient must be given face mask oxygen.

Case study 3

A primigravida patient has still not delivered after her cervix has been fully dilated for 45 minutes. The fetal head is not palpable abdominally and bulges the perineum when the patient bears down with contractions. A prolonged second stage is diagnosed and the doctor is called to assess the patient.

1. Do you agree with the diagnosis of prolonged second stage?

This will depend on when the patient started to bear down and whether her attempts at bearing down were effective. The diagnosis is correct if she has been bearing down well for 45 minutes.

2. What should your management be if the patient has been bearing down well for 45 minutes?

As the head is not palpable abdominally and is distending the perineum, an episiotomy should be done. Thereafter, if the infant has not been delivered after a few contractions with the patient bearing down well, a doctor must be called to evaluate the patient for an assisted delivery.

3. Should an episiotomy be done at the delivery of all primigravidas?

No. Only if there is a definite indication for an episiotomy. In this case an episiotomy is indicated as the second stage is prolonged and delivery would probably be rapidly achieved with an episiotomy.

4. The infant is delivered just before an episiotomy is done and after the birth it is noticed that the patient has a second-degree perineal tear. Would it have been preferable to have done an episiotomy?

No. A second-degree tear should not be seen as a complication as it is preferable to an episiotomy. A second-degree tear is easier to repair, heals faster and causes less pain and discomfort than an episiotomy.

5. How would you have managed this patient if the prolonged labour was due to poor co-operation and ineffective attempts at bearing down by the patient?

Good communication between the staff and the patient during the first stage of labour should have established a trusting relationship. The patient should have been told exactly what she should do during the second stage. She should also have been supported, encouraged and praised.

Case study 4

A multigravida patient weighing 110 kg progresses to full cervical dilatation. After 30 minutes in the second stage of labour, the infant's head is delivered with difficulty. The head is held back and does not fall forward on the perineum while rotation of the head does not occur.

1. What complication has occurred during the second stage of labour?

Impaction of the shoulders (i.e. shoulder dystocia).

2. How could this complication have been predicted?

An overweight patient is at risk for developing impacted shoulders as infants born to these patients are often very big.

3. How should this patient be further managed?

The patient's buttocks must be moved to the edge of the bed so that good posterior traction can be applied to the infant's head. This can be done quickly if the end of the bed can be removed or if the patient can be swung around across the bed. The patient's hips and knees should be flexed so that her knees almost reach her shoulders. The infant's head should be firmly held between both hands and pulled downwards (posteriorly) while an assistant, at the same time, presses down over the suprapubic area. The amount of downward traction applied should be gradually increased until a reasonable amount of traction is used.

4. What should the further management be if these attempts to deliver the shoulders are not successful?

An immediate attempt must be made to deliver the infant's posterior arm. The person conducting the delivery must place a hand posterior to the fetus in the vagina, flex the infant's posterior arm at the elbow and pull it out anteriorly over the chest. When the arm is pulled out the posterior shoulder will automatically be delivered as well. The anterior shoulder can now be released by pulling the infant's head downwards.

Skills: Performing and repairing an episiotomy

Objectives

When you have completed this skills chapter you should be able to:

- Perform a mediolateral episiotomy.
- Repair an episiotomy.

Performing an episiotomy

A. The purpose of an episiotomy

1. To aid the delivery of the presenting part when the perineum is tight and causing poor progress in the second stage of labour.
2. To prevent third-degree perineal tears.
3. To allow more space for operative or manipulative deliveries, e.g. forceps or breech deliveries.
4. To shorten the second stage of labour, e.g. with fetal distress.

B. Preparation for an episiotomy

If you anticipate that an episiotomy may be needed, you should inject local anaesthetic into the perineum. An episiotomy should not be done without adequate analgesia. Usually 10–15 ml 1% lignocaine (Xylotox) supplies adequate analgesia for performing an episiotomy. Be very careful that the local anaesthetic is not injected into the presenting part of the fetus.

C. Types of episiotomy

There are two methods of performing an episiotomy:

1. Mediolateral or oblique.
2. Midline.

The midline episiotomy has the danger that it can extend into the rectum to become a third-degree tear while the mediolateral episiotomy often results in more bleeding. This skills chapter will only deal with the mediolateral episiotomy because it is used most frequently, is safe, and requires the least experience.

D. Performing a mediolateral episiotomy

The incision should only be started during a contraction when the presenting part is stretching the perineum. Doing the episiotomy too early may cause severe bleeding and will not immediately assist the delivery. The incision is started in the midline with the scissors pointed 45° away from the anus. It is usually directed to the patient's left but can also be to the right. 2 fingers of the left hand are slipped between the perineum and the presenting part when performing a mediolateral episiotomy.

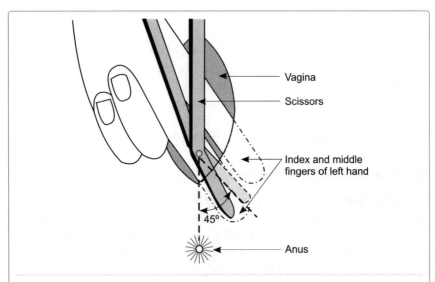

Figure 9A-1: The method of performing a left mediolateral episiotomy

E. Problems with episiotomies

1. The episiotomy is done *too soon*: This can result in excessive bleeding as the presenting part is not pressing on the perineum. An episiotomy will not help the descent of a high head.
2. Extension of the episiotomy by *tearing*: This is not only a problem in a midline episiotomy. Mediolateral episiotomies may also tear through the anal sphincter into the rectum. However, extension of mediolateral episiotomies are less likely to occur than a midline episiotomy.
3. Excessive *bleeding* may occur:
   ○ When the episiotomy is done too early.
   ○ From a mediolateral episiotomy.
   ○ After the delivery.

Arterial bleeders may have to be temporarily clamped, while venous bleeding is easily stopped by packing a swab into the wound. Suturing the episiotomy usually stops the venous bleeding but arterial bleeders need to be tied off.

Repairing an episiotomy

F. Preparations for repairing an episiotomy

1. This is an uncomfortable procedure for the patient. Therefore, it is essential to explain to her what is going to be done.
2. The patient should be put into the lithotomy position if possible.
3. It is essential to have a good light that must be able to shine into the vagina. A normal ceiling light usually is not adequate.
4. Good analgesia is essential and is usually provided by local anaesthesia which is given before the episiotomy is performed. As 20 ml of 1% lignocaine may be safely infiltrated, 5–10 ml usually remains to be given in sensitive areas. An episiotomy should not be sutured until there is good analgesia of the site.

5. In order to prevent blood which drains out of the uterus from obscuring the episiotomy site, a rolled pad or tampon should be carefully inserted into the vagina above the episiotomy wound. As this is uncomfortable for the patient, she should be reassured while this is being done.
6. Absorbable suture material should be used for the repair. Three packets of chromic 0 are required. Two on a round (taper) needle for the vaginal epithelium and muscles, and one on a cutting needle for the skin. With smaller episiotomies one packet on a round needle and one on a cutting needle may be sufficient. Non-absorbable suture material such as nylon and dermalon are very uncomfortable and should not be used. Remember that the patient has to sit on her wound.

G. The following important principles apply to the suturing of an episiotomy

1. The apex (highest point) of the episiotomy must be visualised and a suture put in at the apex.
2. Dead space must be closed.
3. The same opposing tissue must be brought together using the skin vaginal epithelium juncture as an anatomical landmark.
4. Tissues must be brought together but not strangulated by excessive tension on the sutures.
5. Haemostasis must be obtained.
6. The needles must be handled with a pair of forceps and not by hand, and should be removed from the operating field as soon as possible.

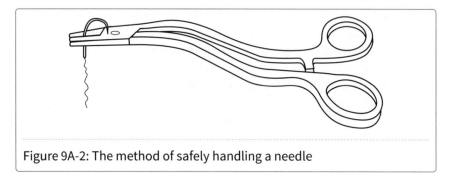

Figure 9A-2: The method of safely handling a needle

H. The method of suturing an episiotomy

Three layers have to be repaired:

1. The vaginal epithelium.
2. The muscles.
3. The perineal skin.

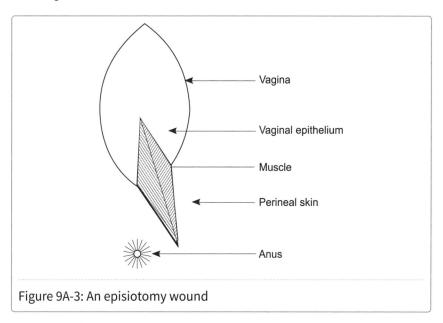

Figure 9A-3: An episiotomy wound

There are four important steps in the repair of an episiotomy wound.

Step 1: Place a suture (stitch) at the apex of the incision in the vaginal epithelium. Then insert one or two more continuous sutures in the vaginal epithelium. Do not complete suturing the vaginal epithelium when the episiotomy is large or deeply cut but leave this suture and do not cut it. When placing the suture at the apex, be very careful not to prick your finger with the needle.

Step 2: Insert interrupted sutures in the muscles. Start at the apex of the wound. The aim is to bring the muscles together firmly and to eliminate any 'dead space', i.e. any spaces between the muscles where blood can collect. Remember that the sutures must be inserted at 90 degrees to the line of the wound.

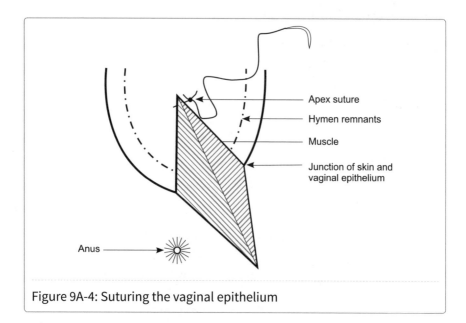

Figure 9A-4: Suturing the vaginal epithelium

When suturing the muscles, be careful not to put the suture through the rectum. If you make sure that the point of the needle is seen when crossing from the one side to the other of the deepest part of the wound, the stitch will not be too deep. 'Figure 8' stitches (double stitches) are used to suture the muscle layer. When the muscles have been correctly sutured the cut edges of the vaginal epithelium and the skin should be lying close together. The markers for correct alignment are:

1. The remains of the hymen.
2. The junction of the skin and the vaginal epithelium. The skin is recognised by the darker pigmentation.

Step 3: Return to the vaginal epithelium and complete the continuous catgut suture, ending at the junction with the skin. Do not pull the sutures tight as they only need to bring the edges of the vaginal epithelium together.

Step 4: Use interrupted sutures with an absorbable suture material to repair the perineal skin. Mattress sutures may be used. Do not pull the sutures tight as they only need to bring the edges of the skin together. Sutures that are too tight become uncomfortable for the patient.

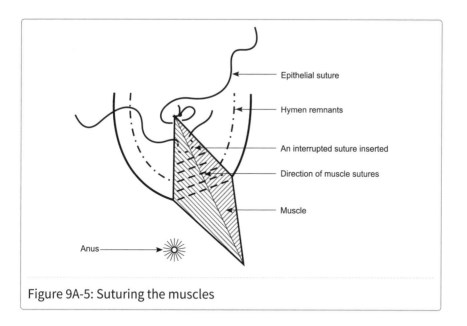

Epithelial suture

Hymen remnants

An interrupted suture inserted

Direction of muscle sutures

Muscle

Anus

Figure 9A-5: Suturing the muscles

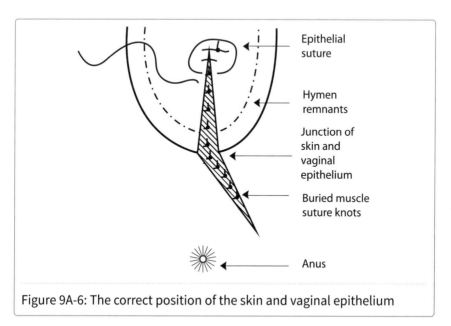

Epithelial suture

Hymen remnants

Junction of skin and vaginal epithelium

Buried muscle suture knots

Anus

Figure 9A-6: The correct position of the skin and vaginal epithelium

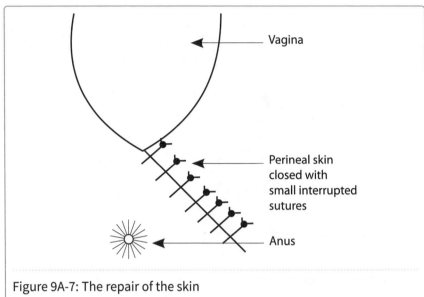

Figure 9A-7: The repair of the skin

When the suturing is complete:

1. Remove the pad from the vagina. Be gentle as this will be uncomfortable for the patient.
2. Put a finger into the rectum and feel if a suture has been placed through the rectal wall by mistake.
3. Make sure that the uterus is well contracted.
4. Get the patient out of the lithotomy position and make sure that she is comfortable.

10

Managing pain during labour

Take the chapter test before and after you read this chapter.

Objectives

When you have completed this unit you should be able to:

- Explain the differences between analgesia, anaesthesia and sedation.
- List the causes of pain in labour.
- List which drugs can be given during labour for analgesia.
- Ensure that a patient has adequate pain relief during labour.
- List the dangers of the drugs which can be used for pain relief.
- Prepare a patient for general anaesthesia.

Pain relief in labour

10-1 What is analgesia?

Analgesia means the relief of pain. Drugs used to relieve pain are called analgesics. Analgesics must not be confused with sedatives which do not relieve pain but only make the patient drowsy.

10-2 What is anaesthesia?

Anaesthesia means the loss of all sensation, including pain. Local anaesthesia causes the loss of all sensation in that region of the body. With general anaesthesia the patient loses consciousness.

10-3 What causes pain during labour?

Pain in labour is caused by:

1. Contractions. They progressively increase in duration and frequency during the first stage of labour and become more painful. Contractions are most painful when the cervix is fully dilated and the patient has an urge to bear down. At first the pain is felt over the abdomen but later, when the cervix is nearly fully dilated, pain is felt in the lower back.
2. Cervical dilatation: This is due to uterine contractions and pressure of the presenting part on the cervix.
3. Vaginal examinations and procedures: Any vaginal examination is uncomfortable and for many patients is also painful. This is particularly so when a forceps delivery, a vacuum extraction, or an episiotomy is performed.

The amount of pain experienced by patients in labour is very variable. Some patients have little pain, while others have severe pain, even during early labour.

10-4 What will make the pain worse?

Anxiety, fear and uncertainty lower the pain threshold. This is particularly noticeable in primigravida patients, especially if they are very young. Pain increases the patient's anxiety, which in turn reduces her ability to tolerate pain.

10-5 What general measures help to reduce pain during labour?

1. Knowledge of what to expect during labour. This important information should be provided during antenatal visits to patients who will be experiencing labour for the first time.
2. A pleasant environment and the support and encouragement of those who are attending to the patient.
3. The help and support of a family member, partner, friend, or doula is of great value.
4. Allowing patients to walk around during labour.

10-6 Why is environmental and emotional support important to a patient in labour?

A patient should be prepared for her labour during the antenatal period. Primigravidas must be told in simple terms what is going to happen during labour. Relaxation exercises and breathing methods can help patients prepare for labour, and should be taught as part of antenatal care.

During labour, particularly during the latent phase and early in the active phase of the first stage, patients may be encouraged to walk around and not spend all the time in bed in the labour ward. This reduces the amount of pain experienced during contractions. In addition, contractions will be more effective, resulting in labour progressing faster.

A calm, considerate and caring attitude from those who are attending the patient in labour is important. Thorough but gentle clinical examinations, rubbing the patient's back and talking to her all do much to relieve the stress of labour and to some extent, the pain.

Most patients find it helpful to have someone with them during labour. A lay person or doula can fulfill this role perfectly well. A patient should be encouraged to have her partner, a family member, or someone else that she knows well to stay with her during labour.

Antenatal preparation and emotional support are important in reducing anxiety and pain during labour.

10-7 Why is it important that labour should be a positive experience?

1. The chances of breastfeeding successfully are increased.
2. Patients will manage their infants with greater confidence and master the art of motherhood quicker.

10-8 Why does a patient get pain relief in labour if her lower back is rubbed?

The nerve impulses that come from the lower back travel to the same spinal segments as the nerves from the uterus and cervix. The nerve impulses from the lower back, therefore partially block those from the uterus and cervix.

As a result, the pain of contractions is experienced as less painful by the patient if her lower back is rubbed.

Use of analgesics in labour

10-9 Why do you need to give a patient analgesia during labour?

1. As health workers, one of our primary responsibilities is to relieve pain and suffering. All too often pain during labour is regarded as part of a normal process. Therefore, during labour patients should frequently be asked whether they need pain relief. If required, the most appropriate and effective form of analgesia available must be given.
2. The relief of pain often allows labour to progress more rapidly by reducing the anxiety which is caused by pain. It is well known that anxiety may cause poor progress during labour.

> The relief of pain is very important and must receive careful attention when a patient is cared for during labour.

10-10 Should all patients receive analgesia?

No. Some patients have little pain in labour and, therefore, may not need an analgesic. Other patients feel that they are able to tolerate the pain of uterine contractions, e.g. by concentrating on their breathing, and choose not to have analgesia. It is important to consider the patient's wishes when deciding whether or not to give analgesia. However, most patients do need analgesia during labour.

10-11 When do you give analgesia to a patient in labour?

1. In the first stage of labour:
   ○ When patients ask for pain relief.
   ○ When patients experience painful uterine contractions during a normal labour.

- When patients have painful contractions and in addition require oxytocin stimulation of labour.
- When patients have painful contractions with slow progress during the active phase of the first stage of labour, e.g. with an occipito-posterior position.

2. In the second stage of labour:
   - When an episiotomy is done.
   - When an instrumental delivery is done.

3. In the third stage of labour:
   - When an episiotomy or perineal tear is repaired.

10-12 What methods of providing analgesia can you use?

1. General measures, as mentioned in sections 10-5 and 10-6.
2. Specific methods:
   - Opiates, e.g. pethidine.
   - Inhalational analgesia, i.e. nitrous oxide with oxygen.
   - Local anaesthesia.
   - Epidural anaesthesia.
   - General anaesthesia.

10-13 Which analgesic drug is commonly used in the first stage of labour?

Pethidine. This drug is a powerful analgesic but commonly causes nausea and vomiting as a side effect. Pethidine also produces some sedation.

10-14 What drug is often given together with pethidine?

Promethazine (Phenergan) or hydroxyzine (Aterax). They combine well with pethidine for three reasons:

1. They have a tranquillising effect which makes the patient feel more relaxed.
2. They have an anti-emetic effect, reducing the nausea and vomiting caused by pethidine.
3. They increase the analgesic effect of pethidine.

The dose of promethazine is 25 mg and hydroxyzine is 100 mg, irrespective of the amount of pethidine given.

10-15 What are the actions of pethidine?

It is a powerful analgesic which causes depression of the central nervous system. Large doses can therefore cause respiratory depression. A drop in blood pressure may also occur. Pethidine crosses the placenta and can cause respiratory depression in the newborn infant who may, therefore, need resuscitation at birth.

Morphine, which is less commonly used, has similar actions and side effects to pethidine.

NOTE
Pethidine and morphine may temporarily affect the cardiotocogram with the fetal heart rate tracing showing loss of beat-to-beat variation.

An overdose of pethidine may cause respiratory depression in both the mother and her infant.

10-16 How is pethidine usually given and how long is its duration of action?

1. The intramuscular route:
   - This is the commonest method of giving pethidine, especially with a cervical dilatation of less than 7 cm.
   - Pain relief will be experienced about 30 minutes after administration and the duration of action will be about 4 hours, although this varies from patient to patient.

2. The intravenous route:
   - This method may be used if the patient requires analgesia urgently and the cervix is already 7 cm or more dilated.
   - Pain relief is experienced within 5 minutes and the duration of action will be about 2 hours.

10-17 What dose of pethidine should be given?

1. The intramuscular route: 2 mg/kg body weight. Therefore, 100 to 150 mg is usually given. Patients weighing less than 50 kg must receive 75 mg.
2. The intravenous route: 1 mg/kg body weight. Therefore, 50 to 75 mg is usually given. Obese patients weighing more than 75 kg must not receive more than 75 mg. An intravenous infusion must first be started before the drug is given.

10-18 How close to full dilatation may pethidine be given?

There is no limit to how late in labour pethidine can be given. If the patient needs analgesia she should be given the appropriate dose. However, if she receives pethidine within 6 hours of delivery, the infant may have respiratory depression at birth.

Pethidine may be given late in labour if needed.

10-19 How often may pethidine be given in labour?

If an adequate dose of intramuscular pethidine is given, it is usually not necessary to repeat the drug within 4 hours. (In South Africa registered nurses are allowed by law to give 100 mg pethidine by intramuscular injection during labour, without a doctor's prescription, and to repeat the injection after an interval of 4 hours or more.)

Naloxone

10-20 How should you treat respiratory depression due to pethidine in a newborn infant?

Naloxone (Narcan) is a specific antidote to pethidine (and morphine) and will reverse the effects of the drug.

If a patient was given pethidine during labour, and delivers an infant who does not breathe well after birth, the infant should be given naloxone (Narcan). The correct dose of naloxone is 0.1 mg/kg (i.e. 0.25 ml/kg). A 1 ml ampoule contains 0.4 mg naloxone. Therefore, an average-sized infant requires 0.75 ml while a large infant up to 1 ml naloxone. Do not give naloxone to asphyxiated infants whose mothers have not received pethidine (or morphine). Naloxone will not reverse the respiratory depression caused by barbiturates (e.g. phenobarbitone), benzodiazepines (e.g. Valium) or a general anaesthetic.

Research has shown that the previously recommended dose (0.01 mg/kg) of neonatal Narcan is tenfold too low. The use of neonatal Narcan must, therefore, be stopped and replaced with adult Narcan.

> Infants who do not breathe well after delivery should only receive naloxone if their mothers were given pethidine or morphine during labour.

10-21 How should naloxone be given?

Usually naloxone is given to a newborn infant by intramuscular injection into the anterolateral aspect of the thigh. The drug will reverse the effects of pethidine. Meanwhile, it is important to continue ventilating the infant. Naloxone can also be given intravenously. The drug acts more rapidly when given intravenously, e.g. into the umbilical vein.

10-22 Is a single dose of naloxone adequate?

Yes. A single dose of naloxone is almost always adequate to reverse the respiratory depression caused by pethidine. The action lasts about 30 minutes. Some infants may become lethargic after 30 minutes and may then require a second dose of naloxone.

Sedation during labour

10-23 Are sedatives useful in labour?

In practice there are very few indications for the use of sedatives in labour. If a patient is restless or distressed, it is almost always because of pain and she therefore needs analgesia. The tranquillising effect of promethazine

(Phenergan) or hydroxyzine (Aterax) together with pethidine will provide sufficient sedation for a restless patient. The dose is 25 mg promethazine (Phenergan) and 100 mg hydroxyzine (Aterax).

There is no role for sedation with diazepam (Valium) and barbiturates. Sedatives may also cross the placenta and sedate the infant. Diazepam (Valium) can cause severe respiratory depression in the infant and this effect is not reversed by naloxone.

Inhalational analgesia

10-24 What inhalational analgesia is available?

The most commonly used inhalational analgesic is Entonox. This is a mixture of 50% nitrous oxide and 50% oxygen. It is usually supplied in cylinders and is breathed in by the patient through a mask when she needs pain relief.

The advantages of Entonox are:

1. It is safe for mother and fetus.
2. It is short acting.
3. It acts quickly.

The disadvantages of Entonox are:

1. It is expensive.
2. It requires special apparatus for administration.
3. It is not always effective because the patient needs to start inhaling the gas as soon as the contraction starts for the analgesic effect to be present during the peak of the contraction. Many patients start the inhalation too late.
4. Patients often hyperventilate and get 'pins and needles' in their face and hands.

10-25 Which patients should preferably use Entonox?

A patient requiring analgesia for the first time in advanced labour, where the delivery is expected within an hour.

10-26 Does Entonox have any serious side effects?

No. Entonox is completely safe and cannot be used in excessive doses.

> Entonox is a completely safe analgesic.

Local anaesthesia

10-27 What is a local anaesthetic?

Local anaesthetics are drugs which are injected into the tissues and which result in a loss of all sensation in the injected area. Local anaesthetics often give a burning sensation which lasts 1 to 2 minutes while they are being injected. The patient should be warned about this before starting the injection.

Lignocaine (Xylocaine) is the local anaesthetic used most commonly. Although available in different concentrations it is best to *only* use the 1% solution. The possibility of giving an overdose will then be reduced.

10-28 When should you use a local anaesthetic?

There are two main indications for local anaesthesia in labour:

1. When performing an episiotomy, or when repairing an episiotomy or perineal tear.
2. When performing a pudendal block. The local anaesthetic acts on the pudendal nerves, and is usually given before an instrumental delivery.

10-29 What are the risks of local anaesthesia?

1. Too much local anaesthetic is dangerous and may cause convulsions. The maximum dose of a 1% solution of lignocaine (Xylocaine) for a patient of average size is 20 ml.
2. A local anaesthetic can cause convulsions if it is injected into a vein in error.

The maximum safe dose of lignocaine is 3 mg/kg body weight. 1 ml of a 1% lignocaine solution contains 10 mg lignocaine.

> An overdose, or intravenous injection, of a local anaesthetic may cause convulsions.

10-30 What is the duration of action of lignocaine?

Lignocaine results in loss of sensation in the infiltrated area for 45 minutes. If the maximum dose has already been given but more local anaesthetic is required, a further 10 ml of 1% lignocaine may be given after 30 minutes.

Epidural anaesthesia

10-31 What are the indications for epidural anaesthesia?

1. When there is poor progress during the active phase of the first stage of labour, e.g. due to an occipito-posterior position.
2. When ineffective uterine contractions are present, prior to starting oxytocin.
3. When it is important to prevent bearing down before a patient's cervix is fully dilated, e.g. with a preterm infant or a breech presentation.
4. Caesarean sections may also be done under epidural anaesthesia.

This is the ideal form of local anaesthesia as it offers the patient complete pain relief. Unfortunately special training and equipment are necessary for giving epidural anaesthesia and, therefore, it is only available in most level 2 and 3 hospitals.

10-32 What special nursing care is required following an epidural anaesthetic?

1. There is a danger of hypotension following the administration of the first and each further dose of the local anaesthetic. The patient's blood pressure must be taken every 5 minutes for 30 minutes following each dose of the local anaesthetic.
2. Depending on the amount of anaesthesia achieved, patients often cannot pass urine. A Foley catheter is therefore often required until the effect of the anaesthesia wears off.

General anaesthesia

10-33 What are the dangers for a pregnant or postpartum patient when receiving a general anaesthetic?

Any pregnant or postpartum patient who receives a general anaesthetic has a very high risk of vomiting and aspirating her stomach contents because:

1. Stomach emptying is delayed.
2. The tone of the sphincter in the lower oesophagus is reduced.
3. The intra-abdominal pressure is increased.

Patients who have been starved must be managed in the same way as patients who have recently eaten. During a general anaesthetic, the risk of the patient vomiting is particularly high during intubation and extubation.

10-34 What precautions must be taken preoperatively that will reduce the dangers of vomiting?

1. A patient who may require a general anaesthetic should be kept nil per mouth (i.e. she should be starved).

2. Metoclopramide (Maxalon) 20 mg (2 ampoules) should be given intravenously 15 minutes before the induction of general anaesthesia. Metoclopramide is an anti-emetic (prevents vomiting) which speeds up the emptying of the stomach and increases the tone of the lower oesophagus. The drug acts for about 2 hours.
3. The gastric acid must be neutralised by an antacid before the induction of general anaesthesia. Usually 30 ml of a 0.3 molar solution of sodium citrate is given. If induction of anaesthesia is not started within 30 minutes of the sodium citrate being given, the 30 ml dose should be repeated.

NOTE
Sodium citrate is cheap and can be made up by any pharmacist. It is an electrolyte solution and therefore preferable to other antacids which contain particles that can cause a chemical pneumonitis if the drug is aspirated.

Case study 1

A patient and her husband present at the maternity hospital. She is 26 years old, gravida 2 para 1 and at term. Her antenatal course has been normal and her routine observations on admission are also normal. The fetal presentation is cephalic with 2/5 of the fetal head palpable above the pelvic brim. The membranes rupture spontaneously and her cervix is found to be 5 cm dilated on vaginal examination. The patient is relaxed and does not find her contractions painful. She is admitted to the labour ward and given 100 mg pethidine and 25 mg promethazine by intramuscular injection as she is already in the active phase of the first stage of labour. Her husband is asked to wait outside the labour ward. It is suggested that he go home for a while as the infant is unlikely to be born during the next 5 or 6 hours.

1. Has the patient been correctly managed?

No. She did not require analgesia. Not all patients need analgesia during labour. Some patients experience little pain during labour while others handle the pain of contractions with no difficulty.

2. What would have been the correct management of this patient?

The patient should have been reassured that her labour was progressing normally. She should have been encouraged to walk about and not spend all the time in bed. Analgesia need not be given routinely to all patients in active labour.

3. Do you agree with the handling of the patient's husband?

No. Most patients prefer to have someone they know well remain with them during labour. Her husband should have been encouraged to stay with her if that was what the patient wanted.

4. What should the husband do if he stays with his wife during labour?

Simply being there is reassuring to the patient. He can help to keep her relaxed and comfortable. Furthermore, he can be shown how to rub her back during contractions.

5. Is it of any value to rub a patient's back during contractions, or is it only an 'old wives' tale' that has no place in modern midwifery?

Rubbing a patient's lower back is of great help as the nerve impulses that come from the skin over the lower back travel to the same spinal segments as the nerve impulses from the cervix and uterus. The nerve impulses from the lower back partially block those from the uterus and cervix. As a result, the pain of contractions is experienced as less painful by the patient if the lower back is rubbed.

Case study 2

A 16-year-old patient presents in labour at term after a normal pregnancy. She is very anxious, does not co-operate with the labour ward staff and complains of unbearable pain during contractions. She bears down with every contraction even though the cervix is only 4 cm dilated. The patient is told to behave herself. She is informed that the worst part of labour is still to come and is scolded for becoming pregnant. As she is a primigravida, she is promised analgesia when her cervix reaches 6 cm dilatation.

1. Why is the patient frightened?

Because she is unprepared for labour and does not know what to expect. In addition, she is in a strange environment and the staff are unfriendly and aggressive. Being anxious results in her experiencing her contractions as very painful while the pain in turn makes her even more anxious.

2. What should have been done during the antenatal period to avoid the present situation?

Receiving good information about the process of labour at antenatal visits, attending antenatal exercise classes and visiting the labour ward during the last weeks of pregnancy would have resulted in a far more relaxed patient in labour.

3. What should have been done in the labour ward to reduce her anxiety?

She should have experienced a pleasant atmosphere in the labour ward with understanding and encouragement from the staff. They should have reassured her that everything was under control and that there was no reason for her to be frightened. The staff themselves should appear confident, relaxed and caring. It is important that a family member or friend of the patient's remain with her.

4. Should the doctor be informed about the unmanageable patient and be asked to prescribe 10 mg of intravenous diazepam (Valium)?

No. Sedatives, especially diazepam, should be used very rarely because they may result in severe respiratory depression in the infant at birth. This complication is not reversed by the commonly available drugs at delivery.

5. What would have been the correct management of labour for this patient, beside reassurance?

She should have been encouraged to concentrate on her breathing during contractions. In addition she should have been given adequate analgesia as soon as possible.

6. What form of analgesia should have been given to this patient?

The ideal form of analgesia for this patient would have been an epidural anaesthetic as it provides complete pain relief. Alternatively she should have been given pethidine and promethazine (Phenergan) or hydroxyzine (Aterax) by intramuscular injection. The tranquillising effect of promethazine or hydroxyzine would have helped to lessen her anxiety.

Case study 3

Cervical dilatation in a multigravida patient in labour at term progresses from 3 cm to 8 cm in 4 hours. Now for the first time she complains that her contractions are very painful. The midwife informs her that she is progressing fast and that her cervix will soon be fully dilated. She adds that the patient must just continue without analgesia for the last 2 hours as the delivery will soon be over.

1. Do you agree with the patient's management?

No. The patient needs analgesia and the most appropriate form of analgesia should be offered to her.

2. What would be the best form of analgesia to offer this patient?

Entonox (nitrous oxide with oxygen) as it works rapidly and is completely safe. She also only needs analgesia for a short time as her cervix will soon be fully dilated.

3. If Entonox is not available or if the patient is unable to use Entonox correctly, what other form of analgesia should be considered?

Pethidine and promethazine (Phenergan) or hydroxyzine (Aterax).

4. What would be the best route of administering the pethidine to this patient?

The pethidine should preferably be given intravenously. Pain relief will then be obtained in 5 minutes and the effect of the drug should last 2 hours.

5. The infant is delivered 45 minutes after the pethidine is given. What complication of the drug may be present in the infant at delivery?

The infant may have respiratory depression and as a result may not breathe adequately at birth.

6. How should the infant be managed if the breathing is inadequate (i.e. the infant has asphyxia)?

The infant must be resuscitated with oxygen and artificial respiration provided via a face mask or endotracheal tube. Naloxone (Narcan) must be given to the infant to reverse the effect of the pethidine. Naloxone is usually given by intramuscular injection. However, it acts more rapidly if it is injected into the umbilical vein.

Case study 4

A multigravida patient, who has had two previous Caesarean sections, is booked for an elective Caesarean section under general anaesthesia at 39 weeks gestation. The patient is admitted to hospital at 07:00, having had nothing to eat since 24:00 the previous night. She is prepared for surgery at 08:00. As the patient has been kept nil per mouth, no drug to prevent vomiting during intubation and extubation is given. Only an intravenous infusion is started and a Foley catheter passed before she is moved to theatre.

1. Do you agree that a drug to prevent vomiting is not needed as the patient has had nothing to eat or drink for 8 hours?

No. All pregnant patients are at risk of vomiting during general anaesthesia even if they have taken nothing by mouth during the past few hours.

2. Why should a pregnant patient who has not eaten overnight still be at risk of vomiting during a general anaesthetic?

Because her stomach has a delayed emptying time, the lower oesophageal tone is reduced and she has a raised intra-abdominal pressure.

3. What preventative measures should have been carried out during the pre-operative preparation of the patient for theatre?

Metoclopramide (Maxalon) 20 mg (2 ampoules) should have been given intravenously 15 minutes before the induction of anaesthesia. It is anti-emetic, it increases the stomach emptying time, and raises the sphincter tone of the lower oesophagus. These effects will reduce the danger of vomiting. An antacid should also be given before the general anaesthetic. The drug of choice is 30 ml of a 0.3 molar solution of sodium citrate.

4. Both these drugs are given at 07:45. However, due to a delay, the patient is only taken to theatre at 08:30. Is it necessary to repeat either of these drugs?

The metoclopramide (Maxalon) acts for 2 hours so need not be repeated. However, the sodium citrate only acts for 30 minutes and, therefore, must be repeated before the start of the anaesthetic.

The third stage of labour

Take the chapter test before and after you read this chapter.

Objectives

When you have completed this unit you should be able to:

- Define the third stage of labour.
- Manage the third stage of labour.
- List the observations needed during the third stage of labour.
- Examine a placenta after delivery.
- Manage a patient with a prolonged third stage of labour.
- Manage a patient with a retained placenta.
- List the causes of postpartum haemorrhage.
- Manage a patient with postpartum haemorrhage.
- Prevent infection of the staff with HIV at delivery.

The normal third stage of labour

11-1 What is the third stage of labour?

The third stage of labour starts immediately after the delivery of the infant and ends with the delivery of the placenta and membranes.

11-2 How long does the normal third stage of labour last?

The normal duration of the third stage of labour depends on the method used to deliver the placenta. It usually lasts less than 30 minutes, and mostly only 2 to 5 minutes.

11-3 What happens during the third stage of labour?

1. Uterine contractions continue, although less frequently than in the second stage.
2. The uterus contracts and becomes smaller and, as a result, the placenta separates.
3. The placenta is squeezed out of the upper uterine segment into the lower uterine segment and vagina. The placenta is then delivered.
4. The contraction of the uterine muscle compresses the uterine blood vessels and this prevents bleeding. Thereafter, clotting (coagulation) takes place in the uterine blood vessels due to the normal clotting mechanism.

11-4 Why is the third stage of labour important?

Excessive bleeding is a common complication during the third stage of labour. Therefore, the third stage, if not correctly managed, can be an extremely dangerous time for the patient. Postpartum haemorrhage is the commonest cause of maternal death in some developing countries.

> The third stage of labour can be a very dangerous time and, therefore, must be correctly managed.

Managing the third stage of labour

11-5 How should the third stage of labour be managed?

There are two ways of managing the third stage of labour:

1. The active method.
2. The passive method.

Whenever possible, the active method should be used. However, a midwife working on her own may need to use the passive method.

Midwives who choose to use the passive method of managing the third stage of labour *must* also be able to confidently use the active method, as this method may have to be used in some patients.

11-6 What is the active management of the third stage of labour?

1. Immediately after the delivery of the infant, an abdominal examination is done to exclude a second twin.
2. An oxytocic drug is given if no second twin is present.
3. When the uterus contracts, controlled cord traction must be applied:
   - Keep steady tension on the umbilical cord with one hand.
   - Place the other hand just above the symphysis pubis and push the uterus upwards.

NOTE
Controlled cord traction is also called the Brandt-Andrews method (manoeuvre).

4. Placental separation will take place when the uterus contracts. When controlled cord traction is applied the placenta will be delivered from the upper segment of the uterus.
5. Once this occurs, continuous light traction on the umbilical cord will now deliver the placenta from the lower uterine segment or vagina.
6. If placental separation does not take place during the first uterine contraction after giving the oxytocic drug, wait until the next contraction occurs and then repeat the manoeuvre.

11-7 Which oxytocic drug is usually given during the third stage of labour?

One of the following two drugs is generally given:

1. Oxytocin (Syntocinon) 10 units. This is given intramuscularly. It is not necessary to protect this drug against direct light. Although the drug must also be kept in a refrigerator, it has a shelf life of 1 month at room temperature.
2. Syntometrine. This is given by intramuscular injection after the delivery of the infant. Syntometrine is supplied in a 1 ml ampoule which contains a mixture of 5 units oxytocin and 0.5 mg ergometrine maleate. The drug must be protected from direct light at all times and must be kept in a

refrigerator. At all times the ampoules must, therefore, be kept in an opaque container in the refrigerator.

Oxytocin (Syntocinon) is the drug of choice. However, as Syntometrine is still generally prescribed, the correct use thereof will also be explained.

NOTE
The latest information in the Cochrane Library indicates that the best drug and dosage to use is oxytocin 10 units.

11-8 What are the actions of the two components of Syntometrine?

1. Oxytocin causes physiological uterine contractions which start 2 to 3 minutes after an intramuscular injection and continue for approximately 1 to 3 hours.
2. Ergometrine causes a tonic contraction of the uterus which starts 5 to 6 minutes after an intramuscular injection and continues for about 3 hours.

11-9 What are the contraindications to the use of Syntometrine?

Syntometrine contains ergometrine and, therefore, should not be used if:

1. The patient is hypertensive. Ergometrine causes vasospasm which may result in a severe increase in the blood pressure.
2. The patient has heart valve disease. Tonic contraction of the uterus pushes a large volume of blood into the patient's circulation, which may cause heart failure with pulmonary oedema.

Make sure that there are no contraindications before using Syntometrine.

11-10 What oxytocic drug should be used if there is a contraindication to the use of Syntometrine?

Oxytocin (Syntocinon) should be used. An intravenous infusion of 10 units oxytocin in 200 ml normal saline is given at a rate of 30 drops per minute (20 drops per ml dropper) or 10 units oxytocin are given by intramuscular injection.

11-11 What is the passive method of managing the third stage of labour?

1. After delivery of the infant the signs of placental separation are waited for.
2. When the signs of placental separation appear, the patient is asked to bear down and the placenta is delivered spontaneously, by maternal effort only.
3. Only after the placenta has been delivered is an oxytocic drug given.

11-12 What are the signs of placental separation?

1. Uterine contraction.
2. The fundus of the uterus rises in the abdomen, when the placenta moves from the upper segment of the uterus to the lower segment and vagina.
3. Lengthening of the umbilical cord. This sign is most easily seen if the cord is clamped with forceps at the vulva. Any lengthening of the umbilical cord above the forceps is then easily noticed.
4. An amount of blood suddenly escapes from the vagina.

Separation of the placenta can now be confirmed by applying suprapubic pressure. The placenta has definitely separated if the umbilical cord does not shorten when the uterus is pushed up (no cord retraction).

11-13 What are the advantages and disadvantages of the active method of managing the third stage of labour?

Advantages:

1. Blood loss is less than when the passive method is used.
2. There is less possibility that oxytocin will be needed to contract the uterus following the third stage of labour.

Disadvantages:

1. The person actively managing the third stage of labour must not leave the patient. Therefore, an assistant is needed to give the oxytocic drug and examine the newborn infant, while the person conducting the delivery continues with the management of the third stage of labour.

2. The risk of a retained placenta is increased if the active method is not carried out correctly, especially if the first two contractions after the delivery of the infant are not used to deliver the placenta.
3. Excessive traction on the umbilical cord can result in inversion of the uterus, especially if the fundus of the uterus is not supported by placing a hand above the bladder on the abdomen.

11-14 What are the advantages and disadvantages of the passive method of managing the third stage of labour?

Advantages:

1. No assistant is needed.
2. A retained placenta is less common than with the active method.

Disadvantages:

1. Blood loss is greater than with the active method.
2. The active method may be needed anyway, if:
   ○ there is excessive bleeding before delivery of the placenta.
   ○ the placenta does not separate spontaneously.

11-15 When should the active method be used and when should the passive method be used in the management of the third stage of labour?

The *active* method:

1. Midwives and doctors working in level 2 and 3 hospitals usually use the active method, as an assistant is generally available at delivery.
2. This method should be used when dealing with intermediate- and high-risk patients.

The *passive* method:

1. Midwives working in a peripheral clinic or level 1 hospital may find this method useful, when they do not have an assistant while conducting a delivery.
2. This method is safe in most low-risk patients managed in clinics and hospitals.

11-16 How long can you safely wait for signs of placental separation, if the passive method of managing the third stage is used?

If the signs of placental separation have still not appeared 30 minutes after the start of the third stage of labour, then an oxytocic drug must be given and the active management of the third stage must be used.

11-17 Should the umbilical cord be allowed to bleed before the placenta is delivered or should the forceps be left in place on the umbilical cord?

1. The umbilical cord must *not* be allowed to bleed after the delivery of the first infant in a multiple pregnancy. In identical twins with a single placenta (monochorionic placenta), the undelivered second twin may bleed to death if the umbilical cord of the firstborn infant is allowed to bleed.
2. The umbilical cord should be allowed to bleed if the patient's blood group is Rhesus negative (Rh negative) with a single fetus. This will reduce the risk of fetal blood crossing the placenta to the mother's circulation and, thereby, sensitising the patient. Nevertheless, anti-D immunoglobulin must always be given to these patients.
3. Allowing the umbilical cord to bleed during the third stage of labour reduces the placental volume and, thereby, speeds up the separation of the placenta. As a general rule, the umbilical cord should be allowed to bleed once a multiple pregnancy has been excluded.

11-18 What recordings must always be made during and after the third stage of labour?

1. Recordings made about the third stage of labour:
   ○ Duration of the third stage.
   ○ The amount of blood lost.
   ○ Medication given.
   ○ The condition of the perineum and the presence of any tears.
2. Recordings made immediately after the delivery of the placenta:
   ○ Whether the uterus is well contracted or not.
   ○ Any excessive vaginal bleeding.

- A short note on the suturing of an episiotomy or perineal tear.
- The patient's pulse rate, blood pressure and temperature.
- The completeness of the placenta and membranes, and any placental abnormality.

3. Recordings made during the first hour after the delivery of the placenta:
   - During this time (sometimes called the fourth stage of labour) it is important to record whether the uterus is well contracted and whether there is any excessive bleeding. During the first hour after the completion of the third stage of labour, there is a high risk of postpartum haemorrhage.
   - If the third stage of labour and the observations were normal, the patient's pulse rate and blood pressure should be measured again an hour later.
   - If the third stage of labour was not normal, the observations must be repeated every 15 minutes, until the patient's condition is normal. Thereafter, the observations should be repeated every hour for a further 4 hours.

> During the first hour after the delivery it is essential to ensure that the uterus is well contracted and that there is no excessive bleeding.

11-19 When should the infant be given to the mother to hold and put to the breast?

If the labour and delivery were normal and the infant appears to be healthy and normal, the infant should be put to the breast immediately after delivery. The nipple stimulation causes uterine contractions which may help placental separation.

Examination of the placenta after birth

11-20 How should you examine the placenta after delivery?

Every placenta must be examined for:

1. Completeness.
2. Make sure that both the placenta and the membranes are complete after the delivery of the placenta:
   - The membranes are examined for completeness by holding the placenta up by the umbilical cord so that the membranes hang down. You will see the round hole through which the infant was delivered. Examine the membranes carefully to determine whether they are complete.
   - The placenta is now held in both hands and the maternal surface is inspected after the membranes are folded away. A missing part of the placenta, or cotyledon, is thus easily noticed.
3. Abnormalities.
   - Cloudy membranes, or a placenta that smells offensive, suggests the presence of chorioamnionitis.
   - Clots of blood which adhere to the maternal surface suggest that abruptio placentae has occurred.
4. Size.

   The weight of the placenta increases with gestational age and is usually 1/6 the weight of the infant, i.e. 450–650 g at term.

   If the placenta is abnormally large, the following possibilities must be considered:

   - A heavy, oedematous placenta is suggestive of congenital syphilis.
   - A heavy, pale placenta is suggestive of Rhesus haemolytic disease.
   - A placenta which is heavier than would be expected for the weight of the infant, but with a normal appearance, is suggestive of maternal diabetes.
   - A placenta which is lighter than would be expected for the weight of the infant, is suggestive of fetal intra-uterine growth restriction (IUGR).

5. Umbilical cord.
6. Two arteries and a vein should be seen on the cut end of the umbilical cord. If only one umbilical artery is present, the infant must be carefully examined for other congenital abnormalities.

NOTE
Infarcts can be recognised as firm, pale areas on the maternal surface of the placenta. Calcification on the maternal surface is normal.

All placentas must be carefully examined for completeness and abnormalities after delivery.

The abnormal third stage of labour

11-21 What is a prolonged third stage of labour?

If the placenta has still not been delivered after 30 minutes, the third stage is said to be prolonged.

11-22 How should a prolonged third stage of labour be managed?

If the active or passive method has been applied and failed:

- An infusion with 20 units of oxytocin in 1000 ml Balsol or normal saline must be started and run in rapidly.
- Once the uterus is well contracted, try again to deliver the placenta by controlled cord traction.

11-23 What should be done if the placenta is still not delivered, after the routine management of a prolonged third stage of labour?

A vaginal examination must be done:

1. If the placenta or part of the placenta is palpable in the vagina or lower segment of the uterus, this confirms that the placenta has separated. By pulling on the umbilical cord with one hand, while pushing the fundus

of the uterus upwards with the other hand (i.e. controlled cord traction), the placenta can be delivered.

2. If the placenta or part of the placenta is not palpable in the vagina or lower segment of the uterus and only the umbilical cord is felt, then the placenta is still in the upper segment of the uterus and a diagnosis of retained placenta must be made.

11-24 What is the management of a retained placenta?

1. Continue with the intravenous infusion of oxytocin and make sure that the uterus is well contracted. This will reduce the risk of postpartum haemorrhage.
2. While waiting for the theatre to be ready for transfer of the patient, check continuously whether the uterus remains well contracted and for excessive vaginal bleeding. The blood pressure and pulse must be measured and recorded every 30 minutes.
3. If the patient is at a clinic or a level 1 hospital without an operating theatre, she must be transferred to a level 2 or 3 hospital, for manual removal of the placenta under general anaesthesia.
4. Keep the patient nil per mouth.

Managing postpartum haemorrhage

11-25 What is a postpartum haemorrhage?

1. Blood loss of more than 500 ml within the first 24 hours after delivery of the infant.
2. Any bleeding after delivery, which appears excessive.

Any excessive bleeding after delivery should be considered to be a postpartum haemorrhage and managed as such.

11-26 What should be done if a patient has a postpartum haemorrhage?

The management will depend on whether the placenta has been delivered or not.

11-27 What is the management of a postpartum haemorrhage if the placenta has not been delivered?

1. If the active method has been used to manage the third stage of labour, a rapid intravenous infusion of 20 units oxytocin in 1000 ml Balsol or normal saline must be started, to ensure that the uterus is well contracted. A further attempt should now be made to deliver the placenta. Immediately after the delivery of the placenta, make sure that the uterus is well contracted, by rubbing up the fundus.
2. If the passive method has been used to manage the third stage of labour, a rapid intravenous infusion of 20 units oxytocin in 1000 ml Balsol or normal saline must be given. The placenta is delivered by controlled cord traction, i.e. the active method is used.
3. If the attempt to deliver the placenta fails, the patient has a retained placenta and should be managed correctly.

The management of a patient with a postpartum haemorrhage before the delivery of the placenta is summarised in Figure 11-1.

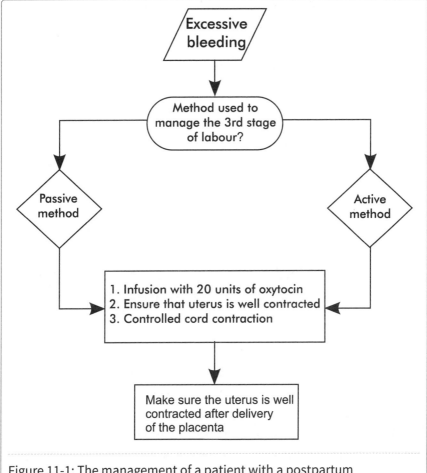

Figure 11-1: The management of a patient with a postpartum haemorrhage before the delivery of the placenta

11-28 What is the management of a patient with a postpartum haemorrhage, if the placenta has already been delivered?

This is a dangerous complication which must be rapidly and correctly managed according to a clear plan:

Step 1: Call for help. One cannot manage a postpartum haemorrhage alone. Someone needs to get the oxytocin, cannulas, infusion sets and intravenous fluids while the other person is controlling the bleeding.

Step 2: The uterus must immediately be rubbed up, (massaged). This will cause the uterus to contract and stop bleeding.

Step 3: A rapid intravenous infusion of 20 units oxytocin in 1000 ml Balsol or normal saline must be started. Once again, make sure that the uterus is well contracted by massaging it.

Step 4: The patient's bladder must be emptied. A full bladder causes the uterus to contract poorly, with resultant haemorrhage.

These four steps must always be carried out, irrespective of the cause of the postpartum haemorrhage. The cause of the haemorrhage must now be diagnosed.

> A postpartum haemorrhage is a dangerous complication and must be managed according to a definite plan.

11-29 What are the main causes of postpartum haemorrhage?

The cause of the haemorrhage must now be diagnosed. The two main causes of postpartum haemorrhage must be differentiated from one another:

1. Haemorrhage due to an atonic (poorly contracted) uterus.
2. Haemorrhage due to trauma, usually in the form of tears (lacerations).

It is very important that the two causes are differentiated from one another as this will determine the correct management.

> The two main causes of postpartum haemorrhage are an atonic uterus and trauma.

The management of a patient with a postpartum haemorrhage after the delivery of the placenta is summarised in Figure 11-2.

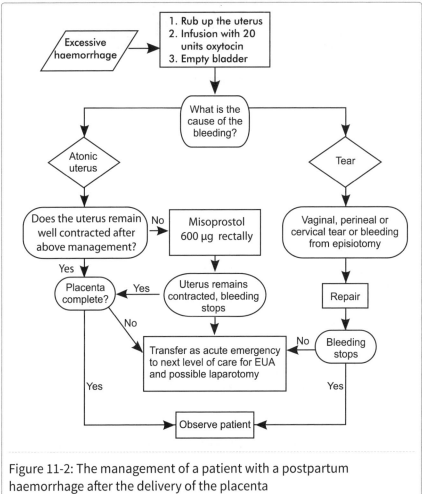

Figure 11-2: The management of a patient with a postpartum haemorrhage after the delivery of the placenta

11-30 What clinical signs indicate that the bleeding is caused by an atonic uterus?

1. The uterus is atonic (feels soft and spongy), or tends to become atonic after it is rubbed up or after an oxytocin infusion is given.
2. The bleeding is intermittent and consists mainly of dark red clots.
3. If the uterus is rubbed up and becomes well contracted, a large amount of dark red blood clots escapes from the vagina.

> Bleeding from an atonic uterus occurs in episodes and consists of dark red blood clots.

11-31 What are the possible causes of an atonic uterus?

1. A uterus full of blood clots is the commonest cause.
2. A full bladder.
3. Retained placental cotyledons.
4. Factors during the pregnancy, which resulted in an abnormally large uterus:
   - A large infant.
   - A multiple pregnancy.
   - Polyhydramnios.
5. A prolonged first stage of labour.
6. The intravenous infusion of oxytocin during the first stage of labour.
7. General anaesthesia.
8. Grande multiparity.
9. Abruptio placentae.

> The commonest causes of an atonic uterus are a uterus full of blood clots and a full bladder.

11-32 What is the correct management of postpartum haemorrhage if the clinical signs indicate bleeding from an atonic uterus?

1. Rub up the uterus, empty the patient's bladder and start a fast intravenous infusion of 20 units oxytocin in 1000 ml Basol or normal saline.
2. If the uterus still tends to relax, examine the placenta again to check whether it is complete.
3. If the placenta is not complete, manage the patient as detailed in section 11-33.
4. If the placenta is complete and the uterus remains poorly contracted, a doctor must be called urgently to examine the patient. If no doctor is available, the patient must be referred to a hospital with theatre

facilities. This is an extremely serious complication, which could result in the patient's death. While waiting for the doctor, or arranging transfer, the following management must be followed:

- Start a second, rapidly running, intravenous infusion and take a sample of blood for urgent cross-matching. A blood transfusion must be started as soon as possible.
- The uterus must be manually compressed between a hand over the uterus abdominally and the other hand, palm upwards, in the anterior fornix of the vagina. This should control the bleeding, until a doctor can attend to the patient or until she reaches a level 2 hospital.
- Lie the patient flat, or in the head-down position and give oxygen by means of a face mask.

5. Place 3 misoprostol (Cytotec) tablets (1 tablet = 200 µg) in the patient's rectum.

NOTE
Further management includes an intravenous infusion of prostaglandin F2 alpha to stimulate uterine contractions. The need for a total abdominal hysterectomy may have to be considered.

11-33 What should be done if the membranes or placenta are not complete after delivery and the patient is not bleeding?

1. Incomplete membranes usually do not cause any complications.
2. An incomplete placenta with one or more cotyledons missing can cause a postpartum haemorrhage due to an atonic uterus. Therefore, manage as follows:

- An intravenous infusion of 20 units oxytocin in 1000 ml Balsol or normal saline must be started to make sure that the uterus is well contracted.
- Inform a doctor or transfer the patient to a hospital with theatre facilities to evacuate the uterus.
- Keep the patient nil per mouth, as a general anaesthetic will be necessary.

An evacuation of the uterus under general anaesthesia is required if placental cotyledons are retained in the uterus.

11-34 What can be done to reduce the risk of postpartum haemorrhage?

In patients who are at high risk of postpartum haemorrhage (e.g. multiple pregnancy, polyhydramnios or grande multiparity) the following should be done:

1. An intravenous infusion should be started during the active phase of the first stage of labour.
2. 20 units of oxytocin in 1000 ml Basol or normal saline should be given by rapid infusion after the placenta has been delivered.
3. Make sure that the uterus is well contracted during the first hour after the delivery of the placenta and make sure that the patient empties her bladder frequently.

11-35 What clinical signs indicate that the bleeding is from a tear?

1. The uterus is well contracted.
2. A continuous trickle of bright red blood comes from the uterus in spite of a well-contracted uterus.

> Bleeding from a tear causes a continuous trickle of bright red blood in spite of a well-contracted uterus.

11-36 What is the correct management if the clinical signs indicate that the bleeding is from a tear?

The patient should be placed in the lithotomy position and examined as follows:

1. First the perineum must be examined for a tear and for bleeding from an episiotomy. Repair any tear or episiotomy.
2. Thereafter, the vagina must be examined for a tear using the index finger of each hand to hold the vagina open. If available, a Werdheim's retractor is helpful in examining the vagina. If a tear is found it must be sutured.
3. If a perineal or vaginal tear cannot be found, a cervical tear or even a ruptured uterus may be present. Therefore, a doctor must be called to

examine the patient or she should be transferred to a hospital so that these conditions can be excluded.

11-37 What is the correct management for bleeding from an episiotomy?

1. If the episiotomy has not yet been stitched, it should be repaired. Make sure that all bleeding stops.
2. If the episiotomy has already been repaired, the stitches must be removed and the bleeding vessels must be identified and tied off. Then the episiotomy must be resutured.

11-38 Which patients are at high risk of a cervical tear?

1. Patients who bear down and deliver an infant before the cervix is fully dilated.
2. Patients with a rapid labour when the cervix dilates very quickly (a precipitous delivery).
3. Patients who have an instrument delivery.

11-39 How can you recognise an inverted uterus?

1. The diagnosis must be considered if a patient suddenly becomes shocked during the third stage of labour without excessive vaginal bleeding.
2. No uterus is palpable on abdominal examination.
3. The uterus lies in the vagina or may even hang out of the vagina.

11-40 What is the management of a patient with an inverted uterus?

1. Two fast-running intravenous infusions must be started to treat the shock.
2. The patient must be transferred to a level 2 or 3 hospital as an emergency.

NOTE
Bleeding disorders can also result in postpartum haemorrhage. Abruptio placentae is the commonest cause of a bleeding disorder in the third stage of labour. In this situation it is extremely important to ensure that the uterus is well

contracted after the delivery of the placenta. The powerful contraction of the
uterus plays a greater role than blood clotting in the prevention of bleeding.

Protecting the staff from HIV infection

11-41 What should be done during labour to prevent the staff from becoming infected with the human immunodeficiency virus (HIV)?

All patients should be regarded as being potentially infected with HIV, the
virus which causes AIDS (Acquired Immune Deficiency Syndrome). The
virus is present in blood, liquor and placental tissue. Contamination of the
eyes or cuts on the hands or arms, and pricks by contaminated needles carry
a small risk of causing infection.

Therefore, the following precautions should be taken for all deliveries:

1. The person conducting the delivery should wear gloves, a plastic apron,
   a face mask and goggles. People wearing glasses need only a mask to
   protect their face.
2. Any person who resuscitates the infant or cleans the labour ward after
   the delivery must wear gloves.
3. The umbilical cord must be squeezed to empty it of blood before
   applying the second clamp. This will prevent blood spurting out when
   the cord is cut.
4. Injection needles must be placed in a sharps container *immediately* after
   being used. Needles must not be replaced into their sheaths.
5. When an episiotomy is repaired, the needle must only be held with a
   needle holder and the tissues with a forceps.
6. The needle should be cut loose from the suture material and replaced in
   the dish as soon as possible. When the needle is to be used again, it must
   be held in a safe manner, with forceps.

> Procedures aimed at preventing the infection of staff with HIV
> must be strictly enforced.

Case study 1

Following normal first and second stages of labour, the third stage of labour is actively managed. The patient was not hypertensive during her pregnancy and does not have a history of heart valve disease. Syntometrine is given by intramuscular injection and the patient is observed for signs of placental separation.

1. Were the necessary precautions taken before giving the Syntometrine ?

No. A second twin must be excluded before giving the Syntometrine.

2. Is the third stage of labour being correctly managed by the active method?

No. The placenta must be delivered when the uterus contracts. If the active method of managing the third stage is used, it is incorrect to wait for signs of placental separation.

3. How soon after giving the Syntometrine does the uterus contract?

Syntometrine includes oxytocin which causes uterine contractions 2 to 3 minutes after intramuscular administration.

4. What should have been done as soon as the uterus contracted?

The umbilical cord should have been steadily pulled with one hand while the other hand was pushing upwards on the uterus, i.e. controlled cord traction. Placental separation and then placental delivery occur with the uterine contraction.

5. What should be done if placental separation does not take place with the first uterine contraction?

A second uterine contraction will occur 5 to 6 minutes after giving Syntometrine by intramuscular injection due to the action of the ergometrine. A second attempt must now be made to deliver the placenta by controlled cord traction. Most placentas which are not delivered with the first contraction will be delivered with the second contraction.

Case study 2

A patient with normal first and second stages of labour has been delivered by a midwife working alone at a peripheral clinic. A second twin is excluded on abdominal examination and the passive method is used to manage the third stage of labour. After 30 minutes there has been no sign of placental separation. A diagnosis of retained placenta is made and the patient is referred to the nearest hospital for a manual removal of the placenta.

1. Is the diagnosis of a retained placenta correct?

No. The diagnosis of retained placenta can only be made if the placenta is not delivered after the active method of managing the third stage of labour has been used. The correct diagnosis is a prolonged third stage of labour.

2. What should have been done in this case of a prolonged third stage of labour?

The placenta should have been delivered by the active method of managing the third stage of labour, i.e. by giving oxytocin 10 units intramuscular and using controlled cord traction.

3. What should be done in a peripheral clinic if the placenta is retained?

The patient should be transferred to a hospital with theatre facilities for the manual removal of the placenta under general anaesthesia.

4. What complication is this patient at high risk of developing?

A postpartum haemorrhage due to an atonic uterus.

5. What should have been done in this case to make the patient's transfer to hospital safer?

An intravenous infusion of 20 units oxytocin in 1000 ml Basol or normal saline should have been started. She should also have been carefully observed to make sure that the uterus was well contracted. Make sure that the uterus remains well contracted, and measure the blood pressure and pulse rate every 15 minutes until the patient is transferred.

Case study 3

After normal first and second stages of labour in a grande multipara, the placenta is delivered by the active management of the third stage of labour. There are no complications. Half an hour later you are called to see the patient as she is bleeding vaginally. You immediately measure her blood pressure which indicates that she is shocked.

1. Was the patient's third stage of labour correctly managed?

No. As the patient falls into a high-risk group for postpartum haemorrhage, an intravenous infusion should have been started during the first stage of labour. Twenty units of oxytocin should have been added to the infusion after the placenta was delivered. The patient should also have been carefully observed to make sure that the uterus remained well contracted.

2. Do you agree that the first step in the management of postpartum haemorrhage is to measure the blood pressure?

No. The first step should be to rub up the uterus in order to stop the bleeding.

3. What should be the further management of this patient?

A rapid intravenous infusion of 20 units oxytocin in 1000 ml Basol or normal saline should be started. Make sure that the uterus is well contracted. Then check that the patient's bladder is empty as a full bladder can cause relaxation of the uterus.

4. What additional management is needed for this patient?

The cause of the bleeding must now be found. The two important causes of postpartum haemorrhage are an atonic uterus or a tear.

5. What is the most probable cause of this patient's postpartum haemorrhage?

As she is a grande multipara the most likely cause is an atonic uterus.

6. What are the clinical signs of bleeding due to an atonic uterus?

The uterus will not be well contracted and will tend to relax after it is rubbed up. In addition, the bleeding is not continuous but occurs in episodes, and the blood consists of dark red clots.

Case study 4

A primigravida patient who did not co-operate well during the first stage of labour delivers soon after a vaginal examination. At the examination the cervix was found to be 7 cm dilated and paper thin. When observations were made an hour after delivery of the placenta, the patient was found lying in a pool of blood. Her uterus was well contracted and her bladder was empty.

1. What should be the next step in the management of this patient?

A rapid intravenous infusion of 20 units oxytocin in 1000 ml Balsol or normal saline should be started and you should make sure that the uterus is well contracted.

2. In spite of this management a continuous trickle of bright red blood is observed. What is the most likely cause of the bleeding?

A tear.

3. Why is this patient at high risk of a cervical tear?

Because the infant was delivered through an incompletely dilated cervix.

4. What should be the next step in the management of this patient?

The patient must be placed in the lithotomy position and be examined for a vaginal or perineal tear. Any tear must be sutured.

5. The midwife who is managing this patient does not find either a vaginal or perineal tear. What should be the next step in the management of this patient?

A doctor should examine the patient for a cervical tear. The most likely site of a tear is the cervix as this patient probably delivered before full cervical dilatation.

12

The puerperium

Take the chapter test before and after you read this chapter.

Objectives

When you have completed this unit you should be able to:

- Define the puerperium.
- List the physical changes which occur during the puerperium.
- Manage the normal puerperium.
- Assess a patient at the 6-week postnatal visit.
- Diagnose and manage the various causes of puerperal pyrexia.
- Recognise the puerperal psychiatric disorders.
- Diagnose and manage secondary postpartum haemorrhage.
- Teach the patient the concept of 'the mother as a monitor'.

The normal puerperium

12-1 What is the puerperium?

The puerperium is the period from the end of the third stage of labour until most of the patient's organs have returned to their pre-pregnant state.

12-2 How long does the puerperium last?

The puerperium starts when the placenta is delivered and lasts for 6 weeks (42 days). However, some organs may only return to their pre-pregnant state weeks or even months after the 6 weeks have elapsed (e.g. the ureters). Other organs never regain their pre-pregnant state (e.g. the perineum).

It is important for the midwife or doctor to assess whether the puerperal patient has returned, as closely as possible, to normal health and activity.

> **The puerperium starts when the placenta is delivered and lasts for 6 weeks.**

12-3 Why is the puerperium important?

1. The patient recovers from her labour, which often leaves her tired, even exhausted. There is, nevertheless, a feeling of great relief and happiness.
2. The patient undergoes what is probably the most important psychological experience of her life, as she realises that she is responsible for another human being, her infant.
3. Breastfeeding should be established.
4. The patient should decide, with the guidance of a midwife or doctor, on an appropriate contraceptive method.

12-4 What physical changes occur in the puerperium?

Almost every organ undergoes change in the puerperium. These adjustments range from mild to marked. Only those changes which are important in the management of the normal puerperium will be described here:

1. General condition:
   - Some women experience shivering soon after delivery, without a change in body temperature.
   - The pulse rate may be slow, normal or fast, but should not be above 100 beats per minute.
   - The blood pressure may also vary and may be slightly elevated in an otherwise healthy patient. It should, however, be less than 140/90 mm Hg.
   - There is an immediate drop in weight of about 8 kg after delivery. Further weight loss follows involution of the uterus and the normal diuresis (an increased amount of urine passed), but also depends on whether the patient breastfeeds her infant.

2. Skin:
   - The increased pigmentation of the face, abdominal wall and vulva lightens but the areolae may remain darker than they were before pregnancy.
   - With the onset of diuresis the general puffiness and any oedema disappear in a few days.
   - Marked sweating may occur for some days.

3. Abdominal wall:
   - The abdominal wall is flaccid (loose and wrinkled) and some separation (divarication) of the abdominal muscles occurs.
   - Pregnancy marks (striae gravidarum), where present, do not disappear, but do tend to become less red in time.

4. Gastrointestinal tract:
   - Thirst is common.
   - The appetite varies from anorexia to ravenous hunger.
   - There may be flatulence (excess wind).
   - Many patients are constipated as a result of decreased tone of the bowel during pregnancy, decreased food intake during labour and passing stool when nearly fully dilated or during the second stage of labour. Constipation is common in the presence of an episiotomy or painful haemorrhoids.

5. The routine administration of enemas when patients are admitted in labour is unnecessary and is not beneficial to patients. It also causes constipation during the puerperium.

6. Urinary tract:
   - Retention of urine is common and may result from decreased tone of the bladder in pregnancy and oedema of the urethra following delivery. Dysuria and difficulty in passing urine may lead to complete urinary retention, or retention with overflow incontinence. A full bladder will interfere with uterine contractions.
   - A diuresis usually occurs on the second or third day of the puerperium. In oedematous patients it may start immediately after delivery.
   - Stress incontinence (a leak of urine) is common when the patient laughs or coughs. It may first be noted in the puerperium or follow stress incontinence which was present during pregnancy. Often

stress incontinence becomes worse initially but tends to improve with time and with pelvic floor exercises.

7. Pelvic floor exercises are also known as pinch or 'knyp' exercises. The muscles that are exercised are those used to suddenly stop a stream of urine midway through micturition. These muscles should be tightened, as strongly as possible, 10 times in succession on at least four occasions a day.

NOTE

Normal bladder function is likely to be temporarily impaired when a patient has been given epidural analgesia. Complete retention of urine or retention with overflow may occur.

8. Blood:
   ○ The haemoglobin concentration becomes stable around the fourth day of the puerperium.
   ○ The platelet count is raised and the platelets become more sticky from the fourth to tenth day after delivery. These and other changes in the clotting (coagulation) factors may cause thromboembolism in the puerperium.

9. Breasts:

   Marked changes occur during the puerperium with the production of milk.

10. Genital tract:

    Very marked changes occur in the genital tract during the puerperium.

    ○ Vulva: The vulva is swollen and congested after delivery, but these features rapidly disappear. Tears and/or an episiotomy usually heal easily.
    ○ Vagina: Immediately after delivery the vagina is large, smooth walled, oedematous and congested. It rapidly shrinks in size and rugae return by the third week. The vaginal walls remain laxer than before and some degree of vaginal prolapse (cystocoele and/or rectocoele) is common after a vaginal delivery. Small vaginal tears, which are very common, usually heal in seven to 10 days.
    ○ Cervix: After the first vaginal delivery the circular external os of the nullipara becomes slit-like. For the first few days after delivery the

cervix remains partially open, admitting 1 or 2 fingers. By the seventh day postpartum the cervical os will have closed.

○ Uterus: The most important change occurring in the uterus is involution. After delivery the uterus is about the size of a 20-week pregnancy. By the end of the first week it is about 12 weeks in size. At 14 days the fundus of the uterus should no longer be palpable above the symphysis pubis. After 6 weeks it has decreased to the size of a normal multiparous uterus, which is slightly larger than a nulliparous one. This remarkable decrease in size is the result of contraction and retraction of the uterine muscle. The normally involuting uterus should be firm and non tender. The decidua of the uterus necroses (dies), due to ischaemia, and is shed as the lochia. The average duration of red lochia is 24 days. Thereafter, the lochia becomes straw coloured. Normal lochia has a typical, non-offensive smell. Offensive lochia is always abnormal.

Management of the puerperium

The management of the puerperium may be divided into three stages:

1. The management of the first hour after delivery of the placenta (sometimes called the fourth stage of labour).
2. The management of the rest of the puerperium.
3. The six week postnatal visit.

12-5 How should you manage the first hour after the delivery of the placenta?

The two main objectives of managing the first hour of the puerperium are:

1. To ensure that the patient is, and remains, in a good condition.
2. The prevention of a postpartum haemorrhage (PPH).

To achieve these, you should:

1. Perform certain routine observations.
2. Care for the needs of the patient.
3. Get the patient's co-operation in ensuring that her uterus remains well contracted and that she reports any vaginal bleeding.

The correct management of the first hour of the puerperium is most important as the risk of postpartum haemorrhage is greatest at this time.

12-6 Which routine observations should you perform in the first hour after delivery of the placenta?

1. Immediately after the delivery of the placenta you should:
   - Assess whether the uterus is well contracted.
   - Assess whether vaginal bleeding appears more than normal.
   - Record the patient's pulse rate, blood pressure and temperature.

2. During the first hour after the delivery of the placenta, provided that the above observations are normal, you should:
   - Continuously assess whether the uterus is well contracted and that no excessive vaginal bleeding is present.
   - Repeat the measurement of the pulse rate and blood pressure after 1 hour.
   - If the patient's condition changes, observations must be done more frequently until the patient's condition returns to normal.

Observations during the first hour of the puerperium are extremely important.

12-7 How should you care for the needs of the patient during the first hour of the puerperium?

After the placenta has been delivered the patient needs to be:

1. Washed.
2. Given something to drink and maybe to eat.
3. Allowed to bond with her infant.
4. Allowed to rest for as long as she needs to.

12-8 How can the patient help to prevent postpartum haemorrhage during the first hour of the puerperium?

1. The patient should be shown how to observe:
   - The height of the uterine fundus in relation to the umbilicus.

- The feel of a well-contracted uterus.
- The amount of vaginal bleeding.

2. She should be shown how to 'rub up' the uterus.
3. She should be told that if the uterine fundus rises or the uterus relaxes or if vaginal bleeding increases, she must:
   - Immediately call the midwife.
   - In the meantime rub up the uterus.

These two important steps may help prevent a postpartum haemorrhage.

> **The patient can play a very important role in the prevention of postpartum haemorrhage.**

12-9 When should a postpartum patient be allowed to go home?

This will depend on:

1. Whether the patient had a normal pregnancy and delivery.
2. The circumstances of the hospital or clinic where the patient was delivered.

12-10 When should a patient be allowed to go home following a normal pregnancy and delivery?

A patient who has had a normal pregnancy and delivery may be allowed to go home about 6 hours after the birth of her infant, provided:

1. The observations done on the mother and infant since delivery have been normal.
2. The mother and infant are normal on examination, and the infant is sucking well.
3. The patient is able to attend her nearest clinic on the day after delivery (day 1) and then again on days 3 and 5 after delivery for postnatal care, or be visited at home by a midwife on those days. Primigravidas should be seen again on day seven, especially to ensure that breastfeeding is well established.

4. Patients who received no antenatal care and are delivered without having had any screening tests must have a rapid syphilis test and a rapid Rhesus grouping. Counselling for HIV testing must also be done.
5. A postnatal card needs to be completed for the mother on discharge as this is the only means of communication between the delivery site and the clinic where she will receive postnatal care.

A patient should only be discharged home after delivery if no abnormalities are found when the following examinations are performed:

1. A general examination, paying particular attention to the:
   ○ Pulse rate.
   ○ Blood pressure.
   ○ Temperature.
   ○ Haemoglobin concentration.
2. An abdominal examination, paying particular attention to the state of contraction and tenderness of the uterus.
3. An inspection of the episiotomy site.
4. The amount, colour, and odour of the lochia.
5. A postnatal examination was completed for the mother and infant.

12-11 When should a patient be discharged from hospital following a complicated pregnancy and delivery?

This will depend on the nature of the complication and the method of delivery. For example:

1. A patient with pre-eclampsia should be kept in hospital until her blood pressure has returned to normal or is well controlled with oral drugs.
2. A patient who has had a Caesarean section will usually stay in hospital for three days or longer.
3. A patient who has had a postpartum haemorrhage must be kept in hospital for at least 24 hours to ensure that her uterus is well contracted and that there is no further bleeding.

12-12 How will the circumstances at a clinic or hospital influence the time of discharge?

1. Some clinics have no space to accommodate patients for longer than 6 hours after delivery. Therefore, patients who cannot be discharged safely at 6 hours will have to be transferred to a hospital.
2. Some hospitals manage patients who live in remote areas where follow-up is not possible. These patients will have to be kept in hospital longer before discharge.

12-13 What postnatal care should be given during the puerperium after the patient has left the hospital or clinic?

The following observations must be done on the mother:

1. Assess the patient's general condition.
2. Observe the pulse rate, blood pressure and temperature.
3. Determine the height of the uterine fundus and assess whether any uterine tenderness is present.
4. Assess the amount, colour, and odour of the lochia.
5. Check whether the episiotomy is healing satisfactorily.
6. Ask if the patient passes urine normally and enquire about any urinary symptoms. Reassure the patient if she has not passed a stool by day five.
7. Measure the haemoglobin concentration if the patient appears pale.
8. Assess the condition of the patient's breasts and nipples. Determine whether successful breastfeeding has been established.

The following observations must be done on the infant:

1. Assess whether the infant appears well.
2. Check whether the infant is jaundiced.
3. Examine the umbilical stump for signs of infection.
4. Examine the eyes for conjunctivitis.
5. Ask whether the infant has passed urine and stool.
6. Assess whether the infant is feeding well and is satisfied after a feed.

> The successful establishment of breastfeeding is one of the most important goals of patient care during the puerperium.

12-14 How can you help to establish successful breastfeeding?

By providing patient education and motivation. This should preferably start before pregnancy and continue throughout the antenatal period and after pregnancy. Encouragement and support are very important during the first weeks after delivery. The important role of breastfeeding in lowering infant mortality in poor communities must be remembered.

12-15 Which topics should you include under patient education in the puerperium?

Patient education regarding herself, her infant, and her family should not start during the puerperium, but should be part of any woman's general education, starting at school. Topics which should be emphasised in patient education in the puerperium include:

1. Personal and infant care.
2. Offensive lochia must be reported immediately.
3. The 'puerperal blues'.
4. Family planning.
5. Any special arrangements for the next pregnancy and delivery.
6. When to start coitus again. Usually coitus can be started three to 4 weeks postpartum when the episiotomy or tears have healed.

Patient education is an important and often neglected part of postnatal care.

12-16 When should a patient be seen again after postnatal care has been completed?

The postnatal visit is usually held 6 weeks after delivery. By this time almost all the organ changes which occurred during pregnancy should have disappeared.

The six week postnatal visit

12-17 Which patients need to attend a six week postnatal clinic?

Patients with specific problems that need to be followed up six weeks postpartum, e.g. patients who were discharged with hypertension need to come back to have their blood pressure measured. Patients who are healthy may be referred directly to the mother-and-child health clinics.

12-18 What are the objectives of the six week postnatal visit?

It is important to determine whether:

1. The patient is healthy and has returned to her normal activities.
2. The infant is well and growing normally.
3. Breastfeeding has been satisfactorily established.
4. Contraception has been arranged to the patient's satisfaction.
5. The patient has been referred to a mother-and-child health clinic for further care.
6. The patient has any questions about herself, her infant, or her family.

12-19 How should the six week postnatal visit be conducted?

1. The patient is asked how she and her infant have been since they were discharged from the hospital or clinic.
2. The patient is then examined. On examination pay particular attention to the blood pressure and breasts, and look for signs of anaemia. An abdominal examination is followed by a speculum examination to check whether the episiotomy, vulval, or vaginal tears have healed. A cytology smear of the cervix should be taken if the patient is 30 years or older and has not previously had a normal cervical smear. A cervical smear should also be taken on any woman who has previously had an abnormal smear. A bimanual examination is then done to assess the size of the uterus. The haemoglobin is measured and the urine tested for glucose and protein.

3. Attention must be given to any specific reason why the patient is being followed up, e.g. arrangements for the management of patients who remain hypertensive after delivery.
4. The patient is given health education as set out in section 12-15. It should again be remembered to ask her whether she has any questions she would like to ask.

If the patient and her infant are both well, they are referred to their local mother-and-child health clinic for further follow-up.

> A patient and her infant should only be discharged if they are both well and have been referred to the local mother-and-child health clinic, and the patient has received contraceptive counselling.

Puerperal pyrexia

12-20 When is puerperal pyrexia present?

A patient has puerperal pyrexia if her oral temperature rises to 38 °C or higher during the puerperium.

12-21 Why is puerperal pyrexia important?

Because it may be caused by serious complications of the puerperium. It may interfere with breastfeeding. The patient may become very ill or even die.

> Puerperal pyrexia may be caused by a serious complication of the puerperium.

12-22 What are the causes of puerperal pyrexia?

1. Genital tract infection.
2. Urinary tract infection.
3. Mastitis or breast abscess.

4. Thrombophlebitis (superficial vein thrombosis).
5. Respiratory tract infection.
6. Other infections.

12-23 What is the cause of genital tract infection?

Genital tract infection (or puerperal sepsis) is caused by bacterial infection of the raw placental site or lacerations of the cervix, vagina or perineum.

12-24 How should you diagnose genital tract infection?

1. History

    If one or more of the following is present:

    - Preterm or prelabour rupture of the membranes, a long labour, operative delivery, or incomplete delivery of the placenta or membranes may have occurred.
    - The patient will feel generally unwell.
    - Lower abdominal pain.

2. Examination

    - Pyrexia, usually developing within the first 24 hours after delivery. Rigors may occur.
    - Marked tachycardia.
    - Lower abdominal tenderness.
    - Offensive lochia.
    - The episiotomy wound or perineal or vaginal tears may be infected.

NOTE
If possible, an endocervical swab should be taken for microscopy, culture, and sensitivity tests.

12-25 How should you manage genital tract infection?

1. Prevention
    - Strict asepsis during delivery.

- Reduction in the number of vaginal examinations during labour to a minimum.
- Prevention of unnecessary trauma during labour.
- Isolation of infected patients.

2. Treatment
   - Admit the patient to hospital.
   - Bring down the patient's temperature, e.g. by tepid sponging.
   - Give the patient analgesia, e.g. paracetamol (Panado) 1 g (two adult tablets) orally 6-hourly.
   - Adequate fluid intake with strict intake and output measurement.
   - Broad spectrum antibiotics, e.g. intravenous ampicillin and oral metronidazole (Flagyl). If the patient is to be referred, antibiotic treatment must be started before transfer.
   - The haemoglobin concentration must be measured. A blood transfusion must be given if the haemoglobin concentration is below 8 g/dl.
   - Removal of all stitches if the wound is infected.
   - Drainage of any abscess.
   - If there is subinvolution of the uterus, an evacuation under general anaesthetic must be done.

NOTE

24 hours after starting this treatment the patient's condition should have improved considerably and the temperature should by then be normal. If this is not the case, evacuation of the uterus is required and gentamicin must be added to the antibiotics. A laparotomy and possibly a hysterectomy is indicated, if peritonitis and subinvolution of the uterus are present, and there is no response to the measures detailed above. Transfer the patient to the appropriate level of care for this purpose.

12-26 How must a patient with offensive lochia be managed?

1. If the patient has pyrexia she must be admitted to hospital.
2. If the involution of the patient's uterus is slower than expected and the cervical os remains open, retained placental products are present. An evacuation of the uterus under general anaesthesia must be done.
3. If the patient has a normal temperature and normal involution of her uterus, she can be managed as an outpatient with oral amoxicillin and metronidazole (Flagyl).

Offensive lochia is an important sign of genital tract infection.

12-27 How should you diagnose a urinary tract infection?

1. History
   - The patient may have been catheterised during labour or in the puerperium.
   - The patient complains of rigors (shivering) and lower abdominal pain and/or pain in the lower back over one or both the kidneys (the loins).
   - Dysuria and frequency. However, these are not reliable symptoms of urinary tract infection.

2. Examination
   - Pyrexia, often with rigors (shivering).
   - Tachycardia.
   - Suprapubic tenderness and/or tenderness, especially to percussion, over the kidneys (punch tenderness in the renal angles).

3. Side-room and special investigations
   - Microscopy of a midstream or catheter specimen of urine usually shows large numbers of pus cells and bacteria.
   - Culture and sensitivity tests of the urine must be done if the facilities are available.

The presence of pyrexia and punch tenderness in the renal angles indicate an upper renal tract infection and a diagnosis of acute pyelonephritis must be made.

12-28 How should you manage a patient with a urinary tract infection?

1. Prevention
   - Avoid catheterisation whenever possible. If catheterisation is essential, it must be done with strict aseptic precautions.

2. Treatment
   - Admit the patient to hospital.
   - Take measures to bring down the temperature.
   - Analgesia, e.g. paracetamol (Panado) 1 g orally 6-hourly.

- ○ Adequate fluid intake.
- ○ Intravenous cefuroxime (Zinacef) 750 mg 8-hourly.

Antibiotics should not be given to a patient with puerperal pyrexia until she has been fully investigated.

Thrombophlebitis

12-29 What is superficial vein thrombophlebitis?

This is a non-infective inflammation and thrombosis of the superficial veins of the leg or forearm where an infusion was given. Thrombophlebitis commonly occurs during the puerperium, especially in varicose veins.

12-30 How should you diagnose superficial leg vein thrombophlebitis?

1. History
   - ○ Painful swelling of the leg or forearm.
   - ○ Presence of varicose veins.

2. Examination
   - ○ Pyrexia.
   - ○ Tachycardia.
   - ○ Presence of a localised area of the forearm or leg which is swollen, red and tender.

12-31 How should you manage a patient with superficial vein thrombophlebitis?

1. Give analgesia, e.g. Aspirin 300 mg (1 adult tablet) 6-hourly.
2. Support the leg with an elastic bandage.
3. Encourage the patient to walk around.

Respiratory tract infection

12-32 How should you diagnose a lower respiratory tract infection?

A lower respiratory tract infection, such as acute bronchitis or pneumonia, is diagnosed as follows:

1. History
   - The patient may have had general anaesthesia with endotracheal intubation, e.g. for a Caesarean section.
   - Cough, which may be productive.
   - Pain in the chest.
   - A recent upper respiratory tract infection.

2. Examination
   - Pyrexia.
   - Tachypnoea (breathing rapidly).
   - Tachycardia.

3. Special investigations
   - A chest X-ray is useful in diagnosing pneumonia.

NOTE
Examination of the chest may reveal basal dullness due to collapse, increased breath sounds or crepitations due to pneumonia, or bilateral rhonchi due to bronchitis.

12-33 How should you manage a patient with a lower respiratory tract infection.

1. Prevention
   - Skilled anaesthesia.
   - Proper care of the patient during induction and recovery from anaesthesia.
   - Encourage deep breathing and coughing following a general anaesthetic to prevent lower lobe collapse.

2. Treatment
   - Admit the patient to hospital, unless the infection is very mild.

- Oxygen, if required.
- Amoxicillin orally or ampicillin intravenously depending on the severity of the infection.
- Analgesia, e.g. paracetamol (Panado) 1 g 6-hourly.
- Physiotherapy.

3. Special investigations
   - Send a sample of sputum for microscopy, culture, and sensitivity testing if possible.

12-34 Which other infections may cause puerperal pyrexia?

Tonsillitis, influenza and any other acute infection, e.g. acute appendicitis.

12-35 What should you do if a patient presents with puerperal pyrexia?

1. Ask the patient what she thinks is wrong with her.
2. Specifically ask for symptoms which point to:
   - An infection of the throat or ears.
   - Mastitis or breast abscess.
   - A chest infection.
   - A urinary tract infection.
   - An infected abdominal wound if the patient had a Caesarean section or a puerperal sterilisation.
   - Genital tract infection.
   - Superficial leg vein thrombophlebitis.
3. Examine the patient systematically, including the:
   - Throat and ears.
   - Breasts.
   - Chest.
   - Abdominal wound, if present.
   - Urinary tract.
   - Genital tract.
   - Legs, especially the calves.

4. Perform the necessary special investigations, but always send off a:
   ◦ Endocervical swab.
   ◦ Midstream or catheter specimen of urine.
5. Start the appropriate treatment.

> If a patient presents with puerperal pyrexia the cause of the pyrexia must be found and appropriately treated.

Puerperal psychiatric disorders

12-36 Which are the puerperal psychiatric disorders?

1. The 'puerperal blues'.
2. Temporary postnatal depression.
3. Puerperal psychosis.

12-37 Why is it important to recognise the various puerperal psychiatric disorders?

1. The 'puerperal blues' are very common in the first week after delivery, especially on day 3. The patient feels miserable and cries easily. Although the patient may be very distressed, all that is required is an explanation, reassurance, and a caring, sympathetic attitude and emotional support. The condition improves within a few days.
2. Postnatal depression is much commoner than is generally realised. It may last for months or even years and patients may need to be referred to a psychiatrist. Patients with postnatal depression usually present with a depressed mood that cannot be relieved, a lack of interest in their surroundings, a poor or excessive appetite, sleeping difficulties, feelings of inadequacy, guilt and helplessness, and sometimes suicidal thoughts.
3. Puerperal psychosis is an uncommon but very important condition. The onset is usually acute and an observant attendant will notice the sudden and marked change in the patient's behaviour. She may rapidly pose a threat to her infant, the staff, and herself. Such a patient must be

referred urgently to a psychiatrist and will usually need admission to a psychiatric unit.

Secondary postpartum haemorrhage

12-38 What is secondary postpartum haemorrhage?

This is any amount of vaginal bleeding, other than the normal amount of lochia, occurring after the first 24 hours postpartum until the end of the puerperium. It commonly occurs between the fifth and 15th days after delivery.

12-39 Why is secondary postpartum haemorrhage important?

1. A secondary postpartum haemorrhage may be so severe that it causes shock.
2. Unless the cause of the secondary postpartum haemorrhage is treated, the vaginal bleeding will continue.

12-40 What are the causes of secondary postpartum haemorrhage?

1. Genital tract infection with or without retention of a piece of placenta or part of the membranes. This is the commonest cause.
2. Separation of an infected slough in a cervical or vaginal laceration.
3. Breakdown (dehiscence) of a Caesarean section wound of the uterus.

However, the cause is unknown in up to half of these patients.

NOTE
Gestational trophoblastic disease (hydatidiform mole or choriocarcinoma) and a disorder of blood coagulation may also cause secondary postpartum haemorrhage.

12-41 What clinical features should alert you to the possibility of the patient developing secondary postpartum haemorrhage?

1. A history of incomplete delivery of the placenta and/or membranes.
2. Unexplained puerperal pyrexia.
3. Delayed involution of the uterus.
4. Offensive and/or persistently red lochia.

12-42 How should you manage a patient with secondary postpartum haemorrhage?

1. Prevention
   - Aseptic technique throughout labour, the delivery and the puerperium.
   - Careful examination after delivery to determine whether the placenta and membranes are complete.
   - Proper repair of vaginal and perineal lacerations.

2. Treatment
   - Admission of the patient to hospital is indicated, except in very mild cases of secondary postpartum haemorrhage.
   - Review of the clinical notes with regard to completeness of the placenta and membranes.
   - Obtain an endocervical swab for bacteriology.
   - Give ampicillin intravenously and metronidazole (Flagyl) orally.
   - Give 20 units oxytocin in an intravenous infusion if excessive bleeding is present.
   - Blood transfusion, if the haemoglobin concentration drops below 8 g/dl.
   - Removal of retained placental products under general anaesthesia.

12-43 What may you find on physical examination to suggest that retained pieces of placenta or membranes are the cause of a secondary postpartum haemorrhage?

1. The uterus will be involuting slower than usual.
2. Even though the patient may be more than seven days postpartum, the cervical os will have remained open (a finger can be passed through the cervix).

Self-monitoring

12-44 What is meant by the concept of 'the mother as a monitor'?

This is a concept where the patient is made aware of the many ways in which she can monitor her own, as well as her fetus' or infant's wellbeing, during pregnancy, in labour, and in the puerperium. This has two major advantages:

1. The patient becomes much more involved in her own perinatal care.
2. Possible complications will be reported by the patient at the earliest opportunity.

12-45 How can the patient act as a monitor in the puerperium?

The patient must be encouraged to report the following complications as soon as she becomes aware of them:

1. Maternal complications
   - Symptoms of puerperal pyrexia.
   - Breakdown of an episiotomy.
   - Breastfeeding problems.
   - Excessive or offensive lochia.
   - Recurrence of vaginal bleeding, i.e. secondary postpartum haemorrhage.
   - Prolonged postnatal depression.

2. Complications in the infant
   - Poor feeding or other feeding problems.
   - Lethargy.
   - Jaundice.
   - Conjunctivitis.
   - Infection of the umbilical cord stump.

Each patient must be taught to monitor her own wellbeing, as well as that of her fetus or infant.

HIV positive mothers

12-46 How should HIV positive mothers and their newborn infants be managed during the puerperium?

Women on ARV prophylaxis should continue taking daily FDC until a week after they have stopped breastfeeding. Women who do not breastfeed can stop their ARV prophylaxis after delivery as there is no further risk of mother to child transmission of HIV.

Women who are on ARV treatment should continue their FDC for life whether they choose to breastfeed or not.

At 6 weeks after delivery women on ARV treatment should be reassessed.

Infants of all HIV positive women should receive a dose of nevirapine at birth and then daily until 6 weeks of age. If the mother is on ARV treatment the daily dose of nevirapine to the infant can be stopped at 6 weeks. If the an HIV positive woman is breastfeeding and not on ARV treatment, the daily nevirapine to the infant should be continued until a week after the last breastfeed.

The HIV status and HIV prophylaxis or treatment of the mother as well as the method of infant feeding must be entered on the infant's Road to Health booklet.

The importance of attending a healthy baby clinic at 6 weeks must be emphasised. At this visit an HIV test (HIV DNA PCR test) will be done to determine whether the infant is HIV infected or not. This result will indicate what further treatment is needed.

12-47 What is the nevirapine dose for infants?

Most term infants will need 1.5 ml NVP from birth to six weeks. Thereafter the amount of NVP will increase as the infant gains weight. See table 12-1 for dosing guidelines.

Table 12-1: Nevirapine dosing guidelines for newborns: NVP syrup 10mg/ml

Birth weight	Daily dosage	Quantity
Less than 2.0 kg	First 2 weeks:2mg/kg	0.2ml/kg
	Next 4 weeks:4mg/kg	0.4ml/kg
2.0 – 2.5 kg	Birth to 6 weeks:10mg	1.0ml
More than 2.5 kg	Birth to 6 weeks:15mg	1.5 ml

Case study 1

Following a spontaneous vertex delivery in a clinic, you have delivered the placenta and membranes completely. The maternal and fetal conditions are good and there is no abnormal vaginal bleeding. You are the only staff member in the clinic. You are called away and will have to leave the patient alone for a while.

1. How can you get the patient's help in preventing a postpartum haemorrhage?

The patient should be shown how to observe:

1. The height of the uterine fundus.
2. Whether the uterus is well contracted.
3. The amount of vaginal bleeding.
4. She should also be asked to empty her bladder frequently.

2. What should the patient do if she notices that her uterus relaxes and/or there is vaginal bleeding?

She should rub up the uterus and call you immediately.

3. What should you check on before leaving the patient?

You should make sure that:

1. The patient and her infant's observations are normal and both their conditions are stable.

2. The patient understands what she has to do.
3. You will be able to hear the patient, if she calls you.

Case study 2

A patient returns to a clinic for a visit three days after a normal first pregnancy and delivery. She complains of leaking urine when coughing or laughing, and she is also worried that she has not passed a stool since the delivery. She starts to cry and says that she should not have fallen pregnant. Her infant takes the breast well and sleeps well after each feed. On examination the patient appears well, her observations are normal, the uterus is the size of a 16-week pregnant uterus, and the lochia is red and not offensive.

1. Is her puerperium progressing normally?

Yes. The patient appears healthy with normal observations, and the involution of her uterus is satisfactory.

2. What should be done about the patient's complaints?

Stress incontinence is common during the puerperium. Therefore, the patient must be reassured that it will improve over time. However, pelvic floor exercises must be explained to her as they will hasten improvement of her incontinence. She need not be worried about not having passed a stool as this is normal during the first few days of the puerperium.

3. Why is the patient regretting her pregnancy and crying for no apparent reason?

She probably has the 'puerperal blues' which are common in the puerperium. Listen sympathetically to the patient's complaints and reassure her that she is managing well as a mother. Also explain that her feelings are normal and are experienced by most mothers.

4. What educational topics must be discussed with the patient during this visit?

1. Family size and when she plans to have her next infant.
2. Which contraceptive method she should use and how to use it correctly.
3. The care and feeding of her infant, stressing the importance of breastfeeding.
4. The time that coitus can be resumed.

Also ask about and discuss any other uncertainties which the patient may have.

Case study 3

Following a prolonged first stage of labour due to an occipito-posterior position, a patient has a spontaneous vertex delivery. The placenta and membranes are complete. There is no excessive postpartum blood loss and the patient is discharged home after 6 hours. Within 24 hours of delivery the patient is brought back to the clinic. She has a temperature of 39 °C, a pulse rate of 110 beats per minute and complains of a headache and lower abdominal pain. The uterus is tender to palpation.

1. What does the patient present with?

Puerperal pyrexia.

2. What is the most likely cause of the puerperal pyrexia?

Genital tract infection, i.e. puerperal sepsis. This diagnosis is suggested by the general signs of infection and the uterine tenderness. The patient had a prolonged first stage of labour, which is usually accompanied by a greater than usual number of vaginal examinations and, therefore, predisposes her to genital tract infection.

3. Was the early postnatal management of this patient correct?

No. The patient should not have been discharged home so early as she had a prolonged first stage of labour which places her at a higher risk of infection. She should have been observed for at least 24 hours.

4. How should you manage this patient further in the clinic?

She must be made comfortable. Paracetamol (Panado) 1 g orally may be given for the headache. If necessary, she should be given a tepid sponging. An intravenous infusion should be started and she must then be referred to hospital. If at all possible, the infant must accompany the patient to hospital. The need to start antibiotic treatment, such as intravenous ampicillin and oral metronidazole (Flagyl), before transfer must be discussed with the doctor.

Case study 4

A patient is seen at a clinic on day 5 following a normal pregnancy, labour and delivery. She complains of rigors and lower abdominal pain. She has a temperature of 38.5 °C, tenderness over both kidneys (loins) and tenderness to percussion over both renal angles. A diagnosis of puerperal pyrexia is made and the patient is given oral amoxicillin. She is asked to come back to the clinic on day seven.

1. Are you satisfied with the diagnosis of puerperal pyrexia?

No. Puerperal pyrexia is a clinical sign and not a diagnosis. The cause of the pyrexia must be found by taking a history, doing a physical examination and, if indicated, completing special investigations.

2. What is the most likely cause of the patient's pyrexia?

An upper urinary tract infection as suggested by the pyrexia, rigors, lower abdominal pain and tenderness over the kidneys.

3. Do you agree with the management given to the patient?

No. A urinary tract infection that causes puerperal pyrexia is an indication for admitting the patient to hospital. Intravenous cefuroxime (Zinacef) must be given, as this will lead to a rapid recovery and prevent serious complications.

4. Why is a puerperal patient at risk of a urinary tract infection and how may this be prevented?

Catheterisation is often required and this increases the risk of a urinary tract infection. Catheterisation must only be carried out when necessary and must always be done as an aseptic procedure. Screening and treating asymptomatic bacteriuria at the antenatal clinic will reduce acute pyelonephritis during the puerperium.

13

Medical problems during pregnancy, labour and the puerperium

Take the chapter test before and after you read this chapter.

Objectives

When you have completed this unit you should be able to:

- Diagnose and manage cystitis.
- Reduce the incidence of acute pyelonephritis in pregnancy.
- Diagnose and manage acute pyelonephritis in pregnancy.
- Diagnose and manage anaemia during pregnancy.
- Identify patients who may possibly have heart valve disease.
- Manage a patient with heart valve disease during labour and the puerperium.
- Manage a patient with diabetes mellitus.

Urinary tract infection during pregnancy

13-1 Which urinary tract infections are important during pregnancy?

1. Cystitis.
2. Asymptomatic bacteriuria.
3. Acute pyelonephritis.

13-2 Why are urinary tract infections common during pregnancy and the puerperium?

1. Placental hormones cause dilatation of the ureters.
2. Pregnancy suppresses the function of the immune system.

> A urinary tract infection is the most common infection during pregnancy.

13-3 How should you diagnose cystitis?

1. These severe urinary symptoms suddenly appear:
   - Dysuria (pain on passing urine).
   - Frequency (having to pass urine often).
   - Nocturia (having to get up at night to pass urine).
2. The patient appears generally well with normal observations. The only clinical sign is tenderness over the bladder.
3. Examination of the urine under a microscope shows many pus cells and bacteria.

A midstream urine sample for culture must be collected, if possible, to confirm the clinical diagnosis. Treatment must commence immediately without waiting for the results of the culture.

13-4 How should you manage a patient with cystitis?

Give 4 adult tablets of co-trimoxazole (e.g. Bactrim, Cotrim, Durobac, Mezenol or Purbac) as a single dose. This is also the drug of choice for patients who are allergic to penicillin.

Amoxycillin (Amoxil) 3 g as a single dose orally could also be used but organisms causing cystitis are often resistant to this antibiotic. The treatment will be more successful if 2 amoxycillin capsules (250 mg) are replaced with 2 Augmentin tablets that contain 125 mg clavulanic acid each.

A midstream sample should again be sent for microscopy, culture, and sensitivity at the next antenatal visit to determine whether the management was successful.

Co-trimoxazole can be safely used during pregnancy, including the first trimester.

13-5 What is asymptomatic bacteriuria?

It is significant colonisation of the urinary tract with bacteria, without any symptoms of a urinary tract infection.

13-6 Why is asymptomatic bacteriuria during pregnancy important?

1. Between 6 and 10% of pregnant women have asymptomatic bacteriuria.
2. One third of these patients with asymptomatic bacteriuria will develop acute pyelonephritis during pregnancy.
3. If patients with asymptomatic bacteriuria are diagnosed and correctly managed, their risk of developing acute pyelonephritis will be reduced by 70%.

> The diagnosis and treatment of asymptomatic bacteriuria will greatly reduce the incidence of acute pyelonephritis during pregnancy.

13-7 How and when should patients be screened for asymptomatic bacteriuria?

If possible, bacterial culture of a midstream urine sample should be done at the first antenatal visit to screen patients for asymptomatic bacteriuria.

NOTE
A culture medium prepared by a laboratory, or a commercially prepared culture medium, is inoculated with urine and then incubated for 12 to 24 hours to determine whether bacteriuria is present or not.

> If possible, a screening test for asymptomatic bacteriuria should be done at the first antenatal visit.

13-8 Can reagent strips be reliably used to diagnose asymptomatic bacteriuria?

No. Tests for nitrites (which detect the presence of bacteria) and leukocytes, separately or together, cannot be used to accurately screen for asymptomatic bacteriuria.

13-9 What is the management of a patient with asymptomatic bacteriuria?

The same as the management of a patient with cystitis, i.e. 4 adult tablets of co-trimoxazole (e.g. Bactrim, Cotrim, Durobac, Mezenol or Purbac) as a single dose or amoxycillin (Amoxil) 3 g as a single dose. Patients who are allergic to penicillin should be given co-trimoxazole.

A midstream specimen of urine should again be sent for culture at the next antenatal visit to determine whether the management was successful.

13-10 What symptoms suggest acute pyelonephritis?

1. Most patients have severe general symptoms
   ◦ Headache.
   ◦ Pyrexia and rigors (shivering).
   ◦ Lower backache, especially pain over the kidneys (renal angles).
2. Only 40% of patients have urinary complaints.

13-11 What physical signs are usually found in a patient with acute pyelonephritis?

1. The patient is acutely ill.
2. The patient usually has high pyrexia and a tachycardia. However, the temperature may be normal during rigors.
3. On abdominal examination, the patient is tender over one or both kidneys. The patient is also tender on light percussion over one or both renal angles (posteriorly over the kidneys).

13-12 What is the management of a patient with acute pyelonephritis?

1. The patient must be admitted to hospital.

2. A midstream urine sample for microscopy, culture and sensitivity must be collected, if possible, to confirm the clinical diagnosis, identify the bacteria and determine the antibiotic of choice.
3. An intravenous infusion of Balsol or Ringer's lactate should be started and 1 litre given rapidly over 2 hours. Thereafter, 1 litre of Maintelyte should be given every 8 hours.
4. Broad-spectrum antibiotics must be given, i.e. cefuroxime (Zinacef) 750 mg 8-hourly. All antibiotics must be given intravenously until the patient's temperature has been normal for 24 hours. Oral cefuroxime (Zinnat) can then be given until a course of 10 days of antibiotics has been completed.
5. Pethidine 100 mg is given intramuscularly for severe pain while paracetamol (Panado) two adult tablets can be used for moderate pain.
6. Paracetamol (Panado) two adult tablets, together with tepid sponges, are used to bring down a high temperature.

NOTE
If the bacterial culture from the urine is positive, the antibiotic may need to be changed, depending on the sensitivity of the bacteria.

Patients with acute pyelonephritis during pregnancy must be admitted to hospital for treatment with a broad-spectrum antibiotic.

13-13 Why is acute pyelonephritis a serious infection in pregnancy?

Because serious complications can result:

1. Preterm labour.
2. Septic shock.
3. Perinephric abscess (an abscess around the kidney).
4. Anaemia.

Septic shock usually presents with continuing hypotension in spite of adequate intravenous fluids. There is also failure of the clinical signs of acute pyelonephritis to improve rapidly within the first 72 hours of treatment. If septic shock is diagnosed, intravenous gentamicin 80 mg must be given immediately, followed by a further 80 mg every 8 hours.

Gentamicin (Garamycin) must be added to any other antibiotic already given. The patient must also be transferred to a level 3 hospital.

13-14 What should be done at the first antenatal visit after the patient has been treated for acute pyelonephritis?

1. A midstream urine sample for culture and sensitivity must be collected to determine whether the treatment has been successful.
2. The haemoglobin concentration must be measured as there is a risk of anaemia developing.

Anaemia in pregnancy

13-15 What is the definition of anaemia in pregnancy?

A haemoglobin concentration of less than 11 g/dl.

13-16 What are the dangers of anaemia?

1. Heart failure, which can result from severe anaemia.
2. Shock, which may be caused by a relatively small vaginal blood loss (antepartum haemorrhage, delivery or postpartum haemorrhage) in an anaemic patient.

13-17 What are the common causes of anaemia in pregnancy?

1. Iron deficiency as the result of a diet poor in iron.
2. Blood loss during pregnancy (also during labour or the puerperium).
3. Acute infections (e.g. pyelonephritis), chronic infections (e.g. tuberculosis and HIV), and infestations (e.g. malaria, bilharzia or hook worm) in regions where these occur.
4. Folic-acid deficiency is less common.

> The commonest cause of anaemia in pregnancy is iron deficiency.

A full blood count, which is sent to the laboratory, will usually identify the probable cause of the anaemia.

The size and colour of the red cells indicate the probable cause of the anaemia:

1. Microcytic, hypochromic cells suggest iron deficiency.
2. Normocytic, normochromic cells suggest bleeding or infection.
3. Macrocytic, normochromic cells suggest folate deficiency.

13-18 What is the management of patients with iron deficiency in pregnancy or the puerperium?

1. The management of iron-deficiency anaemia in pregnancy will depend on the haemoglobin concentration and the duration of pregnancy.
   - If the haemoglobin concentration is less than 8 g/dl, the gestational age is less than 36 weeks, and the patient is asymptomatic, she can be treated with 2 tablets of ferrous sulphate 3 times a day and be followed at the antenatal clinic.
   - If the haemoglobin concentration is less than 8 g/dl and the gestational age is 36 weeks or more, the patient must be admitted to hospital for a blood transfusion.
   - All patients with a haemoglobin concentration of less than 8 g/dl who are short of breath or have a tachycardia of more than 100 beats per minute (signs of heart failure) must be admitted to hospital for a blood transfusion.
   - If the haemoglobin concentration is between 8 g/dl and 10 g/dl, the patient can be treated with 2 tablets of ferrous sulphate 3 times a day. If the haemoglobin concentration does not increase after 2 weeks or the patient is 36 weeks pregnant or more, and a full blood count has not yet been done, then a full blood count must be done to decide whether the cause of the anaemia is iron deficiency.
   - If the haemoglobin concentration is 10 g/dl or more, but less than 11 g/dl, the patient can be treated with 1 tablet of ferrous sulphate 3 times a day.

   In the case of the first three points above, a full blood count must be done. The size and colour of the red blood cells will help in determining the cause of the anaemia.

2. The management of a patient with iron-deficiency anaemia during the puerperium will depend on whether the patient is bleeding or not.
   - If the patient is not bleeding, if she has no signs of heart failure, and her haemoglobin concentration is 6 g/dl or more, she can be treated with oral iron tablets. 1 tablet of ferrous sulphate 3 times daily for a month is sufficient.
   - If the patient is not bleeding and she has signs of heart failure, or if her haemoglobin concentration is less than 6 g/dl, she must be

admitted to hospital and given a blood transfusion to be followed by oral iron for a month.

○ If the patient is bleeding, she should be managed for a postpartum haemorrhage.

The management of a patient with iron-deficiency anaemia during the puerperium is summarised in Figure 13-1.

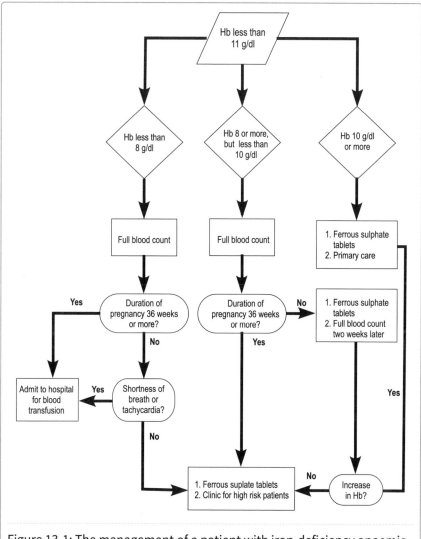

Figure 13-1: The management of a patient with iron-deficiency anaemia in pregnancy

13-19 Should all patients receive iron supplements in pregnancy?

1. Well-nourished patients who have a healthy diet and a haemoglobin concentration of 11 g/dl or more, must take 1 tablet daily.

2. Patients who are poorly nourished, have a poor diet or have a haemoglobin concentration of less than 11 g/dl need iron supplements.
3. Patients from communities where iron deficiency is common, or where socio-economic circumstances are poor, should receive iron supplements.

Iron tablets are dangerous to small children as even 1 tablet can cause serious iron poisoning. Therefore, patients must always keep their iron tablets in a safe place where children cannot reach them.

13-20 How are iron supplements given in pregnancy?

As 200 mg ferrous sulphate tablets.

1. Patients with a haemoglobin concentration of 11 g/dl or higher must take *1* tablet daily.
2. Patients who are anaemic must be correctly managed.

13-21 What side effects can be caused by ferrous sulphate tablets?

Nausea and even vomiting due to irritation of the lining of the stomach.

13-22 How should you manage a patient who complains of side effects due to ferrous sulphate tablets?

1. The tablets should be taken with meals. Although less iron will be absorbed, the side effects will be less.
2. If the patient continues to complain of side effects, she should be given 300 mg ferrous gluconate tablets instead. They cause fewer side effects than ferrous sulphate tablets.

Heart valve disease in pregnancy and the puerperium

Heart valve disease consists of damage to, or abnormality of, one or more of the valves of the heart. Usually the mitral valve is damaged. The cause of heart valve disease in a developing country is almost always rheumatic fever during childhood.

13-23 Why is it important during pregnancy to identify patients with heart valve disease in pregnancy?

1. A correct diagnosis of the type of heart valve disease and good management of the problem reduces the risk to the patient during her pregnancy.
2. Undiagnosed heart valve disease and inadequate treatment may result in serious complications (e.g. heart failure causing pulmonary oedema) which may threaten the patient's life.
3. A clear family-planning plan must be made during the pregnancy. The patient may have a reduced lifespan and cannot risk having a large family.

Correct diagnosis and good management reduce the risk to the patient of heart valve disease in pregnancy.

13-24 Which symptoms in a patient's history suggest that she may have heart valve disease?

1. Shortness of breath on exercise or even with limited effort.
2. Coughing up blood (haemoptysis).
3. Often the patient has previously been told by a doctor that she has a 'leaking heart'.
4. Some patients with heart valve disease give a history of previous rheumatic fever. However, most patients are not aware that they have suffered from previous rheumatic fever.

The cause of heart valve disease in a developing country is almost always previous rheumatic fever. However, these patients usually do not know that they have had one or more attacks of rheumatic fever during childhood.

During the examination of the cardiovascular system, a cardiac murmur will be heard if the patient has heart valve disease.

13-25 How should a patient with heart valve disease in pregnancy be managed?

1. The patient must be referred to the high-risk antenatal clinic.

2. At the high-risk antenatal clinic the type of lesion and correct management will be determined.
3. The follow-up visits will also be at the high-risk antenatal clinic. However, the patient may be referred to the primary-care antenatal clinic for some 'in between' visits. Take care to follow the instructions from the high-risk clinic carefully.
4. Patients who are not hospitalised should stop work earlier and rest more than usual.
5. The patient must be told to report immediately if she experiences any symptoms of heart failure, e.g. worsening shortness of breath or tiredness.
6. The patient must be delivered at least in a secondary level hospital where specialist care is available.

13-26 How should patients with heart valve disease be managed in the first stage of labour?

1. All patients must be delivered in hospital because of the risk of pulmonary oedema.
2. The patient should lie on her side with her upper body raised with pillows to 45 degrees.
3. Good analgesia is important to ensure that the patient does not become exhausted.
4. A slow intravenous infusion of 200 ml saline should be started, using a minidropper to make sure that not too much fluid is given.
5. Ampicillin 1 g and gentamicin 80 mg are given intravenously as prophylaxis against infective endocarditis. These antibiotics should be repeated 8-hourly for another 2 doses. Patients who are allergic to penicillin should be given erythromycin 500 mg instead of ampicillin.

13-27 How should patients with heart valve disease be managed in the second stage of labour?

1. The patient must be managed with her upper body raised with pillows to 45 degrees.
2. There should be good progress with effective maternal effort to ensure a short and easy second stage. Otherwise, an assisted delivery must be done.

3. If indicated, an episiotomy should be done to ensure a short and easy second stage.
4. The patient's legs must not be placed in the normal lithotomy position as this may cause pulmonary oedema. If the lithotomy position is needed, the patient should place her feet on two chairs which are at a lower level than the bed.

13-28 How should patients with heart valve disease be managed in the third stage of labour?

This is a very dangerous time for a patient with heart valve disease as there is an increased risk of pulmonary oedema. Therefore, careful attention must be paid to the following:

1. Syntometrine or ergometrine must *not* be given as they increase the risk of pulmonary oedema.
2. Oxytocin may be given. 10 units are given intramuscularly.
3. The third stage of labour should be actively managed.

Any drug containing ergometrine is absolutely contraindicated in the third stage of labour and the first 24 hours of the puerperium if the patient has heart valve disease.

13-29 What is important in the puerperium in patients with heart valve disease?

The risk of pulmonary oedema during the first 24 hours of the puerperium is great. Therefore, attention must be paid to the following:

1. During the first 24 hours of the puerperium the patient must be carefully observed for signs of pulmonary oedema, i.e. tachypnoea (breathing fast), dyspnoea (shortness of breath) and crepitations in the lungs.
2. The course of prophylactic antibiotics must be completed.

There is a high risk of pulmonary oedema in the third stage of labour and for the first 24 hours of the puerperium in patients with heart valve disease.

13-30 What form of family planning should be offered to patients with heart valve disease who have completed their families?

A postpartum sterilisation should be done. Because of the risk of heart failure, the procedure must be postponed until the third day after delivery. Patients who are willing and are prepared to return for the procedure, can have a laparoscopic sterilisation done six weeks after delivery. Meanwhile, an injectable contraceptive must be given.

Diabetes mellitus in pregnancy

13-31 Why is it important to diagnose diabetes if it develops in pregnancy?

Diabetes mellitus is a disorder which is caused by the secretion of inadequate amounts of insulin from the pancreas to keep the blood glucose concentration normal. As a result, the blood glucose concentration becomes abnormally high. Diabetes may often present for the first time in pregnancy, and may then recover spontaneously after delivery. The early diagnosis and good management of diabetes in pregnancy will greatly reduce the incidence of complications.

The early diagnosis and good management of diabetes in pregnancy will greatly reduce the incidence of complications.

13-32 What complications may be caused by diabetes in pregnancy if it is not diagnosed early and is not well managed?

1. Throughout the pregnancy infections are common, especially:
   o Candida vaginitis.
   o Urinary tract infection.

2. During the first trimester congenital abnormalities may occur in the developing fetus due to the raised blood glucose concentration.
3. During the third trimester pre-eclampsia and polyhydramnios are common.

4. The fetus may be large if the patient's diabetes has been poorly controlled during the pregnancy, resulting in problems during labour and delivery, mainly:
   o Cephalopelvic disproportion.
   o Impacted shoulders.
5. During the third stage of labour there is an increased risk of postpartum haemorrhage.
6. The newborn infant is at increased risk of many complications, especially hypoglycaemia and hyaline membrane disease.

13-33 How can complications which commonly occur in diabetics during pregnancy and labour be avoided?

These complications can largely be avoided by:

1. Early diagnosis.
2. Good control of the blood glucose concentration.

Early diagnosis and good control of the blood glucose concentration will prevent most of the pregnancy and labour complications caused by diabetes.

13-34 How can diabetes be diagnosed early if it should develop for the first time during pregnancy?

1. At every antenatal visit all patients should routinely have their urine tested for glucose.
2. A random blood glucose concentration must be measured if the patient has 1+ glycosuria or more at any antenatal visit.

Patients with repeated or marked glycosuria during pregnancy must always be investigated further for diabetes.

13-35 Is a reagent strip accurate enough to measure a random blood glucose concentration?

Yes, if an electronic instrument (Glucometer or Reflolux) is used to measure the blood glucose concentration. However, a reagent strip alone may not be accurate enough. Therefore, a sample of blood must be sent to the nearest laboratory for a blood glucose measurement, if an instrument is not available.

13-36 Is it possible that a patient with an initially normal blood glucose concentration may develop an abnormal concentration later in pregnancy?

Yes. This may be possible due to an increase in the amount of placental hormones as pregnancy progresses. Placental hormones tend to increase the blood glucose concentration, explaining why some patients only become diabetic during their pregnancies.

13-37 How should random blood glucose measurements be interpreted and how do the results determine further management?

A random blood glucose measurement is done on a blood sample taken from the patient at the clinic without any previous preparation, i.e. the patient does not have to fast. However, patients who have had nothing to eat during the previous four hours should be encouraged to eat something before the test.

1. A random blood glucose concentration of less than 8 mmol/l is normal. These patients can receive routine primary care. However, if glycosuria is again present, a random blood glucose measurement must be repeated.
2. A random blood glucose concentration of 8 mmol/l or more, but less than 11 mmol/l, may be abnormal and is an indication to measure the fasting blood glucose concentration. The further management of the patient will depend on the result of the fasting blood glucose concentration.
3. A random blood glucose concentration of 11 mmol/l or more is abnormal and indicates that the patient has diabetes. These patients

must be admitted to hospital to have their blood glucose controlled. Thereafter, they must remain on treatment and be followed as high-risk patients.

13-38 How should fasting blood glucose measurements be interpreted and how do the results determine further management?

The patient must have nothing to eat or drink (except water) from midnight. At 08:00 the next day a sample of blood is taken and the fasting blood glucose concentration is measured:

1. A fasting blood glucose concentration of less than 6 mmol/l is normal. These patients can receive routine primary care. If their random blood glucose concentration is again abnormal, the fasting blood glucose concentration should be measured again.
2. Patients with fasting blood glucose concentrations of 6 mmol/l or more but less than 8 mmol/l should be placed on a 7 600 kilojoule (1 800 kilocalorie) diabetic diet. A glucose profile should be determined after 2 weeks and be repeated every 4 weeks until delivery. Usually the glucose profile becomes normal on this low kilojoule diet.
3. Patients with a fasting blood glucose concentration of 8 mmol/l or more have diabetes. They must be admitted to hospital so that their blood glucose concentration can be controlled.

A 7600 kJ diabetic diet consists of a normal diet with reduced refined carbohydrates (e.g. sugar, cool drinks, fruit juices) and added high fibre foods (e.g. beans and wholewheat bread).

A patient with a normal blood glucose concentration early in pregnancy may develop diabetes later during that pregnancy.

13-39 How is a glucose profile obtained?

The patient must have nothing to eat or drink (except water) from midnight. At 08:00 the next day a sample of blood is taken and the fasting blood glucose concentration is measured. Immediately afterwards she has breakfast (which she can bring with her to the clinic). After 2 hours the blood glucose concentration is measured again.

13-40 How should the glucose profile be interpreted and how do the results determine further management?

1. A fasting blood glucose result of less than 6 mmol/l and a 2-hour result of less than 8 mmol/l are normal. These patients can be followed up as intermediate-risk patients.
2. A fasting blood glucose result of 6 mmol/l or more and/or a 2-hour result of 8 mmol/l or more are abnormal. These patients must be admitted to hospital so that they can have their blood glucose concentration controlled.

The management of patients with an abnormal random blood glucose concentration is summarised in flow diagram 13-2.

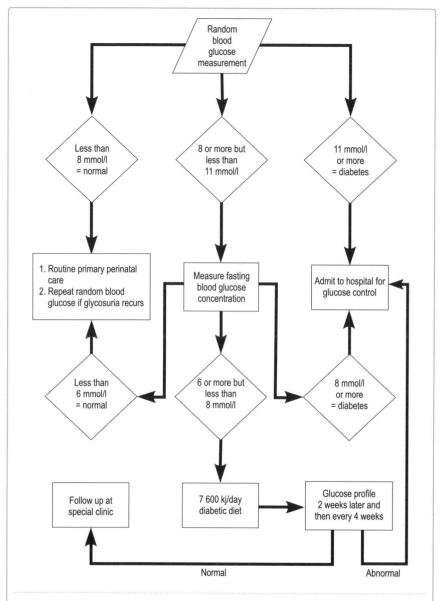

Figure 13-2: The management of a patient with glycosuria who has a random blood glucose concentration measured in pregnancy

Case study 1

A patient presents at 30 weeks gestation and complains of backache, feeling feverish, dysuria and frequency. On examination she has a tachycardia and a temperature of 38.5 °C. A diagnosis of cystitis is made and the patient is given oral amoxicillin to take at home.

1. Do you agree with the diagnosis?

No. The symptoms and signs suggest that the patient has acute pyelonephritis.

2. Is the management of this patient adequate to treat acute pyelonephritis?

No. The patient should be admitted to hospital and be given a broad-spectrum antibiotic intravenously.

3. Why is it necessary to treat acute pyelonephritis in pregnancy so aggressively?

Because severe complications may occur which can be dangerous both to the patient and her fetus.

4. What two complications should you watch for after admitting this patient to hospital?

1. Preterm labour.
2. Septic shock.

5. How will you recognise that the patient has developed septic shock?

The patient will become hypotensive in spite of receiving adequate intravenous fluid.

6. What should be done at the first antenatal visit after the patient is discharged from hospital?

A midstream urine sample should be collected for culture to make sure that the infection has been adequately treated. Her haemoglobin concentration must also be measured as patients often become anaemic after acute pyelonephritis.

Case study 2

A patient is seen at her first antenatal visit. She is already 36 weeks pregnant and has a haemoglobin concentration of 7.5 g/dl. As she is not short of breath and has no history of antepartum bleeding, she is treated with 2 tablets of ferrous sulphate to be taken 3 times a day. She is asked to return to the clinic in 1 week.

1. Do you agree with the management?

No. The patient is already 36 weeks pregnant and, therefore, is at great risk of going into labour before her haemoglobin concentration has had time to respond to the oral iron treatment. Therefore, the patient must be admitted to hospital and be given a blood transfusion.

2. Are any further investigations needed?

Yes. The cause of the anaemia must always be looked for. Blood for a full blood count must be taken before she is given a blood transfusion.

3. Is a full blood count adequate to diagnose the cause of the anaemia, or should other investigations be done?

In most cases a full blood count is adequate. The majority of patients who have anaemia without a history of bleeding are iron deficient. A full blood count will confirm the diagnosis of iron deficiency.

4. What should be done if a patient presents before 36 weeks gestation with a haemoglobin concentration below 8 g/dl?

If the patient is not short of breath and does not have a tachycardia above 100 beats per minute, she may be managed at a high-risk clinic. After blood has been sampled for a full blood count, she should be prescribed 2 ferrous sulphate tablets 3 times a day. With this treatment the patient should have corrected her haemoglobin concentration before she goes into labour.

5. What should be done if a patient presents before 36 weeks gestation with shortness of breath, tachycardia and a low haemoglobin concentration?

The patient must be admitted to hospital for a blood transfusion. This is necessary because the patient has shortness of breath and tachycardia, which suggest heart failure. Again, a full blood count must be done before the transfusion is started.

Case study 3

A patient presents for her first antenatal visit and gives a history that she has a 'leaking heart' due to rheumatic fever as a child. As she has no symptoms and does not get short of breath on exercise, she is reassured and managed as a low-risk patient. As she remains well with no shortness of breath, she is told that she can be delivered by a midwife at the primary perinatal-care clinic.

1. Why is the management incorrect?

With her history of rheumatic fever and a 'leaking heart', the patient must be examined by a doctor to determine whether she has heart valve disease. Undiagnosed heart valve disease can result in serious complications such as pulmonary oedema.

2. What should be done if the patient has a heart murmur due to heart valve disease?

The type of heart valve disease must be diagnosed. If the patient needs medication, the correct drug must be prescribed in the correct dosage. She must be managed as a high-risk patient and should be carefully followed up for symptoms or signs of heart failure.

3. Will most patients with heart valve disease give a history of previous rheumatic fever?

No. Although most heart valve disease is caused by rheumatic fever during childhood, most of these patients are not aware that they have had rheumatic fever.

4. Is it safe to deliver a patient with heart valve disease at a primary perinatal-care clinic?

No. Special management is needed in at least a secondary hospital with specialist care available. The patient must be closely observed for signs of heart failure, good pain relief is needed during labour and prophylactic antibiotics against infective endocarditis must be given. An assisted delivery may be necessary.

5. Is the danger over once the infant is born?

No. The third stage of labour and the first 24 hours of the puerperium are also dangerous. Ergometrine or Syntometrine must not be given and the patient must be closely observed for signs of heart failure. Oxytocin should be given and the third stage must be actively managed.

Case study 4

An obese 35-year-old multiparous patient presents with 1+ glycosuria at 20 weeks gestation. At the previous antenatal visit she had no glycosuria. A random blood glucose concentration is 7.5 mmol/l. She is reassured and followed up as a low-risk patient. At 28 weeks she has 3+ glycosuria. As the random blood glucose concentration at 20 weeks was normal, she is again reassured and asked to come back to the clinic in 2 weeks.

1. Do you agree with the management at 20 weeks gestation?

Yes, the patient was correctly managed when a random blood glucose concentration was measured after she had 2+ glycosuria. When 1+ glycosuria or more is present again, later in pregnancy, a random blood glucose concentration must be measured again.

2. How should the patient have been managed at 28 weeks?

She should have had another random blood glucose concentration measurement. Further management would depend on the result of this test.

3. Why should a patient be investigated if she has 2+ glycosuria of more for the first time?

Because the patient may already be a diabetic with a high blood glucose concentration causing the marked glycosuria.

4. What should the management have been if her random blood glucose was 9.0 mmol/l at 28 weeks gestation?

The patient should be seen the next morning after fasting from midnight. Her fasting blood glucose concentration should then be measured.

5. If the patient has a fasting blood glucose concentration of 7.0 mmol/l, what should her further management be?

The result is abnormal but is not high enough to diagnose diabetes. She should, therefore, be placed on a 7600 kJ per day diabetic diet. A glucose profile must be obtained after 2 weeks and this should be repeated every 4 weeks until delivery.

14

Family planning after pregnancy

Take the chapter test before and after you read this chapter.

Objectives

When you have completed this unit you should be able to:

- Explain the wider meaning of family planning.
- Give contraceptive counselling.
- List the efficiency, contraindications and side effects of the various contraceptive methods.
- List the important health benefits of contraception.
- Advise a postpartum patient on the most appropriate method of contraception.

Contraceptive counselling

14-1 What is family planning?

Family planning is far more than simply birth control, and aims at improving the quality of life for everybody. Family planning is an important part of primary healthcare and includes:

1. Promoting a caring and responsible attitude to sexual behaviour.
2. Ensuring that every child is wanted.
3. Encouraging the planning and spacing of the number of children according to a family's home conditions and financial income.

4. Providing the highest quality of maternal and child care.
5. Educating the community with regard to the disastrous effects of unchecked population growth on the environment.

It is essential to obtain prior community acceptance of, and promote community participation in, any family planning programme if the programme is to succeed in that community.

14-2 Who requires family planning education?

Because family planning aims at improving the quality of life for everybody, every person, female or male, requires family planning education. Such education should ideally start during childhood and be given in the home by the parents. It is then continued at school and throughout the rest of the individual's life.

14-3 Who needs contraceptive counselling?

Every person who is sexually active, or who probably will soon become sexually active, needs contraceptive counselling (i.e. information and advice about birth control). While the best time to advise a woman on contraception is before the first coitus, the antenatal and post-delivery periods are an excellent opportunity to provide contraceptive counselling. Some patients will ask you for contraceptive advice. However, you will often have to first motivate a patient to accept contraception before you can advise her about an appropriate method of contraception.

14-4 How should you motivate a patient to accept contraception after delivery?

A good way to motivate a patient to accept contraception is to discuss with her, or preferably with both her and her partner, the health and socio-economic effects further children could have on her and the rest of the family. Explain the immediate benefits of a smaller, well-spaced family.

It is generally hopeless to try and promote contraception by itself. To gain individual and community support, family planning must be seen as part of total primary healthcare. A high perinatal or infant mortality rate in a community is likely to result in a rejection of contraception.

14-5 How should you give contraceptive advice after delivery?

There are five important steps which should be followed.

Step 1: Discussion of the patient's future reproductive career

Ideally a woman should consider and plan her family before her first pregnancy, just as she would have considered her professional career. Unfortunately in practice this hardly ever happens and many women only discuss their reproductive careers for the first time when they are already pregnant or after the birth of the infant.

When planning her family the woman (or preferably the couple) should decide on:

1. The number of children wanted.
2. The time intervals between pregnancies as this will influence the method of contraception used.
3. The contraceptive method of choice when the family is complete.

Very often the patient will be unable or unwilling to make these decisions immediately after delivery. However, it is essential to discuss contraception with the patient so that she can plan her family. This should be done together with her partner and, where appropriate, other members of her family or friends.

Step 2: The patient's choice of contraceptive method

The patient should always be asked which contraceptive method she would prefer as this will obviously be the method with which she is most likely to continue.

Step 3: Consideration of contraindications to the patient's preferred method

You must decide whether the patient's choice of a contraceptive method is suitable, taking into consideration:

1. The effectiveness of each contraceptive method.
2. The contraindications to each contraceptive method.
3. The side effects of each contraceptive method.
4. The general health benefits of each contraceptive method.

If the contraceptive efficiency of the preferred method is appropriate, if there are no contraindications to it, and if the patient is prepared to accept the possible side effects, then the method chosen by the patient should be used. Otherwise proceed to step 4.

Step 4: Selection of the most appropriate alternative method of contraception

The selection of the most suitable alternative method of contraception after delivery will depend on a number of factors including the patient's wishes, her age, the risk of side effects and whether or not a very effective method of contraception is required.

Step 5: Counselling the patient once the contraceptive method has been chosen

Virtually every contraceptive method has its own side effects. It is a most important part of contraceptive counselling to explain the possible side effects to the patient. Expert family planning advice must be sought if the local clinic is unable to deal satisfactorily with the patient's problem. If family planning problems are not satisfactorily solved, the patient will probably stop using any form of contraception.

> After delivery the reproductive career of each patient must be discussed with her in order to decide on the most appropriate method of family planning to be used.

14-6 What contraceptive methods can be offered after delivery?

1. Sterilisation. Either tubal ligation (tubal occlusion) or vasectomy.
2. Injectables (i.e. an intramuscular injection of depot progestogen).
3. Oral contraceptives. Either the combined pill (containing both oestrogen and progestogen) or a progestogen-only pill (the 'minipill').
4. An intra-uterine contraceptive device (IUCD).
5. The condom.

Breastfeeding, spermicides alone, coitus interruptus and the 'safe period' are all very unreliable. All women should know about postcoital contraception.

> Breastfeeding cannot be relied upon to provide postpartum contraception.

14-7 How effective are the various contraceptive methods?

Contraceptive methods for use after delivery may be divided into very effective and less effective ones. Sterilisation, injectables, oral contraceptives and intra-uterine contraceptive devices are very effective. Condoms are less effective contraceptives.

The effectiveness of a contraceptive method is given as an index which indicates the number of women who would be expected to fall pregnant if 100 women used that method for one year. The ideal efficacy index is 0. The higher the index, the less effective is the method of contraception. The efficacy of the various contraceptive methods for use after delivery is shown in table 14-1.

14-8 How effective is postcoital contraception?

1. Norlevo, E-Gen-C or Ovral are effective within five days of unprotected sexual intercourse, but are more reliable the earlier they are used.
2. A copper intra-uterine contraceptive device can be inserted within six days of unprotected intercourse.
3. Postcoital methods should only be used in an emergency and not as a regular method of contraception.
4. If Norlevo is used, 1 tablet should be taken as soon as possible after intercourse, followed by another 1 tablet after exactly 12 hours.
5. If Ovral or E-Gen-C is used, 2 tablets are taken as soon as possible after intercourse, followed by another 2 tablets exactly 12 hours later.

The tablets for postcoital contraception often cause nausea and vomiting, which reduces their effectiveness. These side effects are less with levonorgestrel (Norlevo and Escapelle) which contains no oestrogen. Therefore levonorgestrel (Norlevo and Escapelle) is a more reliable method and should be used if available. Norlevo and Escapelle as a single dose method is available in South Africa.

14-9 What are the contraindications to the various contraceptive methods?

The following are the common or important conditions where the various contraceptive methods should *not* be used:

1. Sterilisation
   - Marital disharmony.
   - Psychological problems.
   - Forced or hasty decision.
   - Gynaecological problem requiring hysterectomy.

2. Injectables
   - Depression.
   - Pregnancy planned within 1 year.

3. Combined pills
   - A history of venous thromboembolism.
   - Age 35 years or more with risk factors for cardiovascular disease.
   - Anyone of 50 or more years.
   - Oestrogen-dependent malignancies such as breast or uterine cancer.

4. Progestogen-only pill (minipill)
   - None.

5. Intra-uterine contraceptive device
   - A history of excessive menstruation.
   - Anaemia.
   - Multiple sex partners when the risk of genital infection is high.
   - Pelvic inflammatory disease.

A menstrual abnormality is a contraindication to any of the hormonal contraceptive methods (injectables, combined pill or progestogen-only pill) until the cause of the menstrual irregularity has been diagnosed. Thereafter, hormonal contraception may often be used to correct the menstrual irregularity. However, during the puerperium a previous history of menstrual irregularity before the pregnancy is *not* a contraindication to hormonal contraception.

NOTE
If a woman has a medical complication, then a more detailed list of contraindications may be obtained from the standard reference books such as J

Guillebaud: *Your questions answered*. Fifth edition. London: Churchill Livingstone 2009.
The World Health Organisation (WHO) medical eligibility criteria for contraceptive use is also available on a WHO website (www.who.int/reproductive -health/publications/mec/).

14-10 What are the major side effects of the various contraceptive methods?

Most contraceptive methods have side effects. Some side effects are unacceptable to a patient and will cause her to discontinue the particular method. However, in many instances side effects are mild or disappear with time. It is, therefore, very important to counsel a patient carefully about the side effects of the various contraceptive methods, and to determine whether she would find any of them unacceptable. At the same time the patient may be reassured that some side effects will most likely become less or disappear after a few months' use of the method.

The major side effects of the various contraceptive methods used after delivery are:

1. Sterilisation
2. Tubal ligation and vasectomy have no medical side-effects and, therefore, should be highly recommended during counselling of patients who have completed their families. Menstrual irregularities are *not* a problem. However, about 5% of women later regret sterilisation.
3. Injectables
    ○ Menstrual abnormalities, e.g. amenorrhoea, irregular menstruation or spotting.
    ○ Weight gain.
    ○ Headaches.
    ○ Delayed return to fertility within a year of stopping the method. There is no evidence that fertility is reduced thereafter.
    ○ With Nur-Isterate there is a quicker return to fertility, slightly less weight gain and a lower incidence of headaches and amenorrhoea than with Depo-Provera or Petogen.
4. Combined pill
    ○ Reduction of lactation.
    ○ Menstrual abnormalities, e.g. spotting between periods.

- Nausea and vomiting.
- Depression.
- Fluid retention and breast tenderness.
- Chloasma (a brown mark on the face).
- Headaches and migraine.

5. Progestogen-only pill
   - Menstrual abnormalities, e.g. irregular menstruation.
   - Headaches.
   - Weight gain.

6. Copper-containing intra-uterine contraceptive device
   - Expulsion in 3–15 cases per 100 women who use the device for 1 year.
   - Pain at insertion.
   - Dysmenorrhoea.
   - Menorrhagia (excessive and/or prolonged bleeding).
   - Increase in pelvic inflammatory disease.
   - Perforation of the uterus is uncommon.
   - Ectopic pregnancy is not prevented.

7. Progesterone-containing intra-uterine contraceptive devices (Mirena) have lesser side effects and reduce menstrual blood loss. These devices are expensive and not generally available in South Africa

8. Condom
   - Decreased sensation for both partners.
   - Not socially acceptable to everyone.

> **If a couple have completed their family the contraceptive method of choice is tubal ligation or vasectomy.**

Additional contraceptive precautions must be taken when the effectiveness of an oral contraceptive may be impaired, e.g. diarrhoea or when taking antibiotics. There is no medical reason for stopping a hormonal method periodically to 'give the body a rest'.

14-11 What are the important health benefits of contraceptives?

The main objective of all contraceptive methods is to prevent pregnancy. In developing countries pregnancy is a major cause of mortality and morbidity in women. Therefore, the prevention of pregnancy is a very important general health benefit of all contraceptives.

Various methods of contraception have a number of additional health benefits. Although these benefits are often important, they are not generally appreciated by many patients and healthcare workers.

1. Injectables
   ○ Decrease in dysmenorrhoea.
   ○ Less premenstrual tension.
   ○ Less iron-deficiency anaemia due to decreased menstrual flow.
   ○ No effect on lactation.

2. Combined pill
   ○ Decrease in dysmenorrhoea.
   ○ Decrease in menorrhagia (heavy and/or prolonged menstruation).
   ○ Less iron-deficiency anaemia.
   ○ Less premenstrual tension.
   ○ Fewer ovarian cysts.
   ○ Less benign breast disease.
   ○ Less endometrial and ovarian carcinoma.

3. Progestogen-only pill
   ○ No effect on lactation.

4. Condom
   ○ Less risk of HIV infection and other sexually transmitted diseases.
   ○ Less pelvic inflammatory disease.
   ○ Less cervical intra-epithelial neoplasia.

The condom is the only contraceptive method that provides protection against HIV infection.

14-12 What is the most appropriate method of contraception for a patient after delivery?

The most suitable methods for the following groups of patients are:

1. Lactating patients
   - An injectable, but not if a further pregnancy is planned within the next year.
   - A progestogen-only pill (minipill) for 3 months, then the combined pill.
   - An intra-uterine contraceptive device.

2. Teenagers and patients with multiple sexual partners.
   - An injectable, as this is a reliable method even with unreliable patients who might forget to use another method.
   - Additional protection against HIV infection by using a condom is essential. It is important to stress that the patient should only have intercourse with a partner who is willing to use a condom.

3. HIV-positive patients
   - Condoms must be used in addition to the appropriate contraceptive method (dual contraception).

4. Patients whose families are complete
   - Tubal ligation or vasectomy is the logical choice.
   - An injectable, e.g. Depo-Provera or Petogen (12 weekly) or Nur-Isterate (8 weekly).
   - A combined pill until 35 years of age if there are risk factors for cardiovascular disease, or until 50 years if these risk factors are absent.

5. Patients of 35 years or over without risk factors for cardiovascular disease
   - Tubal ligation or vasectomy is the logical method.
   - A combined pill until 50 years of age.
   - An injectable until 50 years of age.
   - A progestogen-only pill until 50 years of age.
   - An intra-uterine contraceptive device until 1 year after the periods have stopped, i.e. when there is no further risk of pregnancy.
6. Patients of 35 years or over with risk factors for cardiovascular disease
   - As above but *no* combination pill.

> **The puerperium is the most convenient time for the patient to have a bilateral tubal ligation performed.**

Every effort should be made to provide facilities for tubal ligation during the puerperium for all patients who request sterilisation after delivery.

Remember that sperms may be present in the ejaculate for up to 3 months following vasectomy. Therefore, an additional contraceptive method must be used during this time.

14-13 What are the risk factors for cardiovascular disease in women taking the combined pill?

The risk of cardiovascular disease increases markedly in women of 35 or more years of age who have one or more of the following risk factors:

1. Smoking.
2. Hypertension.
3. Diabetes.
4. Hypercholesterolaemia.
5. A personal history of cardiovascular disease.

> **Smoking is a risk factor for cardiovascular disease.**

14-14 When should an intra-uterine contraceptive device be inserted after delivery?

It should not be inserted before six weeks as the uterine cavity would not yet have returned to its normal size. At six weeks or more after delivery there is the lowest risk of:

1. Pregnancy.
2. Expulsion.

Postpartum patients choosing this method must be discharged on an injectable contraceptive or progestogen-only pill until an intra-uterine contraceptive device has been inserted.

NOTE
Insertion of an intra-uterine contraceptive device immediately after delivery may be considered if it is thought likely that a patient will not use another contraceptive method and where sterilisation is not appropriate. However, the expulsion rate will be as high as 15 to 20%.

Case study 1

You have delivered the fourth child of an unbooked 36-year-old patient. All her children are alive and well. She is a smoker, but is otherwise healthy. She has never used contraception.

1. Should you counsel this patient about contraception?

Yes. Every sexually active person needs contraceptive counselling. This patient in particular needs counselling as she is at an increased risk of maternal and perinatal complications, should she fall pregnant again, because of her age and parity.

2. Which contraceptive methods would be appropriate for this patient?

Tubal ligation or vasectomy would be the most appropriate method of contraception if she does not want further children. Should she not want sterilisation, either an injectable contraceptive or an intra-uterine contraceptive device would be the next best choice.

3. If the patient accepts tubal ligation, when should this be done?

The most convenient time for the patient and her family is the day after delivery (postpartum sterilisation). Every effort should be made to provide facilities for postpartum sterilisation for all patients who request it.

4. If the couple decides not to have a tubal ligation or vasectomy, how will you determine whether an injectable or an intra-uterine contraceptive device would be the best choice?

Assessing the risk for pelvic inflammatory disease will determine which of the two methods to use. If the patient has a stable relationship, an intra-uterine contraceptive device may be more appropriate. However, if she or her partner has other sexual partners, an injectable contraceptive would be indicated.

5. What other advice must be given to a patient at risk of sexually transmitted infections?

The patient must insist that her partner wears a condom during sexual intercourse. This will reduce the risk of HIV infection.

Case study 2

A 15-year-old primigravida had a normal delivery in a district hospital. She has never used contraception. Her mother asks you for contraceptive advice for her daughter after delivery. The patient's boyfriend has deserted her.

1. Does this young teenager require contraceptive advice after delivery?

Yes, she will certainly need contraceptive counselling and should start on a contraceptive method before discharge from hospital. She needs to learn sexual responsibility and must be told where the nearest family planning clinic to her home is for follow-up. She also needs to know about postcoital contraception.

2. Which contraceptive method would be most the appropriate for this patient?

An injectable contraceptive would probably be the best method for her as she needs reliable contraception for a long time.

3. Why would she need a long-term contraceptive?

Because she should only have her next child when she is fully grown up and able to take care of her children by herself.

4. If the patient prefers to use an oral contraceptive, would you regard this as an appropriate method of contraception for her?

No. A method which she is more likely to use correctly and reliably would be more appropriate. Oral contraceptives are only reliable if taken every day.

5. The patient and her mother are worried that the long-term effect of injectable contraception could be harmful to a girl of 15 years. What would be your advice?

Injectable contraception is extremely safe and, therefore, is an appropriate method for long-term use. This method will not reduce her future fertility.

Case study 3

You have just delivered the first infant of a healthy 32-year-old patient. In discussing contraception with her, she mentions that she is planning to fall pregnant again within a year after she stops breastfeeding. She is a schoolteacher and would like to continue her career after having two children.

1. The patient says that she has used an injectable contraceptive for five years before this pregnancy and would like to continue with this method. What would your advice be?

Injectable contraception would not be appropriate as she plans her next pregnancy within a year, and there may be a delayed return to fertility.

2. If the patient insists on using an injectable contraceptive, which drug would you advise her to use?

An injectable such as Nur-Isterate is preferable, as the return to fertility may be quicker.

3. Following further counselling, the patient decides on oral contraception and is given a combined pill. Do you agree with this management?

No. As she plans to breastfeed, she should be given a progestogen-only pill. Combined oral contraceptive pills may reduce milk production while breastfeeding is being established. Progestogen-only pills have no effect on breastfeeding.

Case study 4

A married primipara from a rural area has just been delivered in a district hospital. She has a stable relationship with her husband and they decide to have their next infant in five years' time. The patient would like to have an intra-uterine contraceptive device inserted.

1. Is this an appropriate method for this patient?

Yes, as the risk of developing pelvic inflammatory disease is low.

2. When should the device be inserted?

Six weeks or more after delivery, as there is an increased risk of expulsion if the device is inserted earlier.

3. Could the patient, in the meantime, rely on breast feeding as a contraceptive method?

No. The risk of pregnancy is too high. She should use reliable contraception, such as injectable contraception or the progestogen-only pill, until the device is inserted.

4. The patient asks if the intra-uterine contraceptive device could be inserted before she is discharged from hospital. Would this be appropriate management?

The expulsion rate and, therefore, the risk of contraceptive failure is much higher if the device is inserted soon after delivery. Therefore, it would be far better if she were to return six weeks later for insertion of the device.

15

Regionalised perinatal care

Take the chapter test before and after you read this chapter.

Objectives

When you have completed this unit you should be able to:

- List the advantages of regionalised perinatal care.
- Describe the functioning of a maternal-care clinic.
- Communicate better with patients and colleagues.
- Safely transfer a patient to hospital.
- Determine the maternal mortality rate.

Regionalised perinatal care

15-1 What is regionalised perinatal care?

Regionalised perinatal care is the care of all pregnant women and their newborn infants in a single health system within a clearly defined region. The responsibility for perinatal care in that region must fall under a single health authority as this standardises care and prevents wasteful duplication of services. The borders of each healthcare region will have to be negotiated with the communities and local health authorities concerned. Similarly, other healthcare services should also be organised on a regional basis.

> All perinatal care provided in a region should be the responsibility of a single health authority.

15-2 Do all women require the same care during their pregnancy, labour and puerperium?

All patients should receive good care. However, all patients do not need the same care as they do not all run the same risk of developing perinatal problems. Patients can be classified into three separate groups:

1. Most patients have only a small chance of developing problems during and after their pregnancy. These women are classified as *low risk*. About 50% of women fall into the low-risk category.
2. About 30% of patients have an increased chance of complications during certain periods of their pregnancy, labour and puerperium only. These patients are said to be at *intermediate risk*. For example, a patient who has had a previous Caesarean section for cephalopelvic disproportion is at low risk during her pregnancy and may, therefore, be cared for at a clinic. However, she is at increased risk during labour and, therefore, must be delivered in a hospital with facilities to perform a Caesarean section.
3. About 20% of women have an increased chance of medical or obstetric problems during their pregnancy and puerperium. They are classified as *high-risk* patients.

15-3 Should all pregnant women be delivered in a hospital?

No. Low-risk patients need primary perinatal care only. This consists of good, basic perinatal care which can be provided at a district hospital or primary-care clinic. Low-risk patients should be delivered at a clinic or district hospital. Patients at high or intermediate risk need more than primary care. They require care at a district hospital with facilities to perform a Caesarean section, secondary level care or tertiary level care. Secondary perinatal care requires additional equipment as well as doctors and nurses with special training. Tertiary perinatal care usually consists of very expensive intensive care which requires highly specialised staff and sophisticated equipment.

> About half of all patients are at low risk of developing clinical problems during pregnancy, labour and the puerperium and, therefore, need primary perinatal care only.

15-4 Should all patients be delivered by a doctor?

No. Patients at low risk who only need primary perinatal care can be safely delivered by a midwife. Patients needing care at a district hospital with facilities to perform a Caesarean section or secondary perinatal care may be delivered by a doctor or a midwife. Patients needing tertiary perinatal care are usually delivered by a doctor who has had specialist training, or a midwife with a doctor immediately available should complications develop. The important feature of tertiary care is the immediate availability of specialist staff and facilities should they be needed.

15-5 What should be the relationship between the various hospitals in a healthcare region?

Each healthcare region will have a regional hospital (level 2) which provides secondary care. Usually two or three regions are supported by a tertiary hospital (level 3). Some tertiary hospitals are attached to a medical school while most have a nursing college. Each region will also have a number of base or district hospitals (level 1) which will provide level 1 care. The regional hospital is responsible for the district hospitals in that region.

The staff at the regional hospital should communicate closely with the staff at the district hospitals. Patients at the district hospitals needing tertiary care should be transferred directly to the tertiary hospital. In turn, the regional hospital staff should provide educational programmes for, and give management advice to, the district hospital staff. Each district hospital usually has a number of primary healthcare centres.

All medical and nursing staff in a health region should regard themselves as members of a team whose goal is to provide good quality care to all the patients in that region. All staff members should, therefore, co-operate and help one another. The responsibility for all mothers and infants in the region is then shared between all the staff working in that region. It is particularly important that the clinic and hospital staff work as a team and do not regard themselves as separate services.

The fragmentation of health services, with various hospitals and clinics falling under different authorities, is a major cause of poor perinatal care in many communities.

15-6 How should the district hospital assist the perinatal clinics in that district?

Each primary-care clinic should be linked to a district hospital (level 1) within the same region. The district hospital is responsible for the perinatal care given at the clinics in that district. The clinic staff should contact this hospital for help or advice, and problem patients should be referred to that hospital when needed. The staff of the district hospital should be able to rotate with the staff at the clinics. This ensures that the standard of care in the clinics is maintained at a high level, and also helps the hospital and clinics staff understand each other's difficulties.

15-7 How should clinic staff communicate with the referral hospital?

1. A telephone or 2-way radio is essential so that the clinic staff and the hospital staff can speak directly to each other.
2. Clear guidelines are needed to indicate which patients should be referred to hospital. If the clinic staff are uncertain whether a patient needs referral, they must discuss the problem with the staff of the referral hospital.
3. The staff at each clinic must know which hospital to contact if they need help. The hospital's telephone number must be displayed next to the clinic's telephone.
4. The clinic staff must collect all the relevant information on the patient before phoning to discuss the patient. Good notes must always accompany the patient as they are one of the most effective methods of communication. Either the complete patient record or at least the antenatal card must be sent with the patient. If the patient is in labour, the partogram must also be sent. It is essential that the clinic staff identify the patient's clinical problems.
5. When speaking to the hospital staff, stress the important information and summarise the problem. State clearly where advice is needed.
6. Always give your name and rank and ask who you are speaking to. If necessary, insist that you speak to a senior staff member if you are not satisfied with the advice you receive.

15-8 How can a referral hospital improve communication with the clinic?

1. A telephone line for incoming calls only (a 'hotline') should be available in the labour ward of the hospital so that the clinic staff can contact the hospital staff without delay.

2. The most senior and experienced nurse or doctor should receive the call. Each day and night someone should be allocated to answer the clinic calls.

3. Listen carefully, be patient, and try to obtain a clear idea of the problem.

4. Ask for important information which has not been provided.

5. It is better to admit the patient if there is any doubt about her condition.

6. Arrange the transfer. Usually this is done by the referring clinic or hospital. However, in an urban region the receiving hospital may prefer to arrange the transport.

7. Indicate any emergency treatment which must be given before or during transport.

8. If possible, inform the clinic after the patient has arrived at the hospital. A reply letter should be used to indicate the patient's condition on arrival, the diagnosis made by the hospital staff and the patient's response to treatment. Feedback to the referring clinic is essential.

9. Ideally, all patients transferred from a clinic should be reviewed every month. This should ideally be done during an outreach visit from the referral hospital. In this way problems with referrals can be identified and corrected.

10. A checklist available at the emergency telephone in the referral hospital helps to ensure that a complete history is obtained and that no important information is forgotten. If the person receiving the call does not know what advice to give, this information is then used when discussing the patient with a more senior colleague. The name and telephone number of the person making the call must always be recorded.

Excellent communication and co-operation between the staff of hospitals and clinics in a region are needed to provide good perinatal care.

The maternal-care clinic

15-9 What is a maternal-care clinic?

A maternal-care clinic (perinatal-care clinic) is a special clinic where midwives provide primary antenatal and postnatal care. Some maternal-care clinics also have facilities to deliver low-risk patients. A maternal-care clinic with a delivery facility is often called a midwife obstetric unit (MOU). These clinics function day and night, and should be situated in or near to the community which it serves. Primary maternal and newborn care (primary perinatal care) is part of *primary healthcare* and, therefore, the facilities of a primary-healthcare centre are often used to provide perinatal care. In practice, the staff providing perinatal care usually provide other forms of primary healthcare as well. A maternal-care clinic may also be run in a level 1 hospital. In large urban or peri-urban communities, there may be maternal-care clinics separate from primary-healthcare centres. Some clinics only offer antenatal care with the mother having to deliver at another clinic further away from her home. These antenatal-care clinics must function as an extension of the maternal-care clinic with a delivery facility as very close co-operation is essential.

At a maternal care clinic midwives provide primary perinatal care to low-risk patients.

15-10 What are the functions of a midwife in a maternal-care clinic where deliveries are done?

The midwife is responsible for all the antenatal care, the care during labour and delivery, and the postnatal care given at the clinic. The midwife should function as an independent nurse-practitioner and meet all the primary perinatal care needs of low-risk patients.

15-11 What are the functions of a doctor in a maternal-care clinic?

The doctor does not fulfil the usual functions of a medical practitioner and should not see every patient who attends the clinic. The functions of the doctor are:

1. To *consult*, i.e. to examine and advise on the management of patients referred by the midwives with various problems.
2. To *teach*. It is essential that the doctor teaches the midwives the essential knowledge and clinical skills which they need to function competently in a maternal-care clinic.
3. To *administer*. Together with the senior midwife, the doctor should plan, implement and evaluate all care given at the maternal-care clinic.
4. To *audit* the number and reasons for referral.

15-12 What is the role of the community in a maternal-care clinic?

The maternal-care clinic should be acceptable to the community as a facility which provides excellent primary perinatal care for patients from that community. Every effort should be made to involve the community in establishing and running the clinic. It is desirable to form a lay organisation (such as 'Friends of the Maternal-Care Clinic') to help meet this role. Representatives from the community, together with medical and nursing staff, should sit on the management board of the clinic. The community can help raise funds for the clinic and can also help provide some of the care, e.g. help run breastfeeding clinics and to be trained as doulas to assist women delivering in clinics or hospitals.

The clinic staff should co-operate and communicate with community members, such as village health workers, traditional birth attendants (TBAs), traditional healers, breastfeeding advisors, social workers and schoolteachers, who can all assist in improving perinatal services in that community.

15-13 What are the advantages of a maternal-care clinic with delivery facilities?

1. The patient remains close to her home and community.
2. More personal care can be given as labour and delivery take place in a relaxed atmosphere.

3. A saving in transfer and hospital costs.
4. The staff often can work close to their homes which saves both time and money. Staff also get great work satisfaction through being able to accept greater responsibility than in a hospital, provided that they receive support from the hospital staff.

The many advantages of delivering low-risk patients in a clinic only apply if the clinic is supported by a level 1 or 2 hospital. The community will not accept care given at a maternal-care clinic if rapid and safe transfer is not available when patients develop complications.

15-14 Why is delivery in a maternal-care clinic safer than a home delivery?

Many low-risk patients can be safely delivered at home. However, many homes do not have good lighting, a telephone, clean water and adequate space for a safe delivery. In addition, many homes are far from the hospital or clinic should problems occur with the mother or infant. In these circumstances it is far safer for the patient to deliver at a maternal-care clinic with a delivery facility where staff and equipment are available to deal with most of the perinatal complications. In densely populated areas midwives working in maternal-care clinics provide a better service to the community.

If patients are delivered at a clinic and then discharged home after an average of six hours, many of the benefits of being close to the family and home surroundings can still be enjoyed.

NOTE
In an affluent community it may be possible to safely deliver carefully selected low-risk patients at home provided a telephone and immediate transport are available in case complications develop.

15-15 Which patients should not be delivered at a maternal-care clinic but must be referred to a hospital?

Every perinatal region must draw up its own detailed and easily understood list of criteria for referring patients from a maternal-care clinic (or level 1 hospital) to either a level 2 or a level 3 hospital. The responsibility for drawing up the list of referral criteria rests with the senior members of the obstetric, neonatal and nursing staff at the regional (level 3) hospital, in consultation with the medical and nursing staff at the level 1 and 2 hospitals and maternal-care clinics. Referral criteria will differ between regions as the criteria will depend on the distance the patient has to be transferred, the facilities and staff available at the clinics, and the quality of the available transport. (A complete set of guidelines for the referral of antenatal patients is listed in Appendix 1.

NOTE
These referral criteria should be frequently reviewed in the light of the number and nature of the clinical problems requiring referral of patients to hospital.

There must be *referral criteria* for the mother as well as for the newborn infant.

> Each maternal-care clinic must have its own list of referral criteria.

15-16 How can communication between the clinic staff and their patients be improved?

1. Make time to speak to the patients.
2. If possible, find a place where the patient can speak to you in private.
3. Be honest when you tell patients about their clinical problems.
4. Listen to what they say and ask.
5. Use simple language.
6. Allow patients to ask questions.
7. Look at the patient when you speak to her.
8. Address the patient by name.
9. Watch, listen and learn when more experienced colleagues speak to patients.
10. Try to understand what the patient is feeling.
11. Be kind and helpful.
12. At the completion of an antenatal visit the patient must be clearly informed if the findings were normal.

15-17 What can be done to simplify note-keeping in a maternal-care clinic?

The patient should carry a hand-held antenatal card or patient record which contains all her antenatal information. This is a simple, cheap and highly effective method of recording patient information when caring for low-risk patients. Most patients look after their cards and take them along to the clinic. It is uncommon for patients to lose their cards. This system avoids the frustrating situation where the patient presents at a clinic or hospital, but her folder is being kept elsewhere. Using an antenatal card instead of a folder also shortens the time the patient has to wait at the clinic and reduces the workload of the staff. If a hand-held antenatal card or patient record system is used, there is no need to issue patient folders before labour.

Transferring patients safely to hospital

15-18 How should the transfer of a patient from a clinic to a hospital be arranged?

It is essential that the base hospital be contacted *before* the patient is transferred. The clinical problem and the required management must be discussed between the maternal-care clinic staff and the hospital staff. Most patients who are transferred during the antenatal period do not need to get to hospital urgently and, therefore, do not need to be transported by ambulance. However, all patients transferred to hospital during labour will require ambulance transport. Usually the referring clinic or hospital will make the arrangements for transferring the patient. If the clinic arranges transport, the hospital must be notified of these arrangements.

> Always contact the referral hospital before transferring a patient.

15-19 What can be done to make the transfer of a patient as safe as possible?

Before an ill patient may be transferred from a primary maternal-care clinic to a hospital, both she and her fetus or newborn infant must first be stabilised. They will then be in the best possible condition to be moved and will have the best chance of arriving safely at the hospital. To achieve these objectives, the following must be done before the patient leaves the maternal-care clinic:

1. The patient and/or the fetus or newborn infant must be fully resuscitated.
2. An intravenous infusion (drip) must be in place.
3. All the necessary drugs must be readily available while the patient is being transferred to hospital.
4. Oxygen and resuscitation equipment in good working order must be available. The latter includes equipment for face-mask ventilation and endotracheal intubation.
5. A person competent in adult and neonatal resuscitation must accompany the patient.

15-20 Who should care for the patient while she is being transported to the hospital?

There are a number of referral criteria where it is quite safe for the patient to travel to hospital with only a lay person accompanying her, e.g. a patient in early labour who has had a previous Caesarean section can use her own or public transport. These conditions must be detailed in the list of referral criteria. In all other circumstances, patients with complications must be accompanied by a qualified person competent in adult and neonatal resuscitation. This may be a midwife, doctor or trained ambulance personnel (ambumedics). To send an ill patient or newborn infant to hospital without being accompanied by such a qualified person is dangerous and is likely to result in serious complications or even the death of the patient and/or her infant.

15-21 What documentation should be sent with the patient?

All the clinical notes of the patient (and her newborn infant) must be sent with her to the hospital. Good record-keeping is an essential part of perinatal care. Before transferring a patient you must, therefore, make sure that the patient record gives an accurate account of what has happened to the patient up to the time of transfer. It is very important to include details of the complications and the management. Clearly state why the patient requires transfer to hospital.

15-22 What are the main dangers to the patient while she is being transported to the hospital?

1. Antepartum haemorrhage.
2. Convulsions, i.e. eclampsia.
3. Intracranial haemorrhage due to severe uncontrolled hypertension.
4. Respiratory arrest.
5. Cord prolapse.
6. Delivery before arrival at the hospital.

Maternal mortality

15-23 What is the maternal mortality ratio?

The maternal mortality ratio is the number of women who die during pregnancy, labour, or the puerperium, and is expressed per 100 000 deliveries. Therefore, if 25 women die during pregnancy, labour, or the puerperium in a healthcare region where 50 000 deliveries are done a year, the maternal mortality ratio for that region in that year will be 50 per 100 000 (i.e. 25/50 000 x 100 000).

The maternal mortality ratio in developing countries or poor communities in developed countries is usually 50 or more per 100 000 deliveries. This contrasts with the maternal mortality ratio of less than 10 per 100 000 in most industrialised countries with good health services.

It is important to note that women who die as a result of complications in early pregnancy, e.g. septic miscarriage or ectopic pregnancy, are included under maternal deaths.

> **The maternal mortality rate in developing countries is high.**

15-24 What is the value of knowing the maternal mortality ratio in your region?

It is very important to determine the maternal mortality ratio in *each* region of the country as this ratio reflects the quality of the care provided to women during pregnancy, and during and after delivery. Even in a poor community, the maternal mortality ratio can be reduced by the provision of good perinatal care. Knowing the maternal mortality ratio of a region also allows comparisons to be made with other regions or comparisons between patients delivered in different years in a region. As the quality of perinatal care improves, the maternal mortality ratio should decrease.

By determining the causes of maternal death, preventable causes, such as postpartum haemorrhage, may be identified. Measures to prevent these complications can then be introduced throughout the region.

Information on maternal deaths should be collected by the health authorities in each region and be interpreted by specialists at the tertiary hospital. A maternal mortality notification form must be used for the data collection.

NOTE
Since October 1997 it has been compulsory to notify all maternal deaths in South Africa to the provincial Maternal, Child and Women's Health (MCWH) Directorate. Maternal death notification forms, as well as an explanatory document on the way the forms have to be completed, must be available at all institutions dealing with pregnant women.

A photostat copy of the patient's entire folder must accompany the maternal death notification forms, as well as photocopies of the patient's folders from any other hospitals or clinics where the patient had been managed before. All information in these folders will be kept strictly confidential.

15-25 What is the difference between primary and final causes of maternal mortality?

1. The *primary* cause of death is the initiating complication or condition that triggered a sequence of events ultimately resulting in a maternal death.
2. The *final* cause of death is the complication that ultimately resulted in a maternal death.

A woman develops severe pre-eclampsia during pregnancy, her blood pressure is not controlled, and a fatal intracranial haemorrhage occurs. The primary and final causes of the maternal death will be pre-eclampsia and an intracranial haemorrhage respectfully.

15-26 What are the important primary causes of maternal mortality in a developing country?

The commonest *primary* causes of maternal mortality in South Africa are:

1. The complications of HIV/AIDS.
2. The hypertensive disorders of pregnancy, especially uncontrolled hypertension causing intracranial haemorrhage.
3. Haemorrhage, especially postpartum haemorrhage.
4. Infection, often complicating prolonged obstructed labour.

In many developing countries, haemorrhage and infection are responsible for more deaths than the hypertensive disorders of pregnancy. As perinatal services improve, deaths due to haemorrhage and infection will decrease.

In contrast, the commonest causes of maternal mortality in a developed country, such as the United Kingdom, are thromboembolism, the hypertensive disorders of pregnancy, and deaths resulting from complications of anaesthesia.

15-27 Should each maternal death be discussed at a special meeting?

Yes. It is very important that each maternal death is discussed to discover the cause. The aim is not to punish anyone who made an error, but rather to learn from the case report in order to prevent the same mistake being made again. Once the common causes of maternal death in a region are identified, steps must be taken to prevent the problems which lead to those deaths.

Case study 1

A patient is diagnosed as having poor progress of labour at a community healthcare clinic. The clinic functions independently and is not formally attached to a hospital. When the clinic staff attempt to contact the hospital they are unable to get any reply from the hospital's telephone exchange. They, therefore, hire a taxi and send the patient to the hospital with a letter asking for help with the further management of the patient.

1. What is wrong with the administration of this clinic?

Every clinic which provides perinatal care should be attached to a hospital within the same healthcare region. This will greatly improve the communication between a clinic and its referral hospital.

2. How could the communication by telephone between the clinic and the hospital be improved?

A direct telephone line from the clinic to the labour ward is needed. This will avoid problems with the telephone exchange and provide immediate contact between the clinic and hospital staff.

3. Why should the clinic staff always speak to the hospital staff before transferring a patient?

Sometimes the patient can be safely managed at the clinic after the clinical problem has been discussed with the hospital staff. This will prevent having to transfer the patient. The management before and during transfer can be decided with the doctor at the hospital. If the patient has to be transferred, the hospital must be informed so that they can make arrangements for her management at the hospital, e.g. prepare for a Caesarean section.

4. What is the danger of transferring a patient in a taxi?

If a patient is moved to a hospital in a taxi, equipment and a person trained in resuscitation usually are not available to handle an emergency, such as haemorrhage, which may occur while the patient is being transferred.

Case study 2

A patient presents with a minor complaint at a maternal-care clinic. A junior member of the clinic staff sees the patient but does not know how to manage her. The patient is, therefore, referred to a regional hospital (level 2) for further care.

1. Was the patient correctly managed?

No. The most senior and experienced person available at the clinic should have been consulted first. The patient's problems would most probably have been solved at the clinic, making the referral unnecessary.

2. What else could have been done if none of the clinic staff knew how to manage the problem?

The referral hospital for that clinic should have been contacted by telephone so that the patient's problem could have been discussed with the doctor on duty.

3. If the patient did require referral to hospital, which hospital would have been the most appropriate to care for the patient?

The district hospital (level 1) in the same healthcare region as the clinic.

4. Why is it always important to carefully consider the referral before transferring a patient to hospital?

Because unnecessary referral causes great inconvenience to the patient and her family. Transport and hospital fees also add to the patient's health expenses. Furthermore, unnecessary referrals place an extra workload on the already overburdened level 2 and 3 hospitals. These should reserve their resources for patients with serious complications requiring specialist care. Therefore, patients with minor problems should always be cared for at a maternal care clinic or level 1 hospital as this is more convenient for the patient and reduces the cost of healthcare.

Case study 3

All deliveries and maternal deaths are recorded in a healthcare region. During a certain year there were 30 000 deliveries and 20 maternal deaths. The commonest cause of maternal death was postpartum haemorrhage.

1. What is the definition of a maternal death?

The death of a woman during pregnancy, labour, or the puerperium.

2. How is the maternal mortality ratio expressed?

Per 100 000 deliveries.

3. What is the maternal mortality ratio in the above health care region for that year?

20/30 000 x 100 000 = 67 per 100 000 deliveries.

4. Is this maternal mortality ratio typical of a developing or a developed community?

A developing community where the ratio is usually 50 or more per 100 000 deliveries. In contrast, the maternal mortality ratio in a developed community is usually less than 10/100000 deliveries.

5. Are you surprised that the commonest cause of maternal death was postpartum haemorrhage?

No. Haemorrhage is one of the commonest causes of maternal death in many developing communities. Most of these haemorrhages can be prevented by the correct management of the third stage of labour at a maternal-care clinic with delivery facilities.

6. How can the common primary causes of maternal death be identified in a perinatal care region so that steps can be taken to reduce their occurrence?

By arranging regular meetings with representatives of all the staff in the region where each maternal death can be discussed. The primary and final causes of the death should be identified and the management of the patient must be examined. In this way the staff can learn which clinical errors may result in serious complications. Steps can then be taken to avoid these errors in future.

Appendix

Guidelines for the management of patients with risk factors and medical problems during pregnancy, labour and the puerperium

The following tables list most of the risk factors and medical problems which may occur during pregnancy, labour, and the puerperium. They also give the possible adverse effects of these conditions, indicate the actions needed, and suggest the level of care required. The tables should be read, but need not be learned. These tables provide a very useful reference for both midwives and doctors who are caring for a patients with risk factors.

The following list gives risk factors which may occur during pregnancy together with their possible adverse effects and assorted problems, and actions which can lead to the prevention, early diagnosis and correct management of complications. The level of care required by the patient is noted in the last column. The list also serves as a useful guide to management, and can be referred to when risk factors are present or develop during pregnancy. The management of many of the problems is discussed in more detail elsewhere in the Perinatal Education Programme.

The level of care needed is shown as follows:

1 = For low-risk patients.

2 = For intermediate-risk patients.

3 = For high-risk patients.

Risk factors	Possible adverse effects during pregnancy and associated problems	Action	Level of care
Risk factors identified from the patient's history			
Maternal age			
15 years or less	Pregnancy may have a detrimental effect on the development of the patient's personality.	Determine the duration of pregnancy. If 20 weeks or less termination may be indicated.	2
16–19 years	Poor social circumstances. Pre-eclampsia. Anaemia.	Refer to social worker for support. Watch for proteinuria and a rise in blood pressure from 28 weeks. Regular Hb checks.	1
37 years or more	Medical conditions such as hypertension and diabetes are commoner. Chromosome abnormalities are commoner, e.g. Down syndrome	Carefully look for medical problems at the first visit, and at 28 and 34 weeks. Motivate for sterilisation.	
		Determine the duration of pregnancy: If 13 weeks or less, an ultrasound examination for nuchal thickness is done, followed at 22 weeks looking for structural defects.	2*
		If more than 13 weeks, a genetic amniocentesis should be done between 16 and 22 weeks.	2*
		Before referral, make sure that the patient will agree to termination of pregnancy, if this is indicated. *Refer back to level 1 if medical and genetic screening is normal and less than 40 years.	1
General history			
Allergies	Penicillin allergy with an anaphylactic reaction is always dangerous, but rarely occurs.	Allergies must always be clearly documented on the folder and antenatal card.	1

Risk factors	Possible adverse effects during pregnancy and associated problems	Action	Level of care
Body Mass Index (BMI)	Cephalopelvic disproportion and shoulder dystocia. Hypertension and diabetes Use weight, height and attached BMI table. When reading BMI off table: With 1st visit in 2nd trimester, subtract 4 kg With 1st visit in 3rd trimester, subtract 8 kg	Ultrasound examination for accurate gestational age estimation at 18-22 weeks. Monitor for hypertension and glycosuria.	
		BMI below 40	1
		BMI above 40 but below 50	2
		BMI above 50	3
Diabetes mellitus (in the patient)	Pregnancy worsens the diabetes. Insulin requirements increase. Higher incidence of fetal death. Large babies with obstructed labour and birth injuries. Neonatal hypoglycaemia.	Careful control of the diabetes, in order to keep the blood glucose levels as close to normal as possible is absolutely essential.	3
Diabetes mellitus (family history)	There is an increased risk of the patient developing diabetes during pregnancy.	Careful screen for glycosuria:	
		If absent –	1
		If present –	2

Risk factors	Possible adverse effects during pregnancy and associated problems	Action	Level of care
Epilepsy	Convulsions may occur more frequently in pregnancy. Some anticonvulsant drugs may cause congenital abnormalities.	The dose of anticonvulsant drugs may need to be increased. Put the patient on a safe drug before pregnancy (e.g. carbamazepine). The drugs are not changed during pregnancy because of the danger of convulsions.	2
Congenital abnormalities (in the family)	Serious abnormalities tend to recur.	Arrange for ultrasound and amniocentesis at 16 weeks:	
		If normal –	1
		If abnormal –	2
Drugs or medication	Danger of teratogenesis. Points towards a disease not mentioned in the history.	Get accurate details and consult a doctor.	1
HIV	Mother-to-child transmission of HIV. With AIDS the mother's clinical condition may deteriorate.	Join a prevention of mother-to-child transmission programme. Refer to an antiretroviral (ARV) clinic for HAART.	1
		The stage of disease needs to be determined and noted. Check at each visit for symptoms and signs indicating progression at a more advanced stage of disease.	2
Auto-immune diseases	Raised perinatal mortality rate. Early onset of severe pre-eclampsia.	Get detailed information about the disease and medication.	3

Risk factors	Possible adverse effects during pregnancy and associated problems	Action	Level of care
Psychiatric illness	Suicide is commoner. Illness may become worse during pregnancy.	Get detailed information about the disease and medication. Termination of pregnancy may be indicated (if duration of pregnancy is less than 20 weeks).	2
Rubella	Congenital abnormalities.	Ask about fever and a skin rash in the first trimester of pregnancy and also about contact with rubella. Antibody titres can confirm or exclude diagnosis.	1
Thyrotoxicosis (hyperthyroidism)	Thyrotoxicosis and/or goitre in the neonate.	Get detailed information about the illness and medication. Thyroid hormone levels in cord blood.	2

Systematic history

Respiratory System

Risk factors	Possible adverse effects during pregnancy and associated problems	Action	Level of care
Asthma	Prostaglandin F2 alpha is contraindicated. Asthma usually improves during pregnancy.	Ask about medication and symptoms: Asymptomatic and not on steroids – Symptomatic and on steroids –	1 2
Chronic cough more than 21 days. Night sweats and weight loss.	Possible tuberculosis and/or AIDS.	Single X-ray chest with fetus screened off and sputum for acid fast bacilli. A rapid test if HIV status unknown.	1
Active tuberculosis	Spread to other family members and the newborn infant.	If stable and on treatment. The newborn infant must be given isoniazid.	1

Cardiovascular System

Risk factors	Possible adverse effects during pregnancy and associated problems	Action	Level of care
Hypertension: 1. Diastolic 90 mm Hg or more. 2. Antihypertensive treatment.	Pre-eclampsia, abruptio placentae, and IUGR or perinatal death.	Change to alpha methyldopa and stop diuretics:	
		With good control and no proteinuria –	2
		With diastolic 90 mm Hg or more or proteinuria –	3
Dyspnoea and orthopnoea	Symptoms of heart failure.	Underlying heart disease must be excluded or confirmed by the doctor.	2
Rheumatic heart disease	Cardiac output increases with increased risk of cardiac failure and maternal death.	No symptoms or signs of heart failure, and no stenotic heart valve lesions –	2
		Symptoms and signs of heart failure and/or stenotic heart valve lesions –	3
Varicose veins	May indicate previous venous thrombosis. Become worse during pregnancy.	Watch for possible thrombosis. Bed rest and elastic stockings.	1
Thrombo-embolism	Increased incidence in pregnancy with risk of maternal death.	Anticoagulant therapy during pregnancy may have to be considered.	3
Alimentary System			
Haemorrhoids	May get worse in pregnancy. May prolapse and thrombose.	Only conservative management needed.	1
Jaundice	Danger if the patient is a carrier of the hepatitis B virus. Can infect the infant during delivery.	Test for the hepatitis B antigen:	
		If antigen absent –	1
		If antigen present (the infant must be given hyperimmune globulin and be immunised) –	2
HIV positive and on HAART	High risk for serious liver damage	Stop nevirapine and refer to an ARV clinic	2

Risk factors	Possible adverse effects during pregnancy and associated problems	Action	Level of care
Urinary system			
Pyelonephritis	High risk of recurrence.	Midstream urine (MSU) for culture to be sure that the infection is completely treated.	1
Cystitis	Common in pregnancy.	MSU for culture if symptomatic.	1
Surgical History			
Myomectomy	Danger of ruptured uterus.	Elective Caesarean section indicated.	2
Thyroidectomy	Hypothyroidism can develop during pregnancy with the danger of abortion. If hyperthyroidism was the indication for surgery, manage as for thyrotoxicosis.	Look carefully for an operation scar. Thyroid function tests are indicated.	2
Chest surgery	High risk of thrombosis of artificial heart valves in pregnancy.	Warfarin: danger of teratogenesis in the 1st and bleeding in the 3rd trimester. Correct use of anticoagulant therapy.	3
Previous obstetric history			
Abruptio placentae	Tends to recur: 10% chance after previous abruption. 25% chance after 2 previous abruptions.	Advise the patient:	
		Induce labour at 38 weeks.	2
		Deliver at 34 weeks, antenatal steroids for lung maturity must be given.	3
Diabetes mellitus	Recurs in successive pregnancies. Complications already mentioned.	Random blood glucose if there is glycosuria.	2

Risk factors	Possible adverse effects during pregnancy and associated problems	Action	Level of care
Ectopic pregnancy	High risk of recurrence.	Gynaecological examination to confirm intra-uterine pregnancy (ultrasound if uncertain).	1
Grande multiparity (five or more pregnancies have reached viability)	Medical conditions are commoner. Obstetric complications are commoner: IUGR, multiple pregnancy, abnormal lie, obstructed labour and postpartum haemorrhage.	Motivate for sterilisation. Look for medical conditions at the first visit. Look for abnormal lie after 34 weeks.	2
Infertility	Ectopic pregnancy and multiple pregnancy commoner.	Gynaecological examination to confirm intra-uterine pregnancy and the size of the uterus. (Ultrasound examination is indicated.)	2
Caesarean section(s)	Danger of ruptured uterus with previous vertical uterine incision, or with two or more Caesarean sections.	Get details of the indication and type of incision from old records. Elective Caesarean section at 39 weeks if 2 previous Caesarean sections or a vertical incision.	2
Congenital abnormalities	Possible genetic inheritance. High risk of recurrence.	Genetic counselling. Amniocentesis and ultrasound may be useful.	2
Abortion	More than two first trimester abortions. One or more mid-trimester abortions.	Genetic amniocentesis indicated. If history indicates an incompetent cervix, a MacDonald stitch may be indicated (inserted at 14-16 weeks).	2
Perinatal death	Highest risk group for another perinatal death to occur (especially when the cause is unknown).	Get a detailed history and the notes from the previous pregnancy.	2

Risk factors	Possible adverse effects during pregnancy and associated problems	Action	Level of care
Postpartum haemorrhage and retained placenta	Tend to recur in successive pregnancies.	Deliver in hospital.	2
Pre-eclampsia	Two groups:		
	1. Primigravidas with pre-eclampsia close to term.	Low risk of recurrence.	1
	2. Previous pregnancy with pre-eclampsia developing in late 2nd or early 3rd trimester of pregnancy.	High risk of recurrence. Low dose aspirin (Disprin) 75 mg daily from 14 weeks.	2
Primigravida	Higher incidence of pre-eclampsia late in pregnancy.	Careful attention to blood pressure and proteinuria.	1
Vacuum extraction or forceps delivery	May indicate cephalopelvic disproportion.	Careful use of the partogram in labour.	1
Preterm labour	High risk of a recurrence in the same pregnancy.	Assess the cervix regularly from 26 to 32 weeks for changes, more regular bed rest, no intercourse in the second half of pregnancy. If there is cervical incompetence, a MacDonald suture may be indicated.	3
Present obstetric history			
Antepartum haemorrhage	Abruptio placentae and placenta praevia are both serious complications. Local causes, e.g. vaginitis, cervicitis, can also cause bleeding.	If not currently bleeding and there is no fetal distress: 1. Do speculum examination:	
		No local cause.	2
		Treatable local cause present.	1
		2. Sonology shows placenta praevia.	3

Risk factors	Possible adverse effects during pregnancy and associated problems	Action	Level of care
Asymptomatic bacteriuria	33% incidence of pyelonephritis in these patients. High risk of preterm labour.	Course of antibiotics. Repeat urine culture at next antenatal visit.	1
Diastolic blood pressure of 90 mm Hg or more	Hypertension or pre-eclampsia.	Repeat after 30 minutes rest on her side:	
		If diastolic 90-99 mm Hg without proteinuria, start alpha methyldopa.	2
		If diastolic 100 mm Hg or more or proteinuria, admit to hospital.	2
Reduced fetal movements	Fetal distress or intra-uterine death.	Duration of pregnancy 28 weeks or more. Repeat kick charts:	
		Good count without IUGR.	1
		Good count with IUGR.	2
		If count remains poor, admit to hospital.	2
Glycosuria 3+ or more	Probable diabetes.	Random blood glucose estimation:	
		8 to 11 mmol/l – arrange for fasting blood glucose estimation.	1
		11 mmol/l or more = diabetes. Admit to hospital for control if diabetes diagnosed.	2
Glycosuria 1+ and 2+	Possible diabetes.	Arrange for random blood glucose estimation. Less than 8 mm/l is normal.	1
Haemoglobin less than 10 g/dl	Anaemia in pregnancy.	Arrange full blood count. If confirmed anaemia – Refer.	2
Haematuria	Possible cystitis. Bilharzia, if endemic in the area.	Urine microscopy and culture. Treat cystitis.	1

Risk factors	Possible adverse effects during pregnancy and associated problems	Action	Level of care
Multiple pregnancy	Greater risk of preterm labour. High incidence of perinatal death and pre-eclampsia. Anaemia.	Regular vaginal examinations from 26 weeks for cervical effacement and dilatation. Careful monitoring of proteinuria and rising blood pressure. Do Hb more frequently. Ultrasound examination for growth and chorionicity:	
		Monochorionic (one placenta)	3
		Dichorionic (two placentas)	2
Pyelonephritis in current pregnancy	High risk of recurrence.	Follow-up urine culture to ensure that treatment was successful.	2
Polyhydramnios	Congenital abnormalities. Multiple pregnancy. Diabetes mellitus. Rh sensitisation may be present.	Ultrasound examination and random blood glucose estimation are indicated. Check blood groups, and possible sensitisation. Exclude oesophageal atresia in the infant immediately after birth.	2
Proteinuria	Pre-eclampsia or renal disease, e.g. chronic nephritis or nephrosis, may be present.	Exclude urinary tract infection. Test urine for protein:	
		Trace (150 mg/l) can be normal.	1
		1+ (500 mg/l) and blood pressure normal.	2
		More than 1 + indicates pre-eclampsia or serious kidney disease. Admit to hospital.	2
Ruptured membranes	Preterm labour and chorioamnionitis.	If 36 weeks or more admit to hospital, wait until the membranes have been ruptured for hours, then induce labour with oxytocin.	1

Risk factors	Possible adverse effects during pregnancy and associated problems	Action	Level of care
		If 34 weeks or less transfer to level 2 hospital.	2
Rhesus negative	Rh-sensitisation with hydrops fetalis.	If no antibodies, retest for antibodies at 26, 32 and 38 weeks. If antibodies present:	1
		Titre less than 1:16.	2
		Titre above 1:16 or more.	3
Preterm labour	Preterm infant.	If 34 weeks or more deliver in level 2 hospital.	2
		If less than 34 weeks admit to level 3 hospital. Consider suppression of labour with a beta2 stimulant.	3
VDRL and FTA/ TPHA positive, or VDRL titre 1:16 or more	Congenital syphilis.	Patient must receive full treatment.	1
VDRL titre less than 1: 16 and FTA or TPHA not available	No history of full treatment of woman and partner in past 3 months.	Patient must be fully treated.	1
Uterus larger than dates	Multiple pregnancy. Polyhydramnios. Diabetes. Large fetus. Incorrect dates.	Arrange for sonology and random blood glucose estimation. With a large fetus there is a danger of disproportion Be ready for shoulder dystocia.	2
Uterus smaller than dates	IUGR. Oligohydramnios Fetal death. Incorrect dates.	Careful measurement of fundal growth and fetal movement counts:	
		Good growth over a period of 2 weeks.	1
		No growth over a period of 2 weeks.	2
		With few or no fetal movements, admit to hospital.	2

Risk factors	Possible adverse effects during pregnancy and associated problems	Action	Level of care
Abnormal lie	Breech, oblique or transverse lies suggest possible placenta praevia, multiple pregnancy or disproportion.	Less than 34 weeks, not important. If more than 34 weeks: exclude the named complications, and refer to a doctor for external cephalic version at 36 weeks, if there are no contraindications.	
		Successful version.	1
		All others.	2
Social history			
Alcohol	Fetal alcohol syndrome.	Counselling: no alcohol should be drunk during pregnancy.	1
Religion (Customs)	Fear that certain customs will not be fulfilled, e.g. with regard to abortions, placenta, etc.	Counselling: Religious beliefs will be respected.	1
Single mother and/or unwanted pregnancy	Complications of pregnancy are commoner because of usually poorer socio-economic circumstances.	Social support may be needed. Advise about an effective method of family planning. Sterilisation may be indicated in a multipara.	1
Smoking	Danger of IUGR.	Advice to the patient: strongly advise her to stop smoking. Encourage her if she stops. Careful attention to fundal growth.	1
Poor socio-economic circumstances	Pregnancy complications will occur more commonly. Malnutrition, infection, and anaemia also occur commonly.	Social support necessary. Advise on effective method of family planning. Sterilisation may be indicated in a multiparous patient.	1

BMI table

Height → Weight ↓	140 cm	145 cm	150 cm	155 cm	160 cm	165 cm	170 cm	175 cm	180 cm	185 cm	190 cm	195 cm	200 cm	205 cm
48 kg	24.5	22.8	21.3	20.0	18.7	17.6	16.6	15.7	14.8	14.0	13.3	12.6	12.0	11.4
51 kg	26.0	24.3	22.7	21.2	19.9	18.7	17.6	16.7	15.7	14.9	14.1	13.4	12.8	12.1
54 kg	27.6	25.7	24.0	22.5	21.1	19.8	18.7	17.6	16.7	15.8	15.0	14.2	13.5	12.8
57 kg	29.1	27.1	25.3	23.7	22.3	20.9	19.7	18.6	17.6	16.7	15.8	15.0	14.3	13.6
60 kg	30.6	28.5	26.7	25.0	23.4	22.0	20.8	19.6	18.5	17.5	16.6	15.8	15.0	14.3
63 kg	32.1	30.0	28.0	26.2	24.6	23.1	21.8	20.6	19.4	18.4	17.5	16.6	15.8	15.0
66 kg	33.7	31.4	29.3	27.5	25.8	24.2	22.8	21.6	20.4	19.3	18.3	17.4	16.5	15.7
69 kg	35.2	32.8	30.7	28.7	27.0	25.3	23.9	22.5	21.3	20.2	19.1	18.1	17.3	16.4
72 kg	36.7	34.2	32.0	30.0	28.1	26.4	24.9	23.5	22.2	21.0	19.9	18.9	18.0	17.1
75 kg	38.3	35.7	33.3	31.2	29.3	27.5	26.0	24.5	23.1	21.9	20.8	19.7	18.8	17.8
78 kg	39.8	37.1	34.7	32.5	30.5	28.7	27.0	25.5	24.1	22.8	21.6	20.5	19.5	18.6
81 kg	41.3	38.5	36.0	33.7	31.6	29.8	28.0	26.4	25.0	23.7	22.4	21.3	20.3	19.3
84 kg	42.9	40.0	37.3	35.0	32.8	30.9	29.1	27.4	25.9	24.5	23.3	22.1	21.0	20.0
87 kg	44.4	41.4	38.7	36.2	34.0	32.0	30.1	28.4	26.9	25.4	24.1	22.9	21.8	20.7
90 kg	45.9	42.8	40.0	37.5	35.2	33.1	31.1	29.4	27.8	26.3	24.9	23.7	22.5	21.4
93 kg	47.4	44.2	41.3	38.7	36.3	34.2	32.2	30.4	28.7	27.2	25.8	24.5	23.3	22.1
96 kg	49.0	45.7	42.7	40.0	37.5	35.3	33.2	31.3	29.6	28.0	26.6	25.2	24.0	22.8
99 kg	50.5	47.1	44.0	41.2	38.7	36.4	34.3	32.3	30.6	28.9	27.4	26.0	24.8	23.6
102 kg	52.0	48.5	45.3	42.5	39.8	37.5	35.3	33.3	31.5	29.8	28.3	26.8	25.5	24.3
105 kg	53.6	49.9	46.7	43.7	41.0	38.6	36.3	34.3	32.4	30.7	29.1	27.6	26.3	25.0
108 kg	55.1	51.4	48.0	45.0	42.2	39.7	37.4	35.3	33.3	31.6	29.9	28.4	27.0	25.7
111 kg	56.6	52.8	49.3	46.2	43.4	40.8	38.4	36.2	34.3	32.4	30.7	29.2	27.8	26.4
114 kg	58.2	54.2	50.7	47.5	44.5	41.9	39.4	37.2	35.2	33.3	31.6	30.0	28.5	27.1
117 kg	59.7	55.6	52.0	48.7	45.7	43.0	40.5	38.2	36.1	34.2	32.4	30.8	29.3	27.8
120 kg	61.2	57.1	53.3	49.9	46.9	44.1	41.5	39.2	37.0	35.1	33.2	31.6	30.0	28.6
123 kg	62.8	58.5	54.7	51.2	48.0	45.2	42.6	40.2	38.0	35.9	34.1	32.3	30.8	29.3

Test 1: Antenatal care

1. An extra-uterine pregnancy is suggested by:

a. A uterus that is larger than expected for the duration of pregnancy

b. Morning sickness and breast tenderness

c. Lower abdominal pain and vaginal bleeding

d. The absence of fetal movements

2. A woman should book for antenatal care:

a. Before she falls pregnant

b. When she has missed her second menstrual period

c. When she first feels fetal movements

d. When she is 28 weeks pregnant

3. When a patient has had a Caesarean section:

a. The type of uterine incision is of no importance

b. Only those patients who had a vertical lower segment incision may be allowed to have a vaginal labour

c. Only those patients who had a transverse lower segment incision may be allowed to have a vaginal labour

d. Only those patients who had a transverse lower segment incision for a non-recurring indication may be allowed to have a vaginal labour

4. The last normal menstrual period may be used to calculate the duration of pregnancy:

a. If that was the last menstrual period while the patient was on her last packet of oral contraceptive pills

b. If the patient has a regular cycle and she was not on contraceptives.

c. If the last menstrual period had started earlier and had been shorter than the patient would have expected.

d. Patients' information about their last menstrual period is always wrong.

5. **A cervical smear for cytology must be done during the first antenatal visit as part of the gynaecological examination:**
   a. In all women
   b. Only if the cervix appears abnormal.
   c. From all women 30 years or more who have not had a previous smear which had been reported as normal
   d. Only if there is a symptomatic vaginal discharge (e.g. itchiness or burning)

6. **The abdominal examination is a useful assessment of the duration of pregnancy:**
   a. From 8 to 12 weeks
   b. From 10 to 16 weeks
   c. From 13 to 17 weeks
   d. From 18 to 24 weeks

7. **If a patient is 10 weeks pregnant:**
   a. The fundus will be palpable 2 cm above the pelvic symphysis
   b. The fundus is not palpable abdominally and it is, therefore, not possible to determine whether the dates correlate with the size of the uterus
   c. It would be better to ask her to return in 6 weeks' time for booking
   d. The uterine size may be determined vaginally with fair accuracy

8. **The best method of assessing the duration of pregnancy by physical examination at 18 or more weeks is:**
   a. The symphysis-fundus measurement
   b. Bimanual palpation of the uterus on vaginal examination
   c. Palpation of the abdomen
   d. To establish the lie of the fetus and assess the size of the fetal head

9. **If the uterine fundus is just below the umbilicus (20 weeks) and the patient is 18 weeks pregnant by dates:**
   a. The dates must be considered correct and used to determine the duration of pregnancy
   b. The fundal height must be considered correct and used to determine the duration of pregnancy
   c. An ultrasound examination must be requested and the result used to determine the duration of pregnancy
   d. The average duration of 19 weeks must be accepted as the correct duration of pregnancy

10. **A uterus that is smaller than expected may be due to:**
    a. A breech presentation
    b. An intra-uterine death
    c. Polyhydramnios
    d. None of the above

11. **Antenatal ultrasound examination is an accurate method of determining the duration of pregnancy up to:**
a. 28 weeks
b. 24 weeks
c. 20 weeks
d. 16 weeks

12. **During the antenatal period ultrasonography must be done between 18 and 22 weeks:**
a. On very obese patients where determination the duration of pregnancy is difficult
b. On patients needing elective delivery, e.g. those with two previous Caesarean sections
c. On patients with a history of severe pre-eclampsia before 34 weeks gestation
d. In all of the above patients

13. **Which of the following results indicate active syphilis?**
a. A negative RPR (VDRL)
b. A positive RPR (VDRL) plus a negative TPHA
c. A positive RPR (VDRL) plus a positive TPHA
d. A CIN III lesion on cervical cytology smear

14. **A positive RPR (VDRL) indicates the presence of syphilis if:**
a. The titre is 1:4 or more
b. The titre is 1:8 or more
c. The titre is 1:16 or more
d. Any titre is present

15. **Syphilis in pregnancy should be treated with:**
a. Nitrofurantoin (Macrodantin)
b. Benzathine penicillin (Bicillin LA or Penilente LA)
c. Tetracycline
d. Ampicillin

16. **How often should a woman at low risk, who lives near a clinic, visit the antenatal clinic between 28 and 34 weeks?**
a. Weekly
b. Every 2 weeks
c. Once a month
d. No visit is required between these dates

17. **The visit at 34 weeks is important because:**
a. The fetus now becomes viable and the patient must monitor the fetal movements.
b. A vaginal examination must be done on patients who are at risk of preterm labour to determine whether there are cervical changes.
c. The lie and presentation of the fetus are now important and have to be carefully determined.
d. A repeat ultrasound examination must now be done on patients who had ultrasonography at 18 and 22 weeks.

18. **Oesophageal candidiasis suggest which clinical stage of HIV infection?**
a. Stage 1
b. Stage 2
c. Stage 3
d. Stage 4

19. **Antiretroviral prophylaxis should be provided with:**
a. AZT alone
b. Nevirapine alone
c. A fixed combination dose (FCD) pill
d. AZT plus FDC

20. **Antiretroviral treatment is indicated if the woman has:**
a. A CD4 count below 500 cells/mm³
b. A CD4 count below 350 cells/mm³
c. Oral candidiasis (thrush)
d. Vaginal candidiasis

Test 2: Assessment of fetal growth and condition during pregnancy

1. **Which of the following statements about intra-uterine growth restriction is correct?**
   a. The cause of severe intra-uterine growth restriction is usually unknown.
   b. Both maternal and fetal factors may cause intra-uterine growth restriction.
   c. Primary placental insufficiency is a common cause of intra-uterine growth restriction.
   d. Poor maternal weight gain during pregnancy is of great value in the diagnosis of intra-uterine growth restriction.

2. **Which of the following is the best clinical method of determining uterine growth between 18 and 36 weeks of pregnancy?**
   a. An abdominal examination
   b. The distance in centimetres between the upper edge of the symphysis pubis and the fundus of the uterus
   c. Serial ultrasound examinations at each antenatal visit
   d. The abdominal circumference measured with a tape at each antenatal visit

3. **Which of the following symphysis-fundus height measurements suggests intra-uterine growth restriction?**
   a. A slowing of the symphysis-fundus growth until 2 measurements are below the 10th centile
   b. A slowing of the symphysis-fundus growth until one measurement is below the 10th centile
   c. 2 measurements the same irrespective of their positions on the centile lines
   d. A measurement that is less than that recorded two visits before and falls below the 10th centile

4. **With severe intra-uterine growth restriction, the difference between the gestational age and the symphysis-fundus height measurement is:**
   a. 2 weeks or more
   b. 3 weeks or more
   c. 4 weeks or more
   d. 5 weeks or more

5. **If the symphysis-fundus measurement suggests intra-uterine growth restriction at 32 weeks gestation, what is the correct management?**
   a. A vaginal examination must be done to determine whether the patient's cervix is favourable for an induction.
   b. The patient must return to the antenatal clinic at 36 weeks.
   c. Fetal heart rate monitoring must be done at each antenatal visit.
   d. The patient must be transferred to a level 2 hospital for a Doppler umbilical artery blood flow measurement.

6. **The fetal condition can best be determined during the antenatal period by:**
   a. Weighing the patient at every antenatal visit
   b. Measuring the patient's blood pressure
   c. Counting the fetal heart rate
   d. Counting fetal movements

7. **During the antenatal period it is essential to determine the fetal condition from:**
   a. 36 weeks
   b. 34 weeks
   c. 28 weeks
   d. 24 weeks

8. **Which of the following statements about fetal movements is correct?**

a. The date when fetal movements are first felt is a good indication of the gestational age.

b. Good fetal movements do not necessarily indicate fetal wellbeing.

c. From 28 weeks, all patients should be told about the importance of fetal movements.

d. A decrease in fetal movements always indicates that the fetus is distressed.

9. **Which patients should use a fetal-movement chart?**

a. All patients, where there is reason to be worried about the fetal condition

b. All primigravidas

c. All pregnant patients from 28 weeks gestation

d. All patients who have had a previous Caesarean section

10. **When will you be worried that a patient may have a decreased number of fetal movements?**

a. 15–20 movements per hour

b. 10–15 movements per hour

c. 5–10 movements per hour

d. Half as many fetal movements as previously counted

11. **What would you advise if a patient felt only a few fetal movements during an hour?**

a. The patient must go to her nearest clinic immediately and report that her fetus is only moving a little.

b. The patient should lie on her side for a further hour and count the fetal movements.

c. The patient should repeat the fetal movement count in the afternoon.

d. Antenatal fetal heart rate monitoring is indicated and, therefore, she must report to her nearest hospital.

12. **What management would be correct if a patient with reduced fetal movements presents at a hospital that does not have a cardiotocograph (CTG machine)?**

a. The responsible doctor must see the patient immediately as a Caesarean section should be done.

b. Refer the patient urgently to a hospital that has a cardiotocograph.

c. Exclude the possibility of fetal death by listening for the fetal heart with a stethoscope.

d. Fetal movements must be counted again the next day.

13. How should a doctor manage a patient which has decreased fetal movements and a viable fetus, without any signs of intra-uterine growth restriction? The duration of pregnancy is 36 weeks.

a. If the cervix is favourable for induction of labour, the membranes must be ruptured and the fetal heart must be monitored carefully.

b. An emergency Caesarean section must be performed immediately, irrespective of the state of the cervix.

c. If the cervix is unfavourable, a medical induction of labour, using prostaglandin E2, must be performed.

d. Delivery to only take place in a level 2 hospital with neonatal intensive care unit or a level 3 hospital.

14. Which of the following statements about antenatal fetal heart rate monitoring is correct?

a. Fetal heart rate monitoring should be done on all patients with pre-eclampsia, as fetal movements in these patients are an unreliable method of assessing the condition of the fetus.

b. All pregnant patients should routinely have antenatal fetal heart rate monitoring.

c. Antenatal fetal heart rate monitoring should be done on all patients with suspected intra-uterine growth restriction.

d. Antenatal fetal heart rate monitoring should be done on high-risk patients where fetal movements have not been shown to be a reliable method of assessing the fetal condition, such as insulin-dependent diabetics, prelabour rupture of the membranes and pre-eclampsia which is being managed conservatively.

15. (*Questions 15 to 20 need only be answered by students who studied sections 2-27 to 2-37 on antenatal fetal heart rate monitoring.*) **If there is a non-reactive fetal heart rate pattern:**
    a. No decelerations occur despite uterine contractions.
    b. Fetal distress should be suspected and intra-uterine resuscitation must be undertaken.
    c. The test must be repeated after 45 minutes.
    d. The beat-to-beat variability must be assessed to determine the presence or absence of fetal wellbeing.

16. **Why must you repeat the test 45 minutes after a non-reactive fetal heart rate pattern, with poor beat-to-beat variability, is obtained?**
    a. Supine hypotension or spontaneous hyperstimulation of the uterus may be present.
    b. Such a fetal heart rate pattern indicates fetal distress and the test must be repeated immediately.
    c. A sleeping fetus may produce a non-reactive fetal heart rate pattern with poor beat-to-beat variability.
    d. Cardiotocography must be repeated after 45 minutes whenever the fetal heart rate pattern indicates fetal distress.

17. **Which of the following results indicates an abnormal stress test?**
    a. No decelerations after 2 contractions that last at least 30 seconds each
    b. Uterine contractions with late decelerations
    c. A fetal tachycardia with a baseline rate above 160 beats per minute
    d. No accelerations

18. **Which of the following indicates a late deceleration on a cardiotocogram?**
a. The trough of the deceleration occurs at least 60 seconds after the peak of the contraction.
b. The trough of the deceleration occurs at least 45 seconds after the peak of the contraction.
c. The trough of the deceleration occurs at least 30 seconds after the peak of the contraction.
d. A deceleration during a contraction that takes 30 seconds or more after the end of the contraction to return to the baseline.

19. **Which form of management will be correct if a fetal heart rate pattern, which indicates fetal distress, is obtained?**
a. As the test result may be falsely abnormal due to postural hypotension or overstimulation of the uterus, these possibilities must first be ruled out.
b. Repeat the stress test on the same day.
c. Repeat the stress test 4 hours later.
d. Perform an immediate Caesarean section.

20. **What is the correct method of intra-uterine resuscitation?**
a. Suppressing uterine contractions and decreasing the uterine tone
b. Administering oxygen to the fetus by means of an intra-uterine catheter
c. Infusing oxytocin in order to stimulate uterine contractions
d. Rubbing the patient's nipples so as to stimulate uterine contractions

Test 3: Hypertensive disorders of pregnancy

1. **What is the definition of hypertension in pregnancy?**
   a. A diastolic blood pressure of 80 mm Hg or above and/or a systolic blood pressure of 120 mm Hg or above
   b. A diastolic blood pressure of 90 mm Hg or above and/or a systolic blood pressure of 140 mm Hg or above
   c. A diastolic blood pressure of 100 mm Hg or above and/or a systolic blood pressure of 160 mm Hg or above
   d. A rise in diastolic blood pressure of 10 mm Hg.

2. **What is the definition of significant proteinuria in pregnancy?**
   a. A trace of protein
   b. 1+ protein or more
   c. 2+ protein or more
   d. 3+ protein

3. **How should you define pre-eclampsia?**
   a. Hypertension and proteinuria presenting before the start of pregnancy
   b. Hypertension and proteinuria presenting in the first half of pregnancy
   c. Hypertension and proteinuria presenting in the second half of pregnancy
   d. Hypertension and proteinuria presenting any time in pregnancy

4. **What is the correct definition of chronic hypertension?**
   a. Hypertension, without proteinuria, that is present in the first half of pregnancy
   b. Hypertension, together with proteinuria, that is present in the first half of pregnancy
   c. Hypertension that is present in the first half of pregnancy, plus proteinuria that presents in the second half of pregnancy
   d. Hypertension alone which is present at the time of booking at 28 weeks

5. **How common is pre-eclampsia?**
   a. Most pregnant women develop pre-eclampsia.
   b. About 25% of all pregnant women develop pre-eclampsia.
   c. About 5–6% of all pregnant women develop pre-eclampsia
   d. Very rare

6. **Which fetal condition is common in pregnancies complicated by pre-eclampsia?**
   a. Congenital malformations
   b. Heart failure due to hypertension
   c. Haemorrhagic disease of the newborn
   d. Intra-uterine growth restriction

7. **Pre-eclampsia may cause fetal distress because it results in:**
   a. A decrease in placental blood flow
   b. Fetal hypertension
   c. Severe protein loss in the mother's urine
   d. Congenital abnormalities caused by antihypertensive drugs

8. **A patient with pre-eclampsia who develops a diastolic blood pressure of 105 mm Hg and 2+ proteinuria at 36 weeks of pregnancy should be graded as having:**
   a. Pre-eclampsia
   b. Severe pre-eclampsia
   c. Imminent eclampsia
   d. Eclampsia

9. **What is an important sign of imminent eclampsia?**
   a. 3 + proteinuria
   b. Increased tendon reflexes
   c. A diastolic blood pressure of 110 mm Hg or more
   d. Tenderness on palpating the calves

10. **A patient with pre-eclampsia has a diastolic blood pressure of 95 mm Hg and 1+ proteinuria. She complains of flashes of light in front of her eyes and upper abdominal pain. In which of the following grades of pre-eclampsia should you put this patient?**
    a. Pre-eclampsia
    b. Severe pre-eclampsia
    c. Imminent eclampsia
    d. Eclampsia

11. **Which of the following women has the highest risk of pre-eclampsia?**
    a. A patient with a history of pre-eclampsia starting early in the third trimester of a previous pregnancy
    b. A patient with a history of a preterm delivery in her previous pregnancy
    c. Grande multiparas
    d. A patient who previously had a twin pregnancy

12. **Which one of the following may be an early warning sign of pre-eclampsia?**
   a. Weight loss during the last months of pregnancy
   b. Generalised oedema especially of the face
   c. Oedema of the feet at the end of the day
   d. Pain on passing urine

13. **What is the management of a patient with pre-eclampsia ?**
   a. Oral antihypertensive drugs
   b. Diuretics to reduce oedema
   c. Hospitalisation
   d. A loading dose of magnesium sulphate

14. **Which one of the following is the method of delivery usually chosen in a patient with pre-eclampsia?**
   a. Caesarean section
   b. Surgical induction followed by vaginal delivery at 34 weeks
   c. Surgical induction followed by vaginal delivery if 36 weeks gestation has been reached.
   d. Waiting until 42 weeks for a spontaneous onset of labour.

15. **What is an important complication of pre-eclampsia?**
   a. Placenta praevia
   b. Oedema of the face
   c. Glycosuria
   d. Intracerebral haemorrhage

16. **Which of the following is the correct method of treatment for a patient with severe pre-eclampsia?**
   a. The patient should be stabilised first, then be moved to a level 2 hospital for further management.
   b. The patient should immediately be rushed to the nearest level 3 hospital for stabilisation.
   c. The patient should be managed at a level 1 hospital.
   d. The infant must immediately be delivered by Caesarean section at a level 2 hospital.

17. **What drug is used to manage a diastolic blood pressure of 110 mm Hg or more?**
   a. Alpha-methyldopa (Aldomet)
   b. Nifedipine (Adalat)
   c. Diazepam (Valium)
   d. Propranolol (Inderal)

18. **What is an important sign of magnesium sulphate overdosage?**
   a. Vomiting
   b. Hyperventilation
   c. A urine output of less than 20 ml per hour
   d. Depressed tendon reflexes

19. **What drug is used to prevent and manage eclampsia?**
   a. Magnesium sulphate
   b. Magnesium trisilicate
   c. Alpha-methyldopa (Aldomet)
   d. Diazepam (Valium)

20. **How should a patient, who feels well but has a diastolic blood pressure of 90 mm Hg at 36 weeks gestation, be managed? At all her previous antenatal visits, her blood pressure was normal, and she has no proteinuria.**
   a. She must be given an intramuscular injection of dihydralazine (Nepresol).
   b. She must be hospitalised.
   c. Weekly antenatal visits should be arranged with additional visits if necessary.
   d. A full blood count should be done to exclude a low platelet count.

Test 4: Antepartum haemorrhage

1. **What is the definition of an antepartum haemorrhage?**
   a. Any vaginal haemorrhage between conception and delivery
   b. Any vaginal haemorrhage during labour
   c. Any vaginal haemorrhage between 24 weeks gestation and delivery
   d. Any vaginal haemorrhage between 24 weeks and the onset of labour

2. **Antepartum haemorrhage is an important complication of pregnancy because:**
   a. It is a common cause of iron-deficiency anaemia.
   b. The fetus may become anaemic.
   c. It may be due to cervical intra-epithelial neoplasia.
   d. Both the mother and fetus may die.

3. **Which of the following is an important sign of shock due to blood loss?**
   a. A fast pulse rate
   b. A low haemoglobin concentration
   c. Concentrated urine
   d. Pyrexia

4. **Why is a speculum examination done on a patient with an antepartum haemorrhage?**
   a. To see how dilated the cervix is
   b. To exclude a placenta praevia before a digital examination is done
   c. To exclude a local cause of the bleeding from the vagina or cervix
   d. To look for a blood clot in the vagina

5. **An antepartum haemorrhage with no fetal heart heard is usually caused by:**
   a. Placenta praevia
   b. Abruptio placentae
   c. Antepartum haemorrhage of unknown cause
   d. Trichomonal vaginitis

6. **What is the most likely cause of a massive antepartum haemorrhage that threatens the mother's life?**
   a. Abruptio placentae
   b. Rupture of the uterus
   c. Cervical carcinoma
   d. Placenta praevia

7. **Which of the following factors will place a patient at the highest risk of abruptio placentae?**
a. A history of abruptio placentae in a previous pregnancy.
b. Any of the hypertensive disorders of pregnancy.
c. Intra-uterine growth retardation.
d. Cigarette smoking.

8. **Which of the following would suggest an abruptio placentae?**
a. The uterus is tonically contracted and tender.
b. Fetal movements are usually present.
c. The haemoglobin concentration is low.
d. The uterus is relaxed and the fetal parts are easily felt.

9. **Which management would be correct if abruptio placentae with an intra-uterine death was diagnosed?**
a. The fetus must be delivered by Caesarean section.
b. A vaginal examination must not be done because the patient has had an antepartum haemorrhage.
c. A vaginal examination must be done to rupture the membranes and, thereby, obtain a vaginal delivery.
d. The spontaneous onset of labour must be awaited.

10. **Which of the following patients is at an increased risk of placenta praevia?**
a. A patient with one of the hypertensive disorders of pregnancy
b. A patient with a multiple pregnancy
c. A patient with intra-uterine growth retardation
d. A patient who smokes

11. **Vaginal bleeding due to placenta praevia is usually associated with:**
a. Fetal parts that are difficult to feel and an absent fetal heartbeat
b. Engagement of the fetal head
c. A uterus that is relaxed and not tender on palpation
d. Lower abdominal pain

12. **In which of the following patients can placenta praevia be excluded?**
a. A patient with a slight vaginal bleed
b. When 2/5 or less of the fetal head can be palpated above the pelvic brim on abdominal examination
c. A patient with a painless, bright red vaginal bleed
d. A patient with a breech presentation

13. Following a small vaginal bleed at 34 weeks gestation, the diagnosis of placenta praevia is confirmed with ultrasonography. Which of the following will be the correct further management?
   a. The fetus must be delivered immediately by Caesarean section.
   b. A vaginal examination must be done in theatre immediately to confirm the diagnosis.
   c. The patient must be hospitalised and managed conservatively until 36 weeks or until active bleeding starts again.
   d. The membranes must be ruptured to induce labour.

14. An antepartum haemorrhage of unknown cause should be suspected:
   a. When the history and abdominal examination are not suggestive of an abruptio placentae
   b. When local causes of bleeding have been excluded by a speculum examination
   c. When a placenta praevia is excluded
   d. When all of the above causes of an antepartum haemorrhage have been excluded

15. Which of the following will exclude a placenta praevia?
   a. A careful speculum examination
   b. A careful abdominal examination
   c. The presence of fetal distress
   d. A vaginal examination in theatre

16. How should you manage a patient with an antepartum haemorrhage of unknown cause?
   a. The patient must be admitted to hospital where fetal movements should be carefully monitored, especially during the first 24 hours.
   b. Because the risk of an abruptio placentae is so great, an emergency Caesarean section must be done.
   c. Once the diagnosis is made, the patient should be discharged and followed up as a low-risk patient.
   d. The patient must be hospitalised until 38 weeks of gestation, when labour should be induced.

17. **An antepartum haemorrhage of unknown cause should always be regarded as a serious complication of pregnancy because:**
a. Intra-uterine growth restriction is often present.
b. It may be caused by cervical cancer.
c. Abruptio placentae may be present.
d. Placenta praevia may be present.

18. **Which of the following is typical of a 'show'?**
a. A vaginal bleed that soaks a sanitary towel
b. A slight bleed consisting of blood mixed with mucus
c. A vaginal discharge mixed with blood
d. Contact bleeding from the cervix caused by a speculum examination

19. **If a speculum examination is done on a patient with a history suggestive of a blood-stained discharge, what finding would diagnose an antepartum haemorrhage?**
a. Bleeding from a closed cervical os
b. A blood-stained discharge seen in the vagina
c. Contact bleeding when the speculum touches the cervix
d. Bulging membranes through a partially dilated cervix

20. **How should you manage a patient who presents at 30 weeks of gestation with a blood-stained vaginal discharge which is caused by vaginitis?**
a. The urine should be tested with a reagent strip for protein, nitrites and leucocytes.
b. A cytology smear must be taken from the cervix to identify the organism causing the vaginitis.
c. A vaginal examination should be done in theatre as with any other patient who presents with an antepartum haemorrhage.
d. The patient and her partner must be treated with metronidazole (Flagyl).

Test 5: Preterm labour and preterm rupture of the membranes

1. **What is the definition of preterm labour?**
   a. Labour starting 1 hour or more after rupture of the membranes
   b. Labour starting before 40 weeks of gestation
   c. Labour starting before 37 weeks of gestation
   d. Labour starting when the fetus is assessed as weighing less than 2000 g, when the gestational age is unknown

2. **Preterm rupture of the membranes is defined as:**
   a. Membranes that have ruptured at term, and not been followed by the onset of labour within 24 hours
   b. Membranes that rupture before the second stage of labour
   c. Membranes that have ruptured before 37 weeks of gestation, in the absence of contractions
   d. Membranes that have ruptured before the onset of labour at any gestational age

3. **Preterm labour is important because it commonly results in death of the infant due to:**
   a. Abruptio placentae
   b. Birth trauma
   c. Jaundice
   d. Hyaline membrane disease

4. **Chorioamnionitis is usually caused by:**
   a. Bacteria which cross the placenta from the maternal circulation to the fetus
   b. Bacteria which spread from the cervix and vagina
   c. Viral infection of the genitalia
   d. Candida vaginitis

5. **Choose the correct statement regarding chorioamnionitis:**
   a. It causes all cases of preterm labour
   b. It always follows preterm rupture of the membranes
   c. It may cause and complicate preterm rupture of the membranes
   d. It only occurs in patients with vaginitis

6. **Chorioamnionitis usually results in:**
   a. No signs or symptoms in the mother or fetus
   b. Maternal pyrexia and tachycardia
   c. An offensive vaginal discharge
   d. Abdominal tenderness

7. **Clinical chorioamnionitis may present with:**
a. Headache and backache
b. Vaginal bleeding
c. Fetal tachycardia
d. Dysuria and frequency

8. **Antibiotics should be given to:**
a. All patients with preterm rupture of the membranes
b. All infants with preterm labour
c. Patients with clinical signs of chorioamnionitis
d. Patients with ruptured membranes, where the pregnancy is allowed to continue

9. **Which of the following commonly causes preterm labour?**
a. Multiple pregnancy
b. Excessive weight gain during pregnancy
c. A breech presentation
d. No sexual intercourse in the second half of pregnancy

10. **Which patients are at the highest risk of preterm labour?**
a. Patients who book early in pregnancy
b. Multigravidas
c. Patients with a history of preterm labour in a previous pregnancy
d. Patients living in low socio-economic circumstances

11. **Women at increased risk of preterm labour should:**
a. Increase their normal amount of exercise
b. Not take baths
c. Not be examined vaginally at the antenatal clinics
d. Avoid coitus during the second half of their pregnancies

12. **Braxton Hicks contractions:**
a. Are sometimes uncomfortable but are not painful
b. Are regular
c. Are associated with cervical dilatation
d. Increase in duration and frequency

13. **Patients with preterm rupture of the membranes should have:**
a. A digital vaginal examination to assess the state of the cervix
b. A sterile speculum examination only
c. No vaginal examination at all
d. Only a rectal examination

14. **The pH of amniotic fluid is:**
a. Acid
b. Neutral
c. Alkaline
d. Variable

15. **If a patient presents with preterm labour, the first step in the management is to:**
    a. Do a vaginal examination to evaluate cervical dilatation and effacement.
    b. Do an abdominal examination to evaluate the frequency and duration of uterine contractions.
    c. Do a sterile speculum examination to see whether liquor is draining from the cervix.
    d. Rule out fetal distress and estimate the gestational age as accurately as possible.

16. **Nifedipine (Adalat) should not be used in a patient with:**
    a. Asthma
    b. Preterm rupture of the membranes
    c. Multiple pregnancy
    d. Hypertension

17. **The initial dose of salbutamol (Ventolin) to suppress preterm labour, is:**
    a. 50 μg
    b. 100 μg
    c. 250 μg
    d. 500 μg

18. **Indomethacin (Indocid) may be more dangerous to the fetus if given at or beyond:**
    a. 28 weeks
    b. 31 weeks
    c. 34 weeks
    d. 36 weeks

19. **A patient with preterm rupture of the membranes, who is allowed to continue with her pregnancy, must:**
    a. Have an examination at least twice daily for signs of clinical chorioamnionitis
    b. Be admitted to hospital for complete bed rest
    c. Be seen at the antenatal clinic at least weekly, as she has a high-risk pregnancy
    d. Have daily white cell counts

20. **It is recommended that pregnancy be allowed to continue in the presence of preterm rupture of the membranes (unless there are contraindications) until the duration of pregnancy reaches:**
    a. 40 weeks
    b. 37 weeks
    c. 34 weeks
    d. 32 weeks

Test 6: Monitoring the condition of the mother during the first stage of labour

1. **What is a partogram?**
   a. A chart for recording cervical dilatation only
   b. An observation chart to record the clinical findings during the antenatal period
   c. A machine to record the fetal heart rate
   d. A chart to record the progress of labour together with the maternal and fetal condition

2. **During the first stage of labour a partogram must be used:**
   a. On all patients
   b. Only on high-risk patients
   c. Only in level 1 clinics
   d. Only in level 2 and 3 hospitals

3. **Which of the following indicates that the general condition of a patient in the first stage of labour is normal?**
   a. The patient's temperature, pulse rate, and blood pressure are normal
   b. The patient is at ease and relaxed between contractions and does not appear pale
   c. The urine output is normal and ketonuria is not present
   d. The patient's blood pressure is normal and proteinuria is not present

4. **The correct management of a 17-year-old primigravida patient who appears very anxious and complains of painful contractions in early labour is:**
   a. The patient must immediately receive analgesics.
   b. A Caesarean section must be done.
   c. The patient must be comforted and reassured and receive appropriate analgesia. If possible, someone she knows should stay with her.
   d. The membranes must be ruptured to ensure a rapid progress of labour.

5. **What is the normal maternal temperature during labour?**
   a. 35.5–36.0 ℃
   b. 36.0–37.0 ℃
   c. 36.5–37.5 ℃
   d. 37.0–38.0 ℃

6. **Why is maternal pyrexia an important complication during the first stage of labour?**
   a. Maternal pyrexia may cause maternal exhaustion and oliguria.
   b. Maternal pyrexia may cause convulsions.
   c. Maternal pyrexia may cause hypertension during labour.
   d. Maternal pyrexia may be caused by an infection which could be dangerous to the patient.

7. **What is the normal maternal pulse rate during labour?**
   a. 60–80
   b. 80–100
   c. 100–120
   d. 120–140

8. **What causes a rapid maternal pulse during labour?**
   a. Fetal distress
   b. Hypertension
   c. Pyrexia
   d. Ketonuria

9. **How often should the blood pressure be monitored in a low-risk patient during the latent phase of labour?**
   a. Every 15 minutes
   b. Every 30 minutes
   c. Hourly
   d. 2-hourly

10. **Which of the following may cause hypertension during labour?**
   a. Anxiety
   b. Fetal distress
   c. Chorioamnionitis
   d. Anaemia

11. **Which of the following would be the best management if a patient's blood pressure was 90/50 mm Hg while she was lying on her back?**
   a. The patient must change into the lateral position and the blood pressure measurement should be repeated after a further 1 to 2 minutes.
   b. As maternal hypotension may cause fetal distress, the fetal heart rate must be checked immediately.
   c. The patient should be reassured that some patients normally have a low blood pressure and, therefore, there is no need for concern.
   d. As blood loss is the most likely cause for hypotension, active resuscitation must be started immediately.

12. **A common clinical sign of shock is:**
   a. Pyrexia
   b. Bradycardia
   c. Hypertension
   d. A cold and sweaty skin

13. **The definition of oliguria is a urine output of less than:**
   a. 10 ml per hour
   b. 20 ml per hour
   c. 50 ml per hour
   d. 100 ml per hour

14. **Oliguria is an important sign of:**
   a. Dehydration
   b. Pyelonephritis
   c. Anxiety
   d. Heart failure

15. **Which of the following statements is correct?**
   a. All patients should receive an intravenous infusion from the time of admission to the labour ward.
   b. Oral fluids must be given to all patients until full cervical dilatation is reached.
   c. All patients to be delivered vaginally must be encouraged to take oral fluids while in the active phase of labour.
   d. A 50 ml ampoule of 50% dextrose should be given intravenously as soon as ketonuria develops during labour.

16. **Infection of the urinary tract may cause:**
   a. 1+ proteinuria
   b. 2+ proteinuria
   c. 3+ proteinuria
   d. 4+ proteinuria

17. **Ketonuria during labour:**
   a. Is always abnormal and must be treated
   b. Is an important sign of fetal distress
   c. May be seen in normal patients
   d. Is a sign of renal disease

18. **Which of the following is a sign of maternal exhaustion during labour?**
   a. Bradycardia
   b. Proteinuria
   c. A dry mouth and oliguria
   d. Pallor and hypotension

19. **What may cause maternal exhaustion during labour?**
   a. Chorioamnionitis
   b. Preterm labour
   c. Placenta praevia
   d. Prolonged labour

20. **How should you treat a patient with maternal exhaustion?**
   a. Stop the contractions with nifedipine (Adalat).
   b. Give oxygen by face mask.
   c. Give 2 litres of Ringer's lactate with 5% dextrose by intravenous infusion.
   d. Deliver the infant by Caesarean section.

Test 7: Monitoring the condition of the fetus during the first stage of labour

1. **Compression of the fetal head during labour:**
   a. Usually does not harm the fetus
   b. Usually damages the fetal brain
   c. Usually causes blindness in the newborn infant
   d. Usually kills the fetus

2. **What is the commonest cause of a reduced supply of oxygen to the fetus during labour?**
   a. Uterine contractions
   b. Partial placental separation
   c. Placental insufficiency
   d. Infection of the membranes

3. **How does the fetus usually respond to a lack of oxygen during labour?**
   a. There is an increase in fetal movements.
   b. There is a decrease in the fetal heart rate.
   c. There is an increase in the fetal heart rate.
   d. There is a decrease in fetal movements.

4. **How should the fetal heart rate be monitored in labour?**
   a. A cardiotocograph (CTG machine) should preferably be used in all labours.
   b. A doptone is the preferred method in primary-care clinics and hospitals.
   c. A fetal stethoscope is the best method for most labours.
   d. The fetal heart rate does not need to be monitored in all low-risk pregnancies.

5. **The fetal heart rate pattern should be monitored:**
   a. During a contraction
   b. Before a contraction
   c. After a contraction
   d. Before, during, and after a contraction

6. **How often should the fetal heart rate be monitored during the first stage of labour in low-risk pregnancies where there is no meconium staining of the liquor?**
   a. Every 3 hours during the latent phase
   b. Every 2 hours during the latent phase
   c. Every 2 hours during the active phase
   d. Every 15 minutes during the active phase

7. **What is the normal baseline fetal heart rate in labour?**
   a. 100–120 beats per minute
   b. 120–140 beats per minute
   c. 140–160 beats per minute
   d. 100–160 beats per minute

8. **Early decelerations:**
   a. Start at the beginning of a contraction and return to the baseline at the end of a contraction
   b. Start at the beginning of a contraction and end 30 seconds or more after the contraction
   c. Do not have any relation to contractions
   d. Occur during the period of uterine relaxation

9. **Early decelerations are usually caused by:**
   a. Intracranial haemorrhage
   b. Compression of the fetal head
   c. A short umbilical cord
   d. A decreased supply of oxygen to the fetus

10. **What are late decelerations?**
    a. Decelerations that occur after 38 weeks gestation
    b. Decelerations that are only present at the end of the first stage of labour
    c. Decelerations that start 30 seconds or more after the beginning of the contraction
    d. Decelerations that return to the baseline 30 seconds or more after the end of the contraction

11. **Late decelerations:**
    a. Always indicate fetal distress
    b. Only suggest that fetal distress may be present
    c. May be normal
    d. Cannot be diagnosed with a fetal stethoscope

12. **A baseline tachycardia:**
    a. Indicates that the fetus is in good condition
    b. Is common when the mother is given pethidine
    c. May be caused by infection of the placenta and membranes
    d. Indicates that the fetus is dying from lack of oxygen

13. **A baseline bradycardia:**
    a. Is a safe pattern
    b. Is a pattern which indicates an increased risk of fetal distress
    c. Indicates severe fetal distress
    d. Is usually caused by infection of the placenta and membranes

14. **Which fetal heart rate pattern warns that there is an increased risk of fetal distress?**
a. Early decelerations
b. Late decelerations
c. Baseline bradycardia
d. Late decelerations plus a baseline bradycardia

15. **When can you be confident that the fetal condition is good?**
a. When the baseline fetal heart rate is normal and there are no decelerations
b. When the baseline fetal heart rate is normal and there are only early decelerations
c. When fetal tachycardia is present and there are no decelerations
d. All of the above

16. **Meconium staining of the liquor:**
a. Is uncommon
b. Occurs in 10–20% of patients
c. Occurs in 30–40% of patients
d. Occurs in most patients

17. **Meconium staining of the liquor is commonest in:**
a. Patients in post-term labour
b. Patients in term labour
c. Patients in preterm labour
d. Patients whose fetuses move a lot during pregnancy

18. **Which form of meconium in the liquor is most likely to indicate the presence of fetal distress?**
a. Fresh meconium indicates definite fetal distress and is an indication for an emergency Caesarean section.
b. Old meconium indicates that there was a problem but that there is no need to be concerned
c. Yellow meconium is of no clinical importance
d. The management is the same as it does not matter what the consistency or colour of the meconium is

19. **Why does a fetus pass meconium during labour?**
   a. Because there is fetal hypoxia
   b. Because it makes the second stage of labour shorter
   c. Because the mother has been given liquid paraffin
   d. Because it is mature and ready for delivery

20. **What is the correct management when the liquor is meconium stained?**
   a. Monitor the fetal heart rate carefully.
   b. Deliver the fetus immediately by Caesarean section.
   c. Give the patient an oxytocin infusion to shorten labour.
   d. Transfer the patient urgently to a level 3 hospital.

Test 8: Monitoring and management of the first stage of labour

1. The latent phase of the first stage of labour is:
   a. The period of time the cervix takes to dilate from 3 cm to full dilatation
   b. The period of time from the onset of labour to full cervical dilatation
   c. The period of time from the onset of labour to 3 cm cervical dilatation
   d. The period of time during which the cervix becomes effaced

2. What is the name given to the first oblique line on the partogram?
   a. The action line
   b. The alert line
   c. The normal cervical dilatation line
   d. The danger line

3. If a patient's cervix is 2 cm dilated, when should you perform the next vaginal examination?
   a. When there are signs that the patient is in established labour with more regular and painful contractions
   b. After 2 hours
   c. After 8 hours
   d. When the patient wants to bear down

4. A patient presents in the latent phase of labour. After 8 hours she has not progressed to the active phase of labour despite regular contractions. Which of the following is the correct management?
   a. She should be discharged home.
   b. If there have been no cervical changes, the membranes should be ruptured.
   c. If there has been slow dilatation and effacement of the cervix, it may be necessary to rupture the membranes.
   d. An oxytocin infusion should be started.

5. A patient presents in established labour with regular contractions and ruptured membranes. On vaginal examination the cervix is 5 cm dilated. Where should her cervical dilatation be noted on the partogram?

a. On the alert line opposite 5 cm cervical dilatation

b. At the beginning of the latent phase of labour opposite 5 cm cervical dilatation

c. At the end of the latent phase of labour opposite 5 cm cervical dilatation

d. On the vertical line at the beginning of the active phase of labour opposite 5 cm cervical dilatation

6. You should be satisfied with the progress of labour during the active phase when:

a. Cervical dilatation falls on or to the left of the alert line together with less fetal head palpable above the pelvis.

b. The cervix dilates at a rate of 2 cm per hour

c. Cervical dilatation falls on or to the left of the alert line together with improvement in the station of the presenting part as assessed on vaginal examination

d. There is progressive dilatation and effacement of the cervix

7. What should be your first step in the management of a patient who fails to progress in the active phase of the first stage of labour?

a. Make sure that the patient is in the active phase of the first stage of labour and that her membranes are ruptured.

b. Perform a pelvic assessment to determine whether she has a small pelvis.

c. Evaluate the patient by following the rule of the '4 Ps'.

d. Make sure that the patient has adequate analgesia.

8. What should be your second step in the management of a patient who fails to progress in the active phase of the first stage of labour?

a. Determine whether the uterine contractions are adequate.

b. Start an oxytocin infusion.

c. Evaluate the patient by following the rule of the '4 Ps'.

d. Make sure that the patient is adequately hydrated.

9. **When does a patient have adequate and effective uterine contractions?**

a. If she has 2 or more contractions every 10 minutes with each contraction lasting 30 seconds or longer

b. If she has 3 or more contractions every 10 minutes with each contraction lasting 60 seconds or longer

c. If she progresses normally during labour

d. If she has pain with every contraction

10. **If a primigravida has poor progress in labour in spite of good, painful uterine contractions, your diagnosis should be:**

a. Ineffective uterine contractions

b. Cephalopelvic disproportion

c. A small pelvis

d. Braxton Hicks contractions

11. **A patient presents in labour at term with 2 contractions of 35 seconds each every 10 minutes. The cervix is 3 cm dilated and the membranes are bulging. The cervical dilatation is plotted on the alert line of the partogram. After 4 hours the cervix is 4 cm dilated while the other observations are unchanged. What is the correct management?**

a. An oxytocin infusion should be started.

b. A Caesarean section should be done.

c. The patient's membranes should be ruptured.

d. The doctor should be called to examine the patient.

12. **What should you do if the cervical dilatation falls on the action line?**
a. A Caesarean section should be done immediately.
b. The patient should be given the correct dose of oxytocin in an infusion.
c. The patient must be personally assessed by a doctor, and further management must be under the direction and responsibility of the doctor.
d. After making sure that the patient is in the active phase of the first stage of labour and her membranes are ruptured, she should be managed according to the rule of the '4 Ps'.

13. **Cephalopelvic disproportion due to a small pelvic inlet should be diagnosed when:**
a. There is no further dilatation of the cervix
b. There is 3/5 or more of the fetal head palpable above the pelvic brim and 3+ or more moulding is present
c. There is 2/5 or less of the fetal head palpable above the pelvic brim and 1+ moulding is present
d. The measurements of the pelvic inlet are assessed as small during a pelvic examination

14. **A patient at term presents after having been in labour at home for some time. On admission, cephalopelvic disproportion is diagnosed. What is the correct further management of this patient?**
a. An oxytocin infusion should be started.
b. A Caesarean section should be done.
c. The patient should be given pethidine and hydroxyzine (Aterax).
d. The patient should be reassured that she will labour and deliver normally.

15. A primigravida presents in labour at term. She is having 2 contractions of 35 seconds each every 10 minutes. The cervix is 3 cm dilated and the membranes have ruptured. Her cervical dilatation is plotted on the alert line. 4 hours later the cervix is 4 cm dilated and her other observations are unchanged. There are no signs of cephalopelvic disproportion. What is the correct management?
   a. An oxytocin infusion should be started.
   b. A Caesarean section should be done.
   c. She should be given pethidine and hydroxyzine (Aterax).
   d. The doctor should be called to examine the patient.

16. A patient at term progresses slowly during the active phase of labour. During a thorough physical examination, an occipito-posterior position with mild caput and 1+ moulding is diagnosed. What should be the further management?
   a. An oxytocin infusion should be started.
   b. A Caesarean section should be done.
   c. The patient should be given pethidine and hydroxyzine (Aterax).
   d. Oxytocin is contraindicated. Rather, an intravenous infusion should be started and the patient should be given adequate analgesia.

17. Which of the following patients should receive oxytocin if they developed poor progress due to inadequate uterine contractions during the active phase of labour?
   a. A patient with 2+ moulding
   b. A primigravida patient with a vertex presentation and no moulding
   c. A multipara with a vertex presentation and no moulding
   d. A primigravida patient with a breech presentation

18. A patient is being referred from a peripheral clinic to a hospital with the diagnosis of cephalopelvic disproportion. Which of the following is the best management for the patient and her fetus, before the patient is transported?
a. Adequate analgesia, e.g. pethidine and hydroxyzine (Aterax)
b. An infusion with oxytocin to improve uterine contractions
c. 3 nifedipine (Adalat) 10 mg capsules (total 30 mg) should be given orally to suppress labour
d. Oxygen administration with a mask

19. Which one of the following patients is at high risk of cord prolapse?
a. A patient with a breech presentation
b. A patient with a cephalic presentation
c. A patient with a post-term pregnancy
d. A patient who ruptures her membranes when the fetal head is still palpable 3/5 above the pelvic brim

20. What should be done first if a patient, whose cervix is 6 cm dilated, presents with a prolapsed cord?
a. Immediately replace the umbilical cord into the vagina and take steps to lift the presenting part off the cord.
b. An oxytocin infusion should be started in order to deliver the infant as soon as possible.
c. Give the patient oxygen by face mask in order to ensure that the fetus receives enough oxygen.
d. The patient must be rushed to theatre for an emergency Caesarean section.

Test 9: The second stage of labour

1. When does the second stage of labour begin and end?

a. From the time the patient has an urge to bear down until the infant is completely delivered
b. From the time the cervix is fully dilated until the infant is completely delivered
c. From the beginning of the active phase of the first stage of labour until the cervix is fully dilated
d. From the beginning of the active phase of the first stage of labour until the infant is completely delivered.

2. What would suggest that the patient's cervix has reached full dilatation?

a. Uterine contractions become stronger with an increase in duration and frequency.
b. The patient becomes restless.
c. Nausea and vomiting occur.
d. All of the above.

3. When is the fetal head engaged?

a. When the widest transverse diameter of the fetal head (i.e. the biparietal diameter) has passed through the entrance of the birth canal
b. When the greatest diameter of the fetal head (i.e. the suboccipito-bregmatic diameter) has passed through the entrance of the birth canal
c. When the occiput has passed through the entrance of the birth canal
d. When the vertex has passed through the entrance of the birth canal

4. How many fifths of the fetal head will be palpable above the brim of the pelvic when engagement has taken place?

a. 5/5
b. 4/5
c. 3/5
d. 2/5

5. **When should a patient in the second stage of labour start bearing down?**
a. When her cervix is fully dilated
b. When her cervix is fully dilated and 1/5 of the fetal head is still palpable above the pelvic brim
c. When her cervix is fully dilated and 2/5 of the fetal head is still palpable above the pelvic brim
d. When her cervix is fully dilated and 3/5 of the fetal head is still palpable above the pelvic brim

6. **When is it safe not to bear down but to wait for engagement of the fetal head to occur in a patient with a fully dilated cervix?**
a. If there is no fetal distress and no cephalopelvic disproportion
b. If the patient is a multigravida
c. If the patient is a primigravida
d. You should not wait, as patients with a fully dilated cervix must start to bear down straight away

7. **What position should the patient adopt when she delivers?**
a. She should lie on her back (i.e. the dorsal position)
b. She should lie on her side (i.e. the lateral position)
c. She should squat upright (i.e. the vertical position)
d. She should choose whichever position she prefers as long as it is practical under the clinical circumstances.

8. **How should the fetal condition be assessed when the patient bears down during the second stage of labour?**
a. You should listen to the fetal heart rate between contractions only.
b. You should listen to the fetal heart rate immediately after each contraction to determine whether the heart rate remains the same as the baseline rate.
c. You should listen to the fetal heart rate immediately after a contraction every 15 minutes to determine whether the heart rate remains the same as the baseline rate.
d. You should listen to the fetal heart rate immediately after a contraction every 10 minutes to determine whether the heart rate remains the same as the baseline rate.

9. **Which of the following indicates satisfactory progress during the second stage of labour?**
   a. The infant is delivered within 30 minutes of the start of the second stage of labour.
   b. The infant is delivered within 45 minutes of the start of the second stage of labour.
   c. With every contraction where the patient bears down, the fetal head descends further onto the perineum.
   d. The infant is delivered after the patient bears down well with 4 contractions.

10. **What is the correct management if there is no progress in the second stage of labour and there are signs of cephalopelvic disproportion?**
    a. The patient must not bear down but should be evaluated by a doctor as a Caesarean section is needed.
    b. An episiotomy should be done to speed up the delivery.
    c. An oxytocin infusion should be started to increase the strength of the contractions.
    d. The patient should continue bearing down for 30 minutes in a primigravida and 45 minutes in a multigravida before any further management is carried out.

11. **The perineum should be supported during the second stage of labour in order to:**
    a. Prevent the patient from passing faeces
    b. Prevent the fetal head from being delivered too fast
    c. Help the internal rotation of the fetal head
    d. Increase flexion of the fetal head so that only the smallest diameter of the head has to pass through the vagina

12. **In which of the following circumstances should an episiotomy be done?**
    a. An episiotomy should be done routinely in all primigravida patients.
    b. An episiotomy should be done at the delivery of a preterm infant to prevent birth injury.
    c. An episiotomy should be done routinely in all patients who have had a previous episiotomy.
    d. An episiotomy should be done routinely in all patients who have had a previous second-degree tear.